Carotid and Cerebrovascular Disease

Editors

CHRISTOPHER J. WHITE
KENNETH ROSENFIELD

INTERVENTIONAL CARDIOLOGY CLINICS

www.interventional.theclinics.com

Consulting Editors
SAMIN K. SHARMA
IGOR F. PALACIOS

January 2014 • Volume 3 • Number 1

ELSEVIER

1600 John F. Kennedy Boulevard • Suite 1800 • Philadelphia, Pennsylvania, 19103-2899

http://www.theclinics.com

INTERVENTIONAL CARDIOLOGY CLINICS Volume 3, Number 1
January 2014 ISSN 2211-7458, ISBN-13: 978-0-323-26396-2

Editor: Barbara Cohen-Kligerman

Interventional Cardiology Clinics (ISSN 2211-7458) is published quarterly by Elsevier Inc., 360 Park Avenue South, New York, NY 10010-1710. Months of issue are January, April, July, and October. Subscription prices are USD 195 per year for US individuals, USD 305 for US institutions, USD 130 per year for US students, USD 230 per year for Canadian individuals, USD 375 for Canadian institutions, USD 150 per year for Canadian students, USD 295 per year for international individuals, USD 375 for international institutions, and USD 150 per year for international students. To receive student/resident rate, orders must be accompanied by name of affiliated institution, date of term, and the *signature* of program/residency coordinator on institution letterhead. Orders will be billed at individual rate until proof of status is received. Foreign air speed delivery is included in all *Clinics* subscription prices. All prices are subject to change without notice. **POSTMASTER:** Send address changes to *Interventional Cardiology Clinics*, Elsevier Health Sciences Division, Subscription Customer Service, 3251 Riverport Lane, Maryland Heights, MO 63043. **Customer Service: Telephone: 1-800-654-2452** (U.S. and Canada); **1-314-447-8871** (outside U.S. and Canada). **Fax: 1-314-447-8029. E-mail: journalscustomerservice-usa@elsevier.com** (for print support); **journalsonlinesupport-usa@elsevier.com** (for online support).

Reprints. For copies of 100 or more of articles in this publication, please contact the Commercial Reprints Department, Elsevier Inc., 360 Park Avenue South, New York, NY 10010-1710. Tel.: 212-633-3874; Fax: 212-633-3820; E-mail: reprints@elsevier.com.

Printed and bound by CPI Group (UK) Ltd, Croydon, CR0 4YY

Transferred to digital print 2012

Contributors

CONSULTING EDITORS

SAMIN K. SHARMA, MD, FSCAI, FACC
Director of Clinical Cardiology; Director of Cardiac Catheterization Laboratory, Mount Sinai Medical Center, New York, New York

IGOR F. PALACIOS, MD, FSCAI
Director of Interventional Cardiology, Cardiology Division, Heart Center, Massachusetts General Hospital; Associate Professor of Medicine, Harvard Medical School, Boston, Massachusetts

EDITORS

CHRISTOPHER J. WHITE, MD
Professor and Chairman, Department of Medicine and Cardiology, Ochsner Medical Center and Ochsner Clinical School of the University of Queensland; Medical Director, John Ochsner Heart and Vascular Institute; System Chairman, Cardiovascular Diseases, Ochsner Medical Institutions, New Orleans, Louisiana

KENNETH ROSENFIELD, MD, MHCDS
Section of Vascular Medicine and Intervention, Division of Cardiology, Massachusetts General Hospital, Boston, Massachusetts

AUTHORS

ALEX ABOU-CHEBL, MD
Professor of Neurology; Director of Interventional Neurology; Director of Vascular and Interventional Neurology Fellowships, Department of Neurology, University of Louisville School of Medicine, Louisville, Kentucky

JASON M. ANDRUS, MD
Department of Radiology, Alleghony General Hospital, Pittsburgh, Pennsylvania

HERBERT D. ARONOW, MD, MPH
St Joseph Mercy Hospital, Ann Arbor, Michigan

JOSHUA A. BECKMAN, MD, MPH
Vascular Medicine Section, Cardiovascular Division, Brigham and Women's Hospital, Boston, Massachusetts

MARC P. BONACA, MD, MPH
Vascular Medicine Section, Cardiovascular Division, Brigham and Women's Hospital, Boston, Massachusetts

SANJAY GANDHI, MD
Heart and Vascular Center, MetroHealth Campus, Case Western Reserve University, Cleveland, Ohio

BEAU M. HAWKINS, MD
Cardiovascular Section, Department of Internal Medicine, University of Oklahoma Health Sciences Center, Oklahoma City, Oklahoma

MICHAEL R. JAFF, DO
Vascular Medicine Section, Cardiology Division, Massachusetts General Hospital, Boston, Massachusetts

J. STEPHEN JENKINS, MD, FACC, FSCAI, FSVM
Associate Section Head, Interventional Cardiology; Director, Interventional Cardiology Research, John Ochsner Heart and Vascular Institute, New Orleans, Louisiana

ANDREAS KASTRUP, MD
Clinic for Neurology, Klinikum Bremen-Mitte/
Bremen-Ost, Bremen, Germany

SASKO KEDEV, MD, FESC, FACC
Professor of Medicine (Cardiology), Medical
Faculty, Department of Interventional
Cardiology, University Clinic of Cardiology,
University of St Cyril & Methodius, Skopje,
Macedonia

JUN LI, MD
Department of Medicine, Case Western
Reserve University School of Medicine;
Division of Cardiovascular Medicine,
Harrington Heart and Vascular Institute,
University Hospitals Case Medical Center,
Cleveland, Ohio

TIFT MANN, MD, FACC
Department of Cardiology, Rex Heart Center,
North Carolina Heart and Vascular Associates,
Raleigh, North Carolina

**D. CHRISTOPHER METZGER, MD, FSCAI,
FACC**
Medical Director, Cardiac and Peripheral
Catheterization Laboratories; Medical Director,
Clinical Research; Wellmont CVA Heart
Institute, Kingsport, Tennessee

PANAGIOTIS PAPANAGIOTOU, MD
Clinic for Diagnostic and Interventional
Neuroradiology, Klinikum Bremen-Mitte/
Bremen-Ost, Bremen, Germany

SAHIL A. PARIKH, MD, FACC, FSCAI
Assistant Professor of Medicine, Department
of Medicine, Case Western Reserve University
School of Medicine; Director, Experimental
Interventional Cardiology Laboratory; Director,
Interventional Cardiology Fellowship Program,
Division of Cardiovascular Medicine,
Harrington Heart and Vascular Institute,
University Hospitals Case Medical Center,
Cleveland, Ohio

WOLFGANG REITH, MD, PhD
Clinic for Diagnostic and Interventional
Neuroradiology, Saarland University Hospital,
Homburg, Germany

R. KEVIN ROGERS, MD, MSc
Section of Vascular Medicine and Intervention,
Division of Cardiology, University of Colorado,
Aurora, Colorado

KENNETH ROSENFIELD, MD, MHCDS
Section of Vascular Medicine and Intervention,
Division of Cardiology, Massachusetts General
Hospital, Boston, Massachusetts

CHRISTIAN ROTH, MD
Clinic for Diagnostic and Interventional
Neuroradiology, Klinikum Bremen-Mitte/
Bremen-Ost, Bremen, Germany

ROBERT D. SAFIAN, MD
Director, Center for Innovation and Research in
Cardiovascular Diseases (CIRC), Beaumont
Health System; Professor of Medicine,
Oakland University William Beaumont School
of Medicine, Royal Oak, Michigan

RAHUL SAKHUJA, MD, MPP, MSc, FACC
Department of Medicine, Division of
Cardiology, Wellmont CVA Heart Institute,
Kingsport, Tennessee

PETER C. THURLOW, MD
Department of Radiology, Allegheny General
Hospital, Pittsburgh, Pennsylvania

SIDDHARTH A. WAYANGANKAR, MD, MPH
University of Oklahoma Health Sciences
Center, Oklahoma City, Oklahoma

CHRISTOPHER J. WHITE, MD
Professor and Chairman, Department of
Medicine and Cardiology, Ochsner Medical
Center and Ochsner Clinical School of the
University of Queensland; Medical Director,
John Ochsner Heart and Vascular Institute;
System Chairman, Cardiovascular Diseases,
Ochsner Medical Institutions, New Orleans,
Louisiana

MARK H. WHOLEY, MD
Department of Radiology, Allegheny General
Hospital; Director, Center for Vascular and
Neurovascular Interventions, Allegheny Health
Network; Adjunct Professor of Biomedical
Engineering, Carnegie Mellon University,
Pittsburgh, Pennsylvania

Contents

standard-risk patients. However, these improved CAS results apply only to CAS procedures performed by experienced operators at experienced centers. Furthermore, these improved results are due largely to operators' lessons learned, helping with appropriate case selection.

Subjective characteristics for increased risk of carotid artery stenting (CAS) have included thrombus-containing lesions, heavily calcified lesions, very tortuous vessels, and near occlusions. More objective high-risk features include contraindications to dual antiplatelet therapy, a history of bleeding complications, and lack of femoral artery vascular access. Variables that increase the risk of CAS complications are attributed to patient characteristics, anatomic features, or procedural factors. Operator and hospital volume affect the risk of complications occurring with CAS. As the complexity and difficulty of CAS patients increases, the need for more highly skilled operators and teams becomes even more necessary to minimize complications.

In patients with asymptomatic carotid artery stenosis the optimal strategy to reduce the risk for stroke remains controversial. Although carotid endarterectomy was traditionally considered the gold standard for revascularization, emerging data suggest that carotid artery stenting is an appropriate alternative in many asymptomatic patients. This article summarizes the evidence base and related controversies regarding carotid endarterectomy versus carotid artery stenting for the revascularization of carotid disease in asymptomatic patients.

Symptomatic carotid artery stenosis is an important cause of stroke with significant morbidity and mortality. Revascularization with carotid endarterectomy reduces the recurrence of stroke and until recently was considered the gold standard of therapy. Carotid artery stenting has emerged as an alternative method of revascularization in both high-risk and standard-risk patients. This review appraises the role of surgery versus stenting for patients with symptomatic carotid stenosis.

Despite rapid growth in the frequency that carotid artery stenting (CAS) is performed, there remain concerns regarding the steep learning curve associated with this procedure. This article reviews the evidence base supporting operator and institutional CAS learning curves and discusses their implications for the establishment and maintenance of competencies. Attempts are made to delineate minimum volume thresholds to attain these goals and means to enhance procedural safety without compromising patient access.

Stroke is the most common cause of permanent disability, the second most common cause of dementia, and the third most common cause of death in the Western world. The treatment of affected patients is a challenge because intravenous (IV) thrombolysis is often ineffective. IV thrombolysis on its own leads to a favorable clinical outcome in only 15% to 25% in patients with large-artery occlusion. Current reperfusion therapies enable high recanalization rates, high rate of favorable clinical outcome, and low complication rates. However, to achieve good clinical results, appropriate patient selection and the use of optimized stroke management system are obligate.

INTERVENTIONAL CARDIOLOGY CLINICS

DOWNLOAD Free App!

Review Articles THE CLINICS

NOW AVAILABLE FOR YOUR iPhone and iPad

Preface

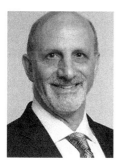

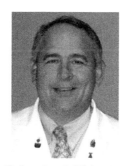

Kenneth Rosenfield, MD, MHCDS   Christopher J. White, MD

Editors

Stroke is the third most common cause of death, and the leading cause of disability, in the United States. Its impact extends beyond health care into every aspect of American society and includes an enormous economic burden. There is no disease that patients fear more than the possibility of having a stroke. As the population ages and people survive other cardiovascular insults, stroke promises to become even more prevalent. Risk factor reduction, treatment of dyslipidemia, and better control of hypertension have all been shown to reduce the incidence of stroke and cerebral vascular disease. Nevertheless, the impact of these factors on stroke prevention has been much less impressive than that seen in cardiovascular disease, where death from myocardial infarction has fallen by 20% to 30% over the past 20 years. We see a great opportunity to close this gap and greatly reduce the burden of cerebral vascular disease over the next 10 years, but it will take a village.

The starting point is increased awareness in the population as a whole, among patients at risk, and in the provider community. It will require more active and systematic efforts to achieve risk factor reduction. Providers who care for cardiovascular and cerebral vascular disease will need to become more knowledgeable about the disease process and team up to develop innovative approaches to prevent and treat stroke, and better systems of care to manage this disease. Processes and algorithms for treating acute stroke must be agreed on, standardized, disseminated, and adopted by health care systems. Finally, we must develop metrics to measure the impact of our interventions and continue to improve on performance and outcome based on the evaluation of these data.

This issue of *Interventional Cardiology Clinics* provides an overview of stroke and cerebral vascular disease. We have chosen to focus predominantly on the vasculogenic stroke; cardiac etiologies are equally as common and much of the information in this issue applies also to cardiogenic stroke. The topics presented address the rapidly changing management paradigm for cerebral vascular disease and provide some insight into where we are today and what are the possibilities as we look to the future.

Drs Bonaca and Beckman begin by providing insights into how best to prevent stroke primarily, medically and with appropriate revascularization. Next, Drs Hawkins and Jaff address the importance of noninvasive imaging in this field and tell us how to approach this from a pragmatic perspective. Drs Kedev and Mann and Dr Metzger then tell us how they actually perform carotid stenting, from "skin to skin," via two different approaches—the more novel radial approach and the conventional femoral approach, respectively. Dr White provides insight into the unique characteristics of each patient that might influence decision-making and outcome of intervention. Drs Li, Sakhuja, and Parikh take on the sometimes controversial issue of deciding whether the symptomatic patient is better served by open surgical endarterectomy or carotid stenting. Drs Rogers, Gandhi, and Rosenfield tackle the same issue for asymptomatic patients. Both sets of authors try to sort through the myriad conflicting data and opinions, in order to provide a balanced,

interventional.theclinics.com

evidence-based assessment. Drs Wayangankar and Aronow enlighten us as to what it takes— what is the learning curve— to become competent and Dr Safian reminds us that complications can occur and that we must be prepared to manage them effectively as we undertake treatments aimed at reducing the incidence and effects of stroke. Dr Jenkins reports on indications, technique, and results for vertebral intervention. We then dive into the details regarding the vascular supply to the brain and how and when to treat the various vessels. Drs Thurlow, Andrus, and Wholey present the variants of carotid and cerebral anatomy that must be considered by the interventionalist when approaching the patient. Dr Abou-Chebl reports on the controversies and technical aspects of intracranial angioplasty and stenting. Finally, Drs Papanagiotou, Reith, Kastrup, and Roth finish by informing us about the reperfusion strategies for acute stroke that are currently employed, and where we are headed in this relatively new and exciting field, particularly with respect to the "game-changing" potential of newer devices and treatment algorithms.

This compendium is by no means designed to be encyclopedic. Rather, it is intended to provide a broad-based and current overview of the field of stroke and cerebral vascular disease. It will introduce the reader to background, justification for treatment, and some of the controversies that exist. It is our hope to increase both the awareness and the knowledge base of the reader and further encourage the medical community to band together to conquer stroke and improve the lives of our collective patients.

We are indebted to our distinguished coauthors, who volunteered their valuable time, energy, knowledge, and wisdom to make high-quality and meaningful contributions. We also extend sincere thanks to Ms Barbara Cohen-Kligerman for her tireless efforts to bring this issue together. We hope this series of articles will provide important, current perspectives that are practical and useful for our interventional colleagues.

Kenneth Rosenfield, MD, MHCDS
Section of Vascular Medicine and Intervention
Division of Cardiology
Massachusetts General Hospital
Boston, MA 02114, USA

Christopher J. White, MD
Department of Medicine and Cardiology
Ochsner Medical Center
Ochsner Clinical School of the University of
Queensland
John Ochsner Heart and Vascular Institute
Ochsner Medical Institutions
1514 Jefferson Highway
New Orleans, LA 70121, USA

E-mail addresses:
krosenfield@fastmail.us (K. Rosenfield)
cwhite@ochsner.org (C.J. White)

Primary Stroke Prevention
Medical Therapy Versus Revascularization

Marc P. Bonaca, MD, MPH, Joshua A. Beckman, MD, MPH*

KEYWORDS

- Carotid artery disease • Asymptomatic carotid disease • Carotid stenosis
- Atherosclerotic vascular disease • Stroke prevention

KEY POINTS

- The finding of asymptomatic carotid artery stenosis should be considered an indicator of heightened cardiovascular risk, and an opportunity for intensified primary prevention.
- Patients should be evaluated broadly for all modifiable risk factors, and educated.
- All patients should be counseled with regard to lifestyle changes and therapeutic targets.
- Maximal medical therapy, including antiplatelet therapy where appropriate, statin therapy, and blood pressure–lowering therapy, should be used as recommended by current consensus guidelines.
- A subset of patients with asymptomatic carotid stenosis may benefit from preventive revascularization to reduce the risk of ipsilateral stroke.
- Careful patient selection is required when considering whether to revascularize as an adjunct to optimal medical therapy.

INTRODUCTION

Primary prevention of ischemic stroke relies on the identification of risk factors indicating that a given patient is at a heightened risk of a first event and subsequent modification of that risk.[1] It is important to recognize that events broadly characterized as ischemic stroke are in fact a heterogeneous group of events that include differing causes such cardioembolic events, artery-to-artery emboli, in situ thrombosis, and small-vessel ischemic changes. Primary preventive strategies must assess patient risk broadly to assess all contributors to risk.[1]

One risk indicator is the finding of a carotid artery stenosis, generally detected by auscultation of bruit on examination or by imaging.[1–4] Significant carotid stenosis is generally defined as more than 50% narrowing of the vessel lumen.[4,5] The most common cause of carotid artery stenosis is atherosclerotic vascular disease with lipid accumulation in the vessel wall and associated remodeling and calcification. Other potential causes include carotid dissection, fibromuscular dysplasia, and inflammation associated with vasculitides.[4] In general (and in this review), the term "carotid artery disease" refers

Disclosures: Dr M.P. Bonaca is an investigator for the TIMI Study Group, which has received research grant support through Brigham and Women's Hospital from Abbott, Amgen, AstraZeneca, Beckman Coulter, BG Medicine, BRAHMS, Bristol-Myers Squibb, Buhlmann, Critical Diagnostics, CV Therapeutics, Daiichi Sankyo Co Ltd, Eli Lilly and Co, GlaxoSmithKline, Genzyme, Merck and Co, Intarcia, Merck, Nanosphere, Novartis Pharmaceuticals, Ortho-Clinical Diagnostics, Pfizer, Randox, Roche Diagnostics, Sanofi-Aventis, Siemens, Singulex, and Takeda. In addition he has received consulting fees from Roche Diagnostics. Dr J.A. Beckman serves as a board member for VIVA Physicians, Inc. Dr J.A. Beckman consults for Astra Zeneca, Ferring Pharmaceutical, Merck, and Novartis. He receives grant support from Bristol-Myers Squibb.
Vascular Medicine Section, Cardiovascular Division, Brigham and Women's Hospital, 75 Francis Street, Boston, MA 02115, USA
* Corresponding author.
E-mail address: jbeckman@partners.org

Intervent Cardiol Clin 3 (2014) 1–11
http://dx.doi.org/10.1016/j.iccl.2013.08.003
2211-7458/14/$ – see front matter © 2014 Elsevier Inc. All rights reserved.

to atherosclerosis of the carotid artery most often apparent at the carotid bulb, but also involving the common, internal, and external carotid arteries.

The question of optimal primary prevention for patients with carotid disease is important.[4] Overall, the prevalence of carotid artery disease is increasing in the setting of an aging population, and the majority of new strokes are ischemic strokes.[6] Ischemic stroke has been described as a highly morbid event that results in permanent disability and loss of independence in a significant proportion of those who survive.[6] A relationship has been described between degree of stenosis associated with carotid atherosclerosis and the subsequent risk of cardiovascular events and ischemic stroke.[5,7,8] This observation has led investigators to target those patients with more severe stenoses in trials of interventions targeted at revascularizing carotid disease and reducing the associated risk of stroke.[9–12] It is estimated that of patients who have carotid atherosclerosis, the estimated prevalence of severe stenoses of more than 60% is low in all adults, but may affect 2% of the Medicare population.[13,14]

It must be recognized, however, that the patient with carotid atherosclerosis suffers from a systemic process with adverse events beyond that attributable to the specific stenosis. In fact, a significant proportion of subsequent ischemic strokes in patients with unilateral carotid disease occur on the contralateral side.[10,12,15] In addition, it is important to recognize shifts in the epidemiology of ischemic stroke that have occurred against the background of an aging population and improving medical therapies, in that it is estimated that currently less than 15% of strokes are due to asymptomatic carotid disease, and that the annualized risk of stroke in patients with asymptomatic carotid disease is approximately 1% and likely decreasing.[14,16–18] Patients with stable carotid disease are at heightened risk for cardiovascular events broadly including other vascular territories, such as acute myocardial infarction (MI).[2–4] Therefore, optimal primary preventive strategies must evaluate the patient first as well as the carotid stenosis.

An important determinant of stroke risk related to carotid stenosis is the clinical status of the lesion and patient.[4] Symptomatic carotid disease, defined as the acute onset of a focal neurologic symptom-referable carotid distribution, is associated with significantly higher rates of related ischemic stroke in comparison with asymptomatic disease.[4,19] Differentiation between the two is critical in determining an appropriate treatment approach. As this article addresses the primary prevention of stroke,

it focuses on the patient with stable or asymptomatic carotid artery atherosclerosis.

This article discusses general approaches to primary preventive strategies for stable patients with atherosclerosis manifesting as asymptomatic carotid disease. Such approaches include strategies generally applicable to all patients with atherosclerotic vascular disease, including lifestyle interventions and medical therapies. In addition, options for carotid revascularization and considerations for appropriate patient selection are reviewed.

TESTING: DIAGNOSIS AND MONITORING
Diagnostic Testing

Although the key focus of this article is the primary prevention of stroke in patients who are found to have carotid artery disease, the question of screening and the follow-up of testing should be addressed. In the literature, there is debate as to whether screening should be performed; however, observational studies have associated the presence of a bruit on examination with cardiovascular risk.[2,3] Although there are differences in recommendations for screening and the population for which it is likely to be most beneficial,[1,14] multispecialty guidelines conclude it is reasonable to perform duplex ultrasonography in patients with auscultated bruits to determine if internal carotid artery stenosis is present.[4] In part, the decision of whether to test should depend on potential therapeutic decision making. Therefore, in patients who are otherwise on optimal medical therapy for reduction of risk associated with atherosclerotic vascular disease and are not candidates for carotid revascularization (see the section on revascularization), the benefit of testing is likely limited. In addition, the detection of atherosclerotic plaque as a mechanism to motivate patients to comply with lifestyle and medical therapy has not been shown to be effective.[20]

Monitoring in Patients with Known Carotid Artery Stenosis

If asymptomatic carotid stenosis is detected, lifestyle changes and optimal medical therapy are recommended regardless of the degree of stenosis. Serial duplex ultrasonographic assessment to assess the progression and stability of findings is reasonable for those in whom revascularization based on degree of stenosis would be considered. In these patients an initial assessment at 6 months followed by annual examinations for stable lesions is reasonable.[4] Indeed, progression of stenosis is a potent marker for heightened risk of stroke, and suggests a time when a risk/benefit assessment is more favorable for revascularization.[21] Data have not supported the routine use of serial ultrasonography in unselected patients with asymptomatic carotid disease.[8]

PRIMARY PREVENTION INTERVENTIONS
Strategies for All Patients

The finding of carotid atherosclerosis in an otherwise healthy patient is a marker of heightened cardiovascular risk. Therefore, all patients should be treated with the goal of risk-factor modification as outlined in **Table 1**.[4]

Education and lifestyle modification
Although testing has not been shown to be efficacious as a means of patient motivation, the finding of carotid atherosclerosis should be used as an opportunity for education and counseling. Consensus

Table 1
General approach to primary prevention of asymptomatic carotid disease

Asymptomatic Stenosis <60%	Asymptomatic Stenosis 60%–99%	Note
Monitoring		
Repeat in 6 mo, if stable repeat annually	Repeat in 6 mo, if stable repeat annually unless revascularizing	Serial imaging only recommended in if there is potential to modify therapy
Assess for Other Cardiovascular Risk Factors		
Measure blood pressure	Measure blood pressure	Goal <140/90 mm Hg
Lipids (LDL)	Lipids (LDL)	Goal <100 mg/dL
Consider diabetes mellitus	Consider diabetes mellitus	
Consider obstructive sleep apnea	Consider obstructive sleep apnea	
Inflammatory biomarkers (hsCRP, Lp-PLA2)	Inflammatory biomarkers (hsCRP, Lp-PLA2)	Effectiveness not well established (Class IIb, level of evidence B)[1]
Lifestyle Modification and Education		
Smoking cessation	Smoking cessation	
Dietary intervention	Dietary intervention	
Cardiovascular exercise	Cardiovascular exercise	
Pharmacotherapy		
Low-dose aspirin (75–100 mg)	Low-dose aspirin (75–100 mg)	In selected patients based on risk. Clopidogrel in patients unable to take aspirin
Lipid-lowering therapy	Lipid-lowering therapy	Statins should be favored and have demonstrated greatest benefit
Blood pressure–lowering therapy	Blood pressure–lowering therapy	ACEi should be considered based on trial data[45]
Revascularization		
Not indicated	Carotid endarterectomy	In selected patients: Life expectancy >5 y Procedural risk <3% Gender considerations Lesion considerations (imaging/TCD)
Not indicated	Carotid stenting	In selected patients: Life expectancy >5 y Acceptable procedural risk High surgical risk Able to take dual-antiplatelet therapy for at least 30 d

Abbreviations: ACEi, angiotensin-converting enzyme inhibitors; hsCRP, high-sensitivity C-reactive protein; LDL, low-density lipoprotein; Lp-PLA2, lipoprotein-associated phospholipase A_2; TCD, transcranial Doppler.

guidelines recommend that all patients with asymptomatic carotid artery stenosis be screened for treatable risk factors.[1] All patients should be educated about risk factors, lifestyle modifications that can reduce risk, and targets for risk reduction (eg, cholesterol and blood pressure goals). General interventions that should be addressed are detailed in multispecialty consensus documents, but in summary should include:

- Smoking cessation[1,4]
- Dietary interventions, including a heart-healthy diet as recommended by consensus guidelines.[1,4] This diet includes moderation of dietary sodium and consideration for potassium supplementation.[1] In addition, recent data have shown that adherence to the Mediterranean diet may reduce the incidence of major cardiovascular events[22]
- Maintenance of a healthy body weight[1]
- Regular cardiovascular exercise[1]
- Identification and treatment of obstructive sleep apnea[1]
- Optimal treatment of other modifiable medical conditions (eg, diabetes mellitus)[1]

Pharmacologic therapy

Pharmacotherapy for the reduction of cardiovascular risk in patients with atherosclerotic vascular disease has advanced markedly over the last 2 decades, with major advances including the development and broad use of statin therapy.[23] Improvement in these therapies has been broadly credited for observed reductions in the risk of cardiovascular events.[18] The pace of improvement in medical therapy has even led some to question whether medical controls in prior randomized trials in this population are still valid.[16,24] Although evidence proving benefit for isolated carotid artery disease varies among therapies, general strategies described herein have proven benefit for risk reduction in patients with atherosclerotic vascular disease.

Antiplatelet therapy

Although antiplatelet therapy with aspirin is generally considered the cornerstone of cardiovascular prevention, data demonstrating benefit in asymptomatic carotid disease for the primary prevention of stroke is limited. Antiplatelet therapy has shown robust efficacy in prevention of adverse cardiovascular events in large meta-analyses of patients at heightened risk of atherosclerotic vascular events.[25,26] However, both the populations and specific therapies included in these studies are variable. Data evaluating the use of aspirin for primary prevention of ischemic stroke are modest.[27] In patients with asymptomatic carotid artery disease, data supporting aspirin use have also been

modest.[28] Overall, single-agent antiplatelet therapy with aspirin is recommended in current consensus guidelines for high-risk patients with carotid artery stenosis at a dose between 75 and 325 mg daily.[1,4] The benefit of aspirin in low-risk patients has not been definitively demonstrated.[1,4] Trials evaluating a range of aspirin doses suggest low-dose aspirin to be as effective as high-dose aspirin in patients presenting with high-risk vascular complications including acute MI.[29]

If patients with an indication for antiplatelet therapy are unable to take aspirin, treatment with an adenosine diphosphate (ADP) receptor blocker such as clopidogrel may be considered.[4] Clopidogrel monotherapy has been studied and shown to be efficacious in stable patients with established atherosclerotic disease (secondary prevention), but has not been studied specifically in patients with asymptomatic carotid artery disease.[30] More intensive antiplatelet therapy with the combination of aspirin and an ADP receptor blockers has not been shown to be efficacious in stable patients with atherosclerotic vascular disease or risk factors, and is not recommended.[31] Newer-generation ADP receptor blockers (eg, prasugrel, ticagrelor) have not been studied in specific randomized trials for primary prevention of events in patients with asymptomatic carotid artery disease. Cilostazol, a phosphodiesterase-3 inhibitor with antiplatelet effects, has been described as having antiproliferative effects, and has been investigated for the prevention of carotid atherosclerosis progression.[32] Additional studies have suggested benefit of cilostazol in patients with carotid disease undergoing procedures for revascularization, or those with restenosis after revascularization.[33,34] Although these findings are of academic interest and are the topic of ongoing investigation, cilostazol is not currently recommended for primary prevention in patients with asymptomatic carotid artery disease.

Lipid-lowering therapy

Measurement and treatment of serum lipids, including low-density lipoprotein cholesterol, is broadly recommended in accordance with National Cholesterol Education Program guidelines.[35,36] Treatment with 3-hydroxy-3-methylglutaryl coenzyme A reductase inhibitors (statins) have the greatest benefit among lipid-lowering therapies in terms of the reduction of cardiovascular events, including robust reductions in major adverse cardiovascular events in primary prevention populations.[37,38] In addition, studies have suggested the potential reverse remodeling in the carotid artery as measured by intima-media thickness through the use of statin therapy,[39,40] as well as reduction in detection of microemboli[40] and a decrease in plaque inflammation.[41]

Blood pressure–lowering therapy

A relationship between blood pressure and the development of carotid artery disease has been described.[42] More importantly, hypertension has been clearly associated with increased risk of ischemic stroke, and antihypertensive therapy has been proved to be beneficial for reduction of risk.[43,44] Although it is clear that blood pressure reduction leads to reduction in stroke risk, it should be recognized that trials of angiotensin-converting enzyme inhibitors (ACEi) have demonstrated benefit in patients with vascular disease, even if not known to have hypertension.[45] Consensus guidelines recommend antihypertensive therapy to reduce blood pressure to lower than 140/90 mm Hg.[1,4] The specific choice of therapy depends in part on additional risk factors, with the preferential use of an ACEi or angiotensin receptor blocker in patients with diabetes mellitus; however, randomized trials have demonstrated benefit in patients with established cerebrovascular disease.[1,4]

REVASCULARIZATION FOR PRIMARY PREVENTION OF STROKE

The question of whether to recommend revascularization for carotid artery stenosis is complex and is the subject of debate, with some arguing that medical therapy alone should be used and revascularization curtailed significantly.[16] The use of optimal medical therapy should be used in all patients, with the decision for adjunctive revascularization for the carotid stenosis made after comprehensive evaluation of the individual. Differences between the available modes of revascularization, surgical carotid endarterectomy (CEA) and carotid artery stenting (CAS), further complicates this decision. The reader is reminded that the following discussion applies to asymptomatic carotid stenosis and not to symptomatic disease.

Patient Selection and Risk Markers

The decision to revascularize requires the acceptance of increased short-term procedural risk with the expectation that long-term risk will be reduced. Randomized trials evaluating revascularization have used the degree of carotid stenosis as a primary determinant of long-term risk and inclusion for study (generally 60%–99%).[9,10,12] As the risk of stroke, MI, and death has decreased in the setting of improving medical therapy, consensus guidelines recommend consideration of additional factors when determining the suitability of revascularization.[1,4] The following factors deserve consideration when evaluating a patient's suitability for revascularization as therapy for asymptomatic carotid artery stenosis.

- Life expectancy. To realize the benefit of revascularization, patients must survive long enough for the risk of an associated event to exceed the risk of the procedure itself (approximately 5 years). The annualized risk of an associated ischemic stroke in patients with stable carotid artery stenosis is low.[17] Accordingly, studies have demonstrated limited benefit for revascularization in patients 80 years or older[46] and those with otherwise limited life expectancy.[47] The benefit of CEA in appropriately selected patients has been described out to 10 years.[11]
- Gender. Although randomized trials of revascularization strategies have not been powered to demonstrate benefit in gender subgroups, emerging data suggest that the benefit of CEA may be attenuated in women relative to men.[48,49]
- Imaging characterization of plaque. Histologic studies have suggested that inflamed plaque with associated thrombosis is associated with a greater risk of stroke.[50] Emerging imaging characteristics may assist in determining whether carotid plaque is inflamed or unstable. This finding has been described both with magnetic resonance (MR) angiography[50,51] and 3-dimensional ultrasonography.[52]
- Asymptomatic embolic activity. Transcranial Doppler (TCD) can detect asymptomatic ipsilateral embolic activity in patients with asymptomatic carotid stenosis, and this activity is associated with the risk of stroke. Several studies including one randomized trial have evaluated TCD for identifying patients with carotid disease who are at heightened risk of stroke.[53–56]
- Advance of plaque stenosis. The progression of carotid stenosis during surveillance has been associated with a 7-fold risk of stroke, with both duplex ultrasonography[21] and MR imaging.[57] Worsening stenosis may indicate a period of plaque instability and heightened risk of plaque rupture.
- Biomarkers. Inflammatory markers, including high-sensitivity C-reactive protein and lipoprotein-associated phospholipase A_2, are discussed in consensus guidelines as a means to identify general heightened risk of cardiovascular events.[1] In addition, investigational markers are being evaluated for prognostic ability in patients with carotid atherosclerosis.[58]

While these markers may portend heightened risk of events in general, they have not at this time been proved useful in terms of patient selection for carotid stenosis revascularization. Measurement of inflammatory markers currently receives a Class IIb, level of evidence B recommendation, noting that their effectiveness is not well established in this population.[1]

Revascularization Procedures

Three major randomized trials have compared surgical revascularization (CEA) with best current medical therapy (at the time of the study) in selected patients with significant carotid artery stenosis (60%–99%) (**Table 2**).[9,10,12] All 3 trials have demonstrated benefit of CEA in appropriately selected patients; however, the magnitude of benefit appears to be less for patients with asymptomatic disease than for those with symptomatic disease.[9,10,12] In addition, the medical therapy comparator arm in these trials differs from contemporary medical therapy, and the background rate of stroke attributable to carotid disease continues to decrease, making modern generalization of these older clinical trial findings complex in the current era.[16,17] Nonetheless, in the absence of disqualifying more recent clinical trials, the available data suggest that it is reasonable to consider revascularization in appropriately selected asymptomatic patients with at least a 70% stenosis in the internal carotid artery, provided the procedure can be done with a low anticipated periprocedural risk.[4,9,10] The 2 generally available revascularization options that exist are CEA and CAS, which are discussed in more detail below; however, CAS is generally recommended in selected patients.[4] In addition, although long-term outcomes between CEA and CAS appear to be similar, there are no randomized trials demonstrating the benefit of either technique relative to contemporary medical therapy.[59–61]

It is important that the availability of and proficiency with CEA and CAS varies according to institution and center volume. Experienced centers participating in trials of CEA report a perioperative risk of stroke or death of less than 3%.[9,10] Centers that perform fewer procedures and those not participating in trials may be associated higher periprocedural risk.[62,63] Integration of local outcomes should be a component of the decision for referral. Likewise, the uptake of CAS has been variable globally. In 2008 in the United States it represented 13% of carotid artery revascularization procedures (down from a peak of 15% in 2006), and will continue to decrease in the absence of approval by the Centers for Medicare and Medicaid Services or new clinical trials and registries.[64,65] Perioperative risk for CAS at experienced institutions appears to be favorable.[66]

Surgical Carotid Endarterectomy

Surgical endarterectomy involves an incision in the neck to expose the carotid artery, clamping of the carotid above and below the area planned for endarterectomy, insertion of a shunt to maintain cerebral blood flow, opening of the vessel and removal of the plaque lining of the artery, and closure of the vessel with removal of the shunt. This procedure has a low risk of periprocedural events in experienced centers.[9,11] Three trials have demonstrated benefit for CEA relative to medical therapy in appropriately selected patients (see **Table 2**). Long-term follow-up has also suggested continued benefit over time.[11] Cost-effectiveness analyses based on the Asymptomatic Carotid Surgery Trial (ACST) concluded that CEA was cost-effective in patients younger than 75 years; however, some have noted that if the background risk of stroke on medical therapy declined to less than 1% per year, CEA would no longer be cost-effective.[67] These investigators do not routinely incorporate the possibility that the same medical therapy that has reduced the stroke risk also reduces the risk of the revascularization procedures. In the ACST, patients on lipid-lowering therapy had both a lower rate of events in the medically treated arm and a lower rate of periprocedural events in the CEA arm.[11] Some contend that the background rate of stroke attributable to asymptomatic carotid disease is now below this threshold, but the majority of patients in these observational cohorts have moderate, but not severe, carotid stenoses.[16]

Carotid Stenting

Carotid stenting is an emerging technology that enables a percutaneous approach to the treatment of carotid stenosis. The arterial system is accessed percutaneously rather than through an incision, the stenosis is characterized with angiography, and the lesion is opened and stabilized with angioplasty balloons and stents. Because of the sensitive nature of the downstream vascular bed, embolic protection is routinely used. In randomized trials, CAS is associated with a periprocedural risk of any stroke or death of 4.1% at 30 days.[68] Patients who are treated with CAS must take dual-antiplatelet therapy for a minimum of 30 days following the procedure and monotherapy afterward.[4] Therefore, patients with contraindications for intensive antiplatelet therapy may not be optimal candidates for this procedure. In addition, the 2 primary randomized trials involving CAS have

Table 2
Major trials comparing surgical revascularization with medical therapy

Authors,[Ref.] Year	Name	Population/Size/Follow-up	Randomization Arms	Primary Findings	Notes
Hobson et al,[12] 1993	VA Trial	Asymptomatic carotid disease with >50% stenosis 444 men Mean follow-up 4 y	Carotid endarterectomy (CEA) vs medical therapy	Ipsilateral stroke 8% CEA vs 20.6% medical $P<.001$	There was no significant benefit on the combined end point of stroke or death. Placebo event rate considered higher than current estimates, and background therapy not considered consistent with current therapy.[16]
Executive Committee for the Asymptomatic Carotid Atherosclerosis Study,[9] 1995	ACAS	Asymptomatic carotid disease with >60% stenosis 1662 patients Median follow-up 2.7 y	CEA vs medical therapy	Ipsilateral stroke or any perioperative stroke or death at 5 y 5.1% CEA vs 11.0% medical $P<.01$	Placebo event rate considered higher than current estimates, and background therapy not considered consistent with current therapy[16]
Halliday et al,[10] 2004	ACST	Asymptomatic carotid disease with >70% stenosis 3120 patients Mean follow-up 3.4 y	CEA vs medical therapy	All stroke (perioperative and nonperioperative) at 5 y 6.4% vs 11.8% $P<.0001$	Placebo event rate considered higher than current estimates, and background therapy not considered consistent with current therapy.[16] Benefit consistent in both genders but less benefit for patients >75 y old

included both symptomatic and asymptomatic patients.[61,68] However, there did not appear to be an interaction when compared with CEA by symptomatic status.[69] Cost-effectiveness and quality of life appear to be similar for CAS and CEA over long-term follow-up.[70]

Which Procedure to Choose?

In general, CAS is considered an alternative to CEA in selected patients. In addition, CAS may be preferred in patients at high surgical risk, such as those with a high carotid artery bifurcation; however, validated risk-prediction models for this purpose do not exist. Overall, trials and meta-analyses suggest similar long-term outcomes with these 2 techniques; however, in the 4 trials of percutaneous compared with surgical revascularization that included asymptomatic patients (CAVATAS, CaRESS, SAPPHIRE, and CREST), the risk of stroke and death or stroke, MI, and death were similar and without significant difference.[59–61,68,71,72] More broadly defined complication rates (MI, stroke, death) have become standard since the primary complication of CEA was noted to be MI in the Mayo Asymptomatic Carotid Endarterectomy (MACE) study in 1992.[73] The major trials organized after the publication of this trial (ACST and CREST) included perioperative MI as component of the primary end point because of its singular importance as a perioperative complication.[69,74] As CREST-2 is now in the planning phase, the value of both surgical and percutaneous revascularization in asymptomatic disease when added to optimal medical therapy will soon be studied, and should provide greater clarity in the selection of procedure.

SUMMARY

The finding of asymptomatic carotid artery stenosis should be considered an indicator of heightened cardiovascular risk and an opportunity for intensified primary prevention. Patients should be evaluated broadly for all modifiable risk factors, and educated. All patients should be counseled with regard to lifestyle changes and therapeutic targets. Maximal medical therapy, including antiplatelet therapy where appropriate, statin therapy, and blood pressure–lowering therapy, should be used as recommended by current consensus guidelines. A subset of patients with asymptomatic carotid stenosis may benefit from preventive revascularization to reduce the risk of ipsilateral stroke. Careful patient selection is required when considering whether to revascularize as an adjunct to optimal medical therapy.

REFERENCES

1. Goldstein LB, Bushnell CD, Adams RJ, et al. Guidelines for the primary prevention of stroke: a guideline for healthcare professionals from the American Heart Association/American Stroke Association. Stroke 2011;42:517–84.
2. Pickett CA, Jackson JL, Hemann BA, et al. Carotid bruits as a prognostic indicator of cardiovascular death and myocardial infarction: a meta-analysis. Lancet 2008;371:1587–94.
3. Pickett CA, Jackson JL, Hemann BA, et al. Carotid bruits and cerebrovascular disease risk: a meta-analysis. Stroke 2010;41:2295–302.
4. Brott TG, Halperin JL, Abbara S, et al. 2011 ASA/ACCF/AHA/AANN/AANS/ACR/ASNR/CNS/SAIP/SCAI/SIR/SNIS/SVM/SVS guideline on the management of patients with extracranial carotid and vertebral artery disease: executive summary: a report of the American College of Cardiology Foundation/American Heart Association Task Force on Practice Guidelines, and the American Stroke Association, American Association of Neuroscience Nurses, American Association of Neurological Surgeons, American College of Radiology, American Society of Neuroradiology, Congress of Neurological Surgeons, Society of Atherosclerosis Imaging and Prevention, Society for Cardiovascular Angiography and Interventions, Society of Interventional Radiology, Society of Neurointerventional Surgery, Society for Vascular Medicine, and Society for Vascular Surgery. Vasc Med 2011;16:35–77.
5. Autret A, Pourcelot L, Saudeau D, et al. Stroke risk in patients with carotid stenosis. Lancet 1987;1:888–90.
6. Roger VL, Go AS, Lloyd-Jones DM, et al. Heart disease and stroke statistics—2012 update: a report from the American Heart Association. Circulation 2012;125:e2–220.
7. Chambers BR, Norris JW. Outcome in patients with asymptomatic neck bruits. N Engl J Med 1986;315:860–5.
8. Lewis RF, Abrahamowicz M, Cote R, et al. Predictive power of duplex ultrasonography in asymptomatic carotid disease. Ann Intern Med 1997;127:13–20.
9. Anonymous. Endarterectomy for asymptomatic carotid artery stenosis. Executive Committee for the Asymptomatic Carotid Atherosclerosis Study. JAMA 1995;273:1421–8.
10. Halliday A, Mansfield A, Marro J, et al. Prevention of disabling and fatal strokes by successful carotid endarterectomy in patients without recent neurological symptoms: randomised controlled trial. Lancet 2004;363:1491–502.
11. Halliday A, Harrison M, Hayter E, et al. 10-year stroke prevention after successful carotid endarterectomy

for asymptomatic stenosis (ACST-1): a multicentre randomised trial. Lancet 2010;376:1074–84.

12. Hobson RW 2nd, Weiss DG, Fields WS, et al. Efficacy of carotid endarterectomy for asymptomatic carotid stenosis. The Veterans Affairs Cooperative Study Group. N Engl J Med 1993;328:221–7.

13. O'Leary DH, Polak JF, Kronmal RA, et al. Distribution and correlates of sonographically detected carotid artery disease in the cardiovascular health study. The CHS Collaborative Research Group. Stroke 1992;23:1752–60.

14. Wolff T, Guirguis-Blake J, Miller T, et al. Screening for carotid artery stenosis: an update of the evidence for the U.S. Preventive Services Task Force. Ann Intern Med 2007;147:860–70.

15. Inzitari D, Eliasziw M, Gates P, et al. The causes and risk of stroke in patients with asymptomatic internal-carotid-artery stenosis. North American Symptomatic Carotid Endarterectomy Trial collaborators. N Engl J Med 2000;342:1693–700.

16. Abbott AL. Medical (nonsurgical) intervention alone is now best for prevention of stroke associated with asymptomatic severe carotid stenosis: results of a systematic review and analysis. Stroke 2009;40:e573–83.

17. Marquardt L, Geraghty OC, Mehta Z, et al. Low risk of ipsilateral stroke in patients with asymptomatic carotid stenosis on best medical treatment: a prospective, population-based study. Stroke 2010;41: e11–7.

18. King A, Shipley M, Markus H, for the ACES Investigators. The effect of medical treatments on stroke risk in asymptomatic carotid stenosis. Stroke 2012;44(2):542–6.

19. Anonymous. Clinical alert: benefit of carotid endarterectomy for patients with high-grade stenosis of the internal carotid artery. National Institute of Neurological Disorders and Stroke Stroke and trauma division. North American Symptomatic Carotid Endarterectomy Trial (NASCET) investigators. Stroke 1991;22:816–7.

20. Wyman RA, Gimelli G, McBride PE, et al. Does detection of carotid plaque affect physician behavior or motivate patients? Am Heart J 2007; 154:1072–7.

21. Olin JW, Fonseca C, Childs MB, et al. The natural history of asymptomatic moderate internal carotid artery stenosis by duplex ultrasound. Vasc Med 1998;3:101–8.

22. Estruch R, Ros E, Salas-Salvado J, et al. Primary prevention of cardiovascular disease with a Mediterranean diet. N Engl J Med 2013;368:1279–90.

23. Rothwell PM, Coull AJ, Giles MF, et al. Change in stroke incidence, mortality, case-fatality, severity, and risk factors in Oxfordshire, UK from 1981 to 2004 (Oxford Vascular Study). Lancet 2004;363: 1925–33.

24. Raman G, Moorthy D, Hadar N, et al. Management strategies for asymptomatic carotid stenosis: a systematic review and meta-analysis. Ann Intern Med 2013;158:676–85.

25. Antithrombotic Trialists' Collaboration. Collaborative meta-analysis of randomised trials of antiplatelet therapy for prevention of death, myocardial infarction, and stroke in high risk patients. BMJ 2002;324:71–86.

26. Antithrombotic Trialists' (ATT) Collaboration, Baigent C, Blackwell L, et al. Aspirin in the primary and secondary prevention of vascular disease: collaborative meta-analysis of individual participant data from randomised trials. Lancet 2009; 373:1849–60.

27. Anonymous. Final report on the aspirin component of the ongoing physicians' health study. Steering committee of the Physicians' Health Study Research Group. N Engl J Med 1989;321:129–35.

28. Cote R, Battista RN, Abrahamowicz M, et al. Lack of effect of aspirin in asymptomatic patients with carotid bruits and substantial carotid narrowing. The asymptomatic cervical bruit study group. Ann Intern Med 1995;123:649–55.

29. CURRENT-OASIS 7 Investigators, Mehta SR, Bassand JP, et al. Dose comparisons of clopidogrel and aspirin in acute coronary syndromes. N Engl J Med 2010;363:930–42.

30. Anonymous. A randomised, blinded, trial of clopidogrel versus aspirin in patients at risk of ischaemic events (CAPRIE). CAPRIE steering committee. Lancet 1996;348:1329–39.

31. Bhatt DL, Fox KA, Hacke W, et al. Clopidogrel and aspirin versus aspirin alone for the prevention of atherothrombotic events. N Engl J Med 2006;354:1706–17.

32. Geng DF, Deng J, Jin DM, et al. Effect of cilostazol on the progression of carotid intima-media thickness: a meta-analysis of randomized controlled trials. Atherosclerosis 2012;220:177–83.

33. Tsutsumi M, Aikawa H, Nii K, et al. Cilostazol reduces periprocedural hemodynamic depression in carotid artery stenting. Neurol Med Chir (Tokyo) 2013;53:163–70.

34. Takigawa T, Matsumaru Y, Hayakawa M, et al. Cilostazol reduces restenosis after carotid artery stenting. J Vasc Surg 2010;51:51–6.

35. Expert Panel on Detection, Evaluation, and Treatment of High Blood Cholesterol in Adults. Executive summary of the third report of the National Cholesterol Education Program (NCEP) expert panel on detection, evaluation, and treatment of high blood cholesterol in adults (adult treatment panel III). JAMA 2001;285:2486–97.

36. Grundy SM, Cleeman JI, Merz CN, et al. Implications of recent clinical trials for the National Cholesterol Education Program Adult Treatment Panel III guidelines. J Am Coll Cardiol 2004;44:720–32.

37. Ridker PM, Danielson E, Fonseca FA, et al. Rosu-vastatin to prevent vascular events in men and women with elevated C-reactive protein. N Engl J Med 2008;359:2195–207.

38. Amarenco P, Labreuche J. Lipid management in the prevention of stroke: review and updated meta-analysis of statins for stroke prevention. Lancet Neurol 2009;8:453–63.

39. Crouse JR 3rd, Raichlen JS, Riley WA, et al. Effect of rosuvastatin on progression of carotid intima-media thickness in low-risk individuals with subclin-ical atherosclerosis: the METEOR trial. JAMA 2007; 297:1344–53.

40. Spence JD, Coates V, Li H, et al. Effects of inten-sive medical therapy on microemboli and cardio-vascular risk in asymptomatic carotid stenosis. Arch Neurol 2010;67:180–6.

41. Tawakol A, Fayad ZA, Mogg R, et al. Intensification of statin therapy results in a rapid reduction in atherosclerotic inflammation: results of a multi-center FDG-PET/CT feasibility study. J Am Coll Cardiol 2013. [Epub ahead of print].

42. Howard G, Manolio TA, Burke GL, et al. Does the association of risk factors and atherosclerosis change with age? An analysis of the combined ARIC and CHS cohorts. The Atherosclerosis Risk in Communities (ARIC) and Cardiovascular Health Study (CHS) investigators. Stroke 1997; 28:1693–701.

43. Lawes CM, Bennett DA, Feigin VL, et al. Blood pressure and stroke: an overview of published reviews. Stroke 2004;35:1024.

44. Neal B, MacMahon S, Chapman N, Blood Pressure Lowering Treatment Trialists' Collaboration. Effects of ACE inhibitors, calcium antagonists, and other blood-pressure-lowering drugs: results of prospec-tively designed overviews of randomised trials. Blood Pressure Lowering Treatment Trialists' Collaboration. Lancet 2000;356:1955–64.

45. Yusuf S, Sleight P, Pogue J, et al. Effects of an angiotensin-converting-enzyme inhibitor, rami-pril, on cardiovascular events in high-risk patients. The Heart Outcomes Prevention Evalu-ation Study investigators. N Engl J Med 2000; 342:145–53.

46. De Rango P, Lenti M, Simonte G, et al. No benefit from carotid intervention in fatal stroke prevention for >80-year-old patients. Eur J Vasc Endovasc Surg 2012;44:252–9.

47. Wallaert JB, De Martino RR, Finlayson SR, et al. Ca-rotid endarterectomy in asymptomatic patients with limited life expectancy. Stroke 2012;43:1781–7.

48. Rothwell PM, Eliasziw M, Gutnikov SA, et al. Sex difference in the effect of time from symptoms to surgery on benefit from carotid endarterectomy for transient ischemic attack and nondisabling stroke. Stroke 2004;35:2855–61.

49. Sangiorgi G, Roversi S, Biondi Zoccai G, et al. Sex-related differences in carotid plaque features and inflammation. J Vasc Surg 2012;57(2):338–44.

50. Spagnoli LG, Mauriello A, Sangiorgi G, et al. Extra-cranial thrombotically active carotid plaque as a risk factor for ischemic stroke. JAMA 2004;292: 1845–52.

51. Millon A, Boussel L, Brevet M, et al. Clinical and histological significance of gadolinium enhance-ment in carotid atherosclerotic plaque. Stroke 2012;43:3023–8.

52. Madani A, Beletsky V, Tamayo A, et al. High-risk asymptomatic carotid stenosis: ulceration on 3D ultrasound vs TCD microemboli. Neurology 2011; 77:744–50.

53. King A, Markus HS. Doppler embolic signals in ce-rebrovascular disease and prediction of stroke risk: a systematic review and meta-analysis. Stroke 2009;40:3711–7.

54. Abbott AL, Chambers BR, Stork JL, et al. Embolic signals and prediction of ipsilateral stroke or tran-sient ischemic attack in asymptomatic carotid ste-nosis: a multicenter prospective cohort study. Stroke 2005;36:1128–33.

55. Horn J, Naylor AR, Laman DM, et al. Identification of patients at risk for ischaemic cerebral complica-tions after carotid endarterectomy with TCD moni-toring. Eur J Vasc Endovasc Surg 2005;30:270–4.

56. Markus HS, King A, Shipley M, et al. Asymptomatic embolisation for prediction of stroke in the Asymp-tomatic Carotid Emboli Study (ACES): a prospec-tive observational study. Lancet Neurol 2010;9: 663–71.

57. Mono ML, Karameshev A, Slotboom J, et al. Pla-que characteristics of asymptomatic carotid ste-nosis and risk of stroke. Cerebrovasc Dis 2012; 34:343–50.

58. Persson J, Folkersen L, Ekstrand J, et al. High plasma adiponectin concentration is associated with all-cause mortality in patients with carotid atherosclerosis. Atherosclerosis 2012;225:491–6.

59. Ederle J, Featherstone RL, Brown MM. Random-ized controlled trials comparing endarterectomy and endovascular treatment for carotid artery ste-nosis: a Cochrane systematic review. Stroke 2009;40:1373–80.

60. Bonati LH, Lyrer P, Ederle J, et al. Percutaneous transluminal balloon angioplasty and stenting for carotid artery stenosis. Cochrane Database Syst Rev 2012;(9):CD000515.

61. Gurm HS, Yadav JS, Fayad P, et al. Long-term results of carotid stenting versus endarterectomy in high-risk patients. N Engl J Med 2008;358: 1572–9.

62. Kansara A, Miller D, Damani R, et al. Variability in carotid endarterectomy practice patterns within a metropolitan area. Stroke 2012;43:3105–7.

63. Wennberg DE, Lucas FL, Birkmeyer JD, et al. Variation in carotid endarterectomy mortality in the Medicare population: trial hospitals, volume, and patient characteristics. JAMA 1998;279: 1278–81.

64. Lee AH, Busby J, Brooks M, et al. Uptake of carotid artery stenting in England and subsequent vascular admissions: an appropriate response to emerging evidence? Eur J Vasc Endovasc Surg 2013;46(3):282–9.

65. Dumont TM, Rughani AI. National trends in carotid artery revascularization surgery. J Neurosurg 2012; 116:1251–7.

66. Dumont TM, Wach MM, Mokin M, et al. Perioperative complications after carotid artery stenting: a contemporary experience from the University at Buffalo neuroendovascular surgery team. Neurosurgery 2013. [Epub ahead of print].

67. Thapar A, Garcia Mochon L, Epstein D, et al. Modelling the cost-effectiveness of carotid endarterectomy for asymptomatic stenosis. Br J Surg 2012;100(2):231–9.

68. Brott TG, Hobson RW 2nd, Howard G, et al. Stenting versus endarterectomy for treatment of carotid-artery stenosis. N Engl J Med 2010;363:11–23.

69. Silver FL, Mackey A, Clark WM, et al. Safety of stenting and endarterectomy by symptomatic status in the Carotid Revascularization Endarterectomy Versus Stenting Trial (CREST). Stroke 2011;42:675–80.

70. Vilain KR, Magnuson EA, Li H, et al. Costs and cost-effectiveness of carotid stenting versus endarterectomy for patients at standard surgical risk: results from the Carotid Revascularization Endarterectomy Versus Stenting Trial (CREST). Stroke 2012;43:2408–16.

71. Yadav JS, Wholey MH, Kuntz RE, et al. Protected carotid-artery stenting versus endarterectomy in high-risk patients. N Engl J Med 2004;351:1493–501.

72. Anonymous. Endovascular versus surgical treatment in patients with carotid stenosis in the carotid and vertebral artery transluminal angioplasty study (CAVATAS): a randomised trial. Lancet 2001;357: 1729–37.

73. Anonymous. Results of a randomized controlled trial of carotid endarterectomy for asymptomatic carotid stenosis. Mayo Asymptomatic Carotid Endarterectomy Study Group. Mayo Clin Proc 1992;67: 513–8.

74. Kinlay S. Fire in the hole: carotid stenting versus endarterectomy. Circulation 2011;123:2522–5.

Non-Invasive Carotid Imaging
A Comparative Assessment and Practical Approach

Beau M. Hawkins, MD[a], Michael R. Jaff, DO[b],*

KEYWORDS

- Carotid stenosis • Ultrasound • Computed tomographic angiography
- Magnetic resonance angiography • Carotid endarterectomy • Carotid stent

KEY POINTS

- Multiple noninvasive imaging methods, including duplex ultrasonography, computerized tomographic angiography, and magnetic resonance angiography, are available to assess the extracranial carotid artery and guide clinical decision making.
- A thorough understanding of noninvasive carotid imaging is imperative to provide efficient, effective, and high-quality care for patients with atherosclerotic carotid artery disease.

INTRODUCTION

Stroke occurs in nearly 800,000 individuals annually, is the fourth most common cause of death, and imparts significant morbidity and functional impairment in survivors.[1] Thromboembolic events associated with atherosclerotic carotid artery disease are a frequent cause of ischemic strokes, comprising roughly 10% of all ischemic events, and nearly 25% of those classified as embolic in origin.[2,3]

Landmark trials completed nearly 2 decades ago demonstrated significant stroke reduction with endarterectomy (CEA) relative to medical therapy,[4,5] and modern studies comparing carotid stenting (CAS) with CEA have shown similar composite outcomes in standard and high-surgical risk patients.[6,7] Revascularization, therefore, in conjunction with medical therapy and risk factor modification, remains an important therapy for patients with carotid artery disease.

The detection and quantification of extracranial carotid artery disease are now readily achievable with several noninvasive imaging modalities including duplex ultrasonography (DUS), computerized tomography angiography (CTA), and magnetic resonance angiography (MRA). In fact, the information obtained from such studies often strongly influences the chosen therapy, particularly that relating to whether revascularization should be considered. Although unique advantages and pitfalls are present with each modality, the use of more than 1 imaging test is often necessary to adequately assess the extracranial carotid circulation and inform clinical decision making. Moreover, noninvasive imaging remains an important surveillance tool following revascularization. This article aims to discuss the available noninvasive imaging

Dr B.M. Hawkins reports no disclosures.

Dr M.R. Jaff is a noncompensated advisor to Abbott Vascular, Cordis, Covidien/ev3, Medtronic Vascular, and is a member of the Board of Directors, VIVA Physicians, Incorporated, a 501c3 not-for-profit education and research organization.

[a] Cardiovascular Section, Department of Internal Medicine, University of Oklahoma Health Sciences Center, 920 Stanton L. Young Blvd, Williams Pavilion 3010, Oklahoma City, OK 73104, USA; [b] Vascular Medicine Section, Cardiology Division, Massachusetts General Hospital, 55 Fruit Street, Warren Building 905, Boston, MA 02115, USA

* Corresponding author.

E-mail address: mjaff@partners.org

Intervent Cardiol Clin 3 (2014) 13–20

http://dx.doi.org/10.1016/j.iccl.2013.08.002

modalities for extracranial carotid artery disease and provide a clinically relevant framework for the use of noninvasive imaging in the care of patients with atherosclerotic carotid artery disease.

CATHETER-BASED ANGIOGRAPHY: THE HISTORICAL GOLD STANDARD

Carotid stenosis severity, most often expressed as a percentage stenosis, is the feature most commonly used to determine whether revascularization should be considered.[6] Multiple techniques have been described to quantify stenosis using catheter-based angiography. In 1 such method, the ECST (European Carotid Surgery Trial), the percent stenosis is calculated as the ratio of the narrowest segment of the stenosis within the internal carotid artery by the diameter of the carotid artery at the site of stenosis.[5] The more widely accepted method, the NASCET (North American Symptomatic Carotid Endarterectomy Trial) method, is defined as the percentage of the ratio of the diameter of the most severe stenosis to the diameter of the normal distal internal carotid artery, usually occurring at the level of the second cervical vertebrae, where the walls become parallel.[4] Importantly, this measurement does not involve the region of poststenotic dilatation of the internal carotid artery or the carotid bulb, and the

caliber of the distal healthy internal carotid is often considerably smaller than these segments. Thus, the calculated stenosis with the NASCET method tends to be much more conservative,[8] and this method is the dominant strategy for assessing the severity of carotid stenosis in modern practice.

DUPLEX ULTRASONOGRAPHY

Based on its safety, cost, reliability, and reproducibility, DUS is generally the first-line test used to screen for extracranial carotid artery disease in symptomatic individuals, those with a cervical bruit detected on physical examination, or in those at risk for carotid stenosis. The typical DUS examination involves imaging of the common, external, internal, and vertebral arteries bilaterally. Direct grayscale imaging of the carotid arteries in longitudinal and transverse planes is performed to identify the presence and morphology of atherosclerotic plaque. Doppler interrogation is also performed to calculate peak systolic and end-diastolic velocities using the Doppler principle. These velocities are used to quantify stenosis severity (**Fig. 1**). In general, peak systolic velocity, end-diastolic velocity, and the ratio of the peak systolic velocity in the internal carotid artery compared with the distal common carotid artery are the measures used to quantify stenosis

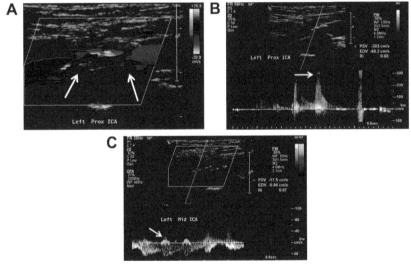

Fig. 1. DUS identification of a severe carotid stenosis in a patient with amaurosis fugax. (*A*) A longitudinal view of the proximal left internal carotid artery demonstrates a long, echogenic plaque (*arrows*) that nearly obstructs the entire lumen. (*B*) Doppler interrogation in this stenotic segment identified a peak systolic velocity of 303 cm/s, consistent with severe stenosis (*arrow*). (*C*) Flow velocity in the midsegment of the left internal carotid is severely (*arrow*) diminished because of the severe stenosis in the adjacent, proximal segment. In addition to the low velocity, note that the Doppler waveform has a slow upstroke, a finding in DUS commonly indicative of more proximal stenosis. Although duplex ultransonography cannot always visualize these more proximal stenoses, particularly if the lesion involves the subclavian or innominate vessels, the Doppler waveform is a valuable tool unique to ultrasound that can be used to identify abnormalities outside of the imaged vessels.

severity. **Table 1** displays commonly used criteria to grade carotid stenosis.[9] Note, however, that there is significant variation regarding the ideal velocity that corresponds to a severe (>70%) stenosis. As an example, 3 separate studies reported that a >70% stenosis corresponds to peak systolic velocities of 220 cm/s, 230 cm/s, and 283 cm/s.[9–11] These differences are likely due to multiple factors including patient population characteristics, interlaboratory variations, technologist skill, and equipment differences.

In general, DUS is an accurate imaging modality, with reported sensitivities and specificities ranging from 62% to 99% and 69% to 100%, respectively.[12] Jahromi and colleagues[13] performed a meta-analysis of published literature and found that a peak systolic velocity of 200 cm/s has a sensitivity of 90% and specificity of 94% for detection of greater than 70% stenosis.

DUS does have some limitations. Severe calcification of the diseased carotid segment may result in acoustic shadowing that can obscure the lumen. Doppler interrogation of these shadowed regions may miss the most diseased areas resulting in underestimation of stenosis severity.[14] In severe contralateral disease, the peak velocities may be falsely elevated, which may lead to stenosis overestimation.[15] This is 1 setting in which the use of internal-to-common carotid velocity ratios may be particularly useful, since common carotid velocities should be elevated in the presence of severe contralateral stenosis or occlusion. Vessel tortuosity, a finding common in the very elderly, may also artificially raise velocities, leading to overestimation of a stenosis. The differentiation between occlusion and near-occlusion, or the so-called string sign, is also often difficult, because it

may not be possible to precisely interrogate and identity a narrow channel of flow through a heavily diseased artery. Finally, the internal carotid segment visualized with DUS is limited; disease distal to the angle of the mandible is not readily accessible with this technique (**Box 1**).[16]

COMPUTED TOMOGRAPHY ANGIOGRAPHY

Technological advances have allowed CTA to become a useful imaging modality for carotid artery disease. In contemporary practice, CTA is a widely available tool, and most studies can be performed quickly, distinguishing it from other axial imaging techniques (ie, MRA). Modern scanners and associated imaging protocols have resulted in the achievement of high spatial resolution, resulting in image quality that is not obtainable with other noninvasive methods. Reported sensitivities and specificities for the detection of carotid stenosis greater than 70% range from 67% to 100% and 82% to 100%, respectively.[12] Koelemay and colleagues[17] performed an analysis of pooled data and reported a sensitivity and specificity of 85% and 93% for stenosis greater than 70% in severity, respectively. For carotid occlusion, the sensitivity and specificity were 97% and 99%, respectively, highlighting the valuable role CTA has in confirming occlusions (**Fig. 2**). In contrast to DUS, CTA also visualizes the intracranial carotid segments in addition to the surrounding osseous and musculoskeletal structures.

Limitations of CTA include its requirement for iodinated contrast, which may cause or exacerbate existing renal impairment. Radiation with its attendant health risks is used during the examination. Vessel and plaque calcification may produce

Table 1
DUS consensus criteria for carotid stenosis

Stenosis (%)	ICA PSV (cm/s)	Plaque Estimate (%)	ICA/CCA PSV Ratio	ICA EDV (cm/s)
Normal	<125	None	<2	<40
<50	<125	<50	<2	<40
50–69	125–230	≥50	2–4	40–100
≥70 but less than near occlusion	>230	≥50	>4	>100
Near occlusion	High, low, or undetectable	Visible	Variable	Variable
Occlusion	Undetectable	Visible, no detectable lumen	Not applicable	Not applicable

Abbreviations: CCA, common carotid artery; EDV, end diastolic velocity; ICA, internal carotid artery; PSV, peak systolic velocity.

From Grant EG, Benson CB, Moneta GL, et al. Carotid artery stenosis: gray-scale and Doppler US diagnosis- Society of Radiologists in Ultrasound consensus conference. Radiology 2003;229:344; with permission.

Box 1
Duplex ultrasonography

- DUS is the first-line imaging test for patients with suspected carotid artery stenosis.
- DUS uses velocity criteria to quantify stenosis severity, and has been demonstrated to be accurate relative to invasive angiography.
- Estimates of DUS-derived stenosis severity may be less reliable in settings of severe calcification, vessel tortuosity, contralateral disease, and near-occlusions.

Box 2
Computed tomography angiography

- CTA is particularly useful in differentiating complete occlusions from severe stenosis (eg, near-occlusions or string signs).
- The requirements of contrast and radiation are the major limitations of CTA.

imaging artifacts that obscure the lumen, leading to overestimation of stenosis (**Box 2**).[18,19]

MAGNETIC RESONANCE ANGIOGRAPHY

In contrast to CTA, MRA does not require radiation or iodinated contrast. Several MRA techniques are available to image the carotid arteries, but the 2 most commonly used include time-of-flight (TOF) and contrast-enhanced (CE) MRA. TOF-MRA does not use gadolinium contrast, and relies on laminar blood flow for image acquisition. As would be anticipated, in areas within and adjacent to severe stenoses, flow may become naturally turbulent or slow, and this may degrade image quality, leading to signal dropout.[16] Such dropout leads to difficulty in deciphering whether an imaged segment is occluded or severely stenotic, and TOF-MRA in fact, is not an appropriate modality for distinguishing these conditions. This has important clinical implications, since revascularization is generally not indicated for carotid occlusion.[12] CE-MRA does use gadolinium contrast, which may cause nephrogenic systemic sclerosis in the setting of renal insufficiency.[20] However, CE-MRA does not depend as readily on laminar

blood flow for image acquisition, and it provides better visualization of the vessel lumen (**Fig. 3**). As such, it more readily differentiates occlusions from severe stenoses.[16]

With the mentioned exception of near-occlusions, MRA is an accurate imaging modality. U-King-Im and colleagues[21] examined the performance of CE-MRA in relation to digital subtraction angiography (DSA). When comparing CE-MRA with DSA-derived stenosis of greater than 70% using the NASCET method, they reported sensitivity of 93% and specificity of 88%. TOF-MRA has been reported to have similarly good performance. In a study comparing TOF-MRA with DSA for greater than 70% stenoses, DeMarco and colleagues[22] reported sensitivity and specificity for TOF-MRA of 94% and 97%, respectively.

MRA does have some additional limitations. Image acquisition time can be lengthy, and this at times is not well tolerated by patients, particularly those with claustrophobia. MRA cannot be performed in the setting of certain implants (eg, certain pacemakers or defibrillators), and surgical clips in the vicinity of the carotid territory may produce artifacts. Despite the reported accuracy of CE-MRA, this technique is known to be prone to stenosis overestimation.[21] In addition to signal dropout, vessel tortuosity can also create artifact, which diminishes accuracy (**Box 3**).[16]

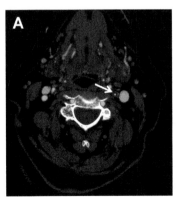 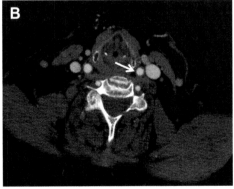

Fig. 2. CTA of the left internal carotid reveals a very severe stenosis. (*A*) A pinpoint lumen that was not detectable with DUS is present (*arrow*). (*B*) The relatively healthy distal left internal carotid is highlighted for reference (*arrow*).

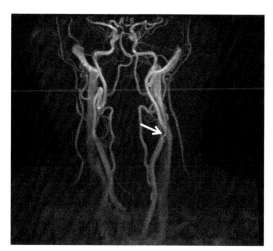

Fig. 3. CE-MRA of the internal carotid demonstrates a severe stenosis (*arrow*).

SPECIAL CLINICAL SCENARIOS
Poststent Surveillance

Appropriate use criteria support the performance of DUS following carotid revascularization,[23] and in practice, this is the most common modality used to image carotid arteries following either CEA or CAS. DUS is advantageous in that it is safe, does not require radiation or contrast, is inexpensive, and is reproducible. DUS can visualize stents, confirm whether intimal hyperplasia is present within the stented lumen, and assess whether de novo disease (proximal or distal to stent) is present. DUS is also capable of identifying stent fracture, a phenomenon that has been reported.[24,25] However, uniform criteria to grade restenosis based on Doppler velocity measurements are less established. Stent placement may distort the diastolic relaxation of the carotid artery and result in a high resistant flow pattern. Doppler interrogation of such stented arteries generally produces velocities that are significantly elevated. In general, a peak systolic velocity of greater than 300 cm/s is usually accepted as indicative of severe restenosis (>70%–80%),[26] and peak systolic velocity has been shown to be a better predictor of restenosis than end-diastolic velocity or the internal-to-common carotid artery velocity ratio.[27] Additionally, there are several helpful characteristics that may assist with the DUS identification of restenosis, including poststenotic turbulence, presence of a color bruit, luminal narrowing within the stent during color imaging, diffuse spectral broadening, and velocity decrement distal to the suspected stenosis.[16]

MRA is not currently an acceptable surveillance modality following CAS. Indwelling stents produce signals that artificially obscure the lumen and may lead to overestimation of stenosis.[28] Technological advances that circumvent this artifact limitation are in progress and may at some point allow for the use of MRA for this purpose.[29] Due to its requirement for radiation, CTA has inherent limitations as a surveillance tool. However, it can image stented carotids,[30] although difficulty in assessing restenosis severity has been reported (**Box 4**).[31]

Revascularization Planning

In contrast to CEA, in which direct inspection and plaque excision of the ICA are performed through open neck dissection, CAS usually mandates navigation of the aortic arch, safe manipulation of catheters into the target carotid vessel, and favorable anatomy to deploy embolic protection. Moreover, in addition to clinical characteristics that increase procedural risk with CAS,[32] anatomic features such as arch type, circumferential calcification, and vessel tortuosity have been shown to increase procedural complexity and CAS risk.[33,34] Innominate and subclavian artery stenoses, as well as disease distal to the carotid bifurcation, may impact percutaneous revascularization strategies. Knowledge of these anatomic considerations is not readily obtainable with DUS, and it is therefore often necessary to perform an additional imaging study to more fully gauge procedural risk, inform clinical decision making, and

---

Box 3
Magnetic resonance angiography

- MRA has comparable, if not superior, accuracy to other noninvasive carotid imaging modalities.

- In contrast to other noninvasive modalities, carotid calcification does not significantly impair MRA performance.

- MRA cannot reliably distinguish between near and complete occlusions in most cases.

Box 4
Poststent surveillance

- DUS is the test of choice for poststent surveillance.

- CTA may be used to image stented carotids, but its requirements for radiation and contrast make it a less ideal surveillance tool.

- MRA is not a reliable surveillance modality because of the artifacts produced by indwelling stents.

guide procedural planning. This strategy is supported by current guidelines.[12]

RECOMMENDATIONS FOR NONINVASIVE CAROTID IMAGING

DUS is the first-line test used to screen for carotid disease owing to its safety, cost advantage, and reliability. DUS may be used in individuals with asymptomatic cervical bruits, those with symptoms of transient ischemic attack (TIA) or stroke, or as a surveillance tool following either CEA or CAS.[12] In acutely symptomatic patients,

CTA and MRA have the added advantage of being able to provide detail regarding the brain parenchyma and assist in determining whether an acute cerebrovascular event has occurred. Regarding asymptomatic patients, proposed imaging algorithms have been previously published (**Fig. 4**).[16,31] In general, if DUS excludes the presence of significant (>50%) disease, no further confirmatory imaging is required. A routine surveillance program should be initiated. However, if DUS reveals findings of significant carotid disease, and intervention is planned, additional imaging with CTA or MRA is recommended.

CAROTID STENOSIS EVALUATION ALGORITHM

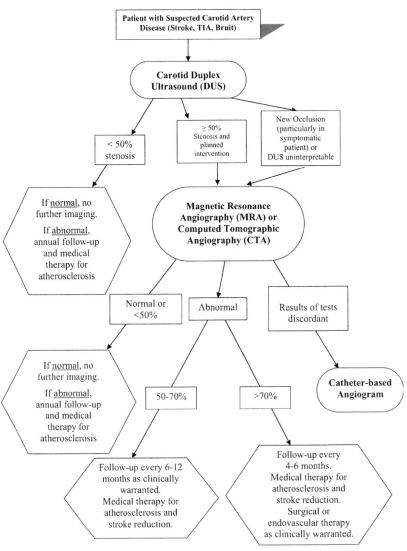

Fig. 4. Proposed algorithm for imaging in asymptomatic patients. (*Reproduced from* The Society of Vascular Medicine, Jaff MR, Goldmakher GV, Lev MH, et al. Imaging of the carotid arteries: the role of duplex ultrasonography, magnetic resonance arteriography, and computerized tomographic arteriography. Vasc Med 2008;13: 283; with permission.)

When results of DUS and CTA or MRA are discordant, catheter-based angiography should be considered.

SUMMARY

Multiple noninvasive imaging tests are available to assess the extracranial carotid circulation. Each modality has unique advantages and limitations, and in this sense, they serve a complementary rather than competitive role in evaluation of the carotid artery. A thorough understanding of noninvasive carotid imaging is imperative to provide efficient, effective, and high-quality care for patients with atherosclerotic carotid artery disease.

REFERENCES

1. Go AS, Mozaffarian D, Roger VL, et al. Heart disease and stroke statistics—2013 update: a report from the American Heart Association. Circulation 2013;127:e6–245.
2. White H, Boden-Albala B, Wang C, et al. Ischemic stroke subtype incidence among whites, blacks, and Hispanics: the Northern Manhattan Study. Circulation 2005;111:1327–31.
3. Gleason S, Furie KL, Lev MH, et al. Potential influence of acute CT on inpatient costs in patients with ischemic stroke. Acad Radiol 2001;8:955–64.
4. Beneficial effect of carotid endarterectomy in symptomatic patients with high-grade carotid stenosis. North American Symptomatic Carotid Endarterectomy Trial Collaborators. N Engl J Med 1991;325: 445–53.
5. Randomised trial of endarterectomy for recently symptomatic carotid stenosis: final results of the MRC European Carotid Surgery Trial (ECST). Lancet 1998;351:1379–87.
6. Brott TG, Hobson RW 2nd, Howard G, et al. Stenting versus endarterectomy for treatment of carotid-artery stenosis. N Engl J Med 2010;363.11–23.
7. Yadav JS, Wholey MH, Kuntz RE, et al. Protected carotid-artery stenting versus endarterectomy in high-risk patients. N Engl J Med 2004;351: 1493–501.
8. Rothwell PM, Gibson RJ, Slattery J, et al. Equivalence of measurements of carotid stenosis. A comparison of three methods on 1001 angiograms. European Carotid Surgery Trialists' Collaborative Group. Stroke 1994;25:2435–9.
9. Grant EG, Benson CB, Moneta GL, et al. Carotid artery stenosis: gray-scale and Doppler US diagnosis–Society of Radiologists in Ultrasound Consensus Conference. Radiology 2003;229:340–6.
10. Heijenbrok-Kal MH, Buskens E, Nederkoorn PJ, et al. Optimal peak systolic velocity threshold at duplex us for determining the need for carotid endarterectomy: a decision analytic approach. Radiology 2006;238:480–8.
11. Saba L, Sanfilippo R, Montisci R, et al. Carotid artery stenosis quantification: concordance analysis between radiologist and semi-automatic computer software by using Multi-Detector-Row CT angiography. Eur J Radiol 2011;79:80–4.
12. Brott TG, Halperin JL, Abbara S, et al. 2011 ASA/ACCF/AHA/AANN/AANS/ACR/ASNR/CNS/SAIP/SCAI/SIR/SNIS/SVM/SVS guideline on the management of patients with extracranial carotid and vertebral artery disease: executive summary. A report of the American College of Cardiology Foundation/American Heart Association Task Force on Practice Guidelines, and the American Stroke Association, American Association of Neuroscience Nurses, American Association of Neurological Surgeons, American College of Radiology, American Society of Neuroradiology, Congress of Neurological Surgeons, Society of Atherosclerosis Imaging and Prevention, Society for Cardiovascular Angiography and Interventions, Society of Interventional Radiology, Society of NeuroInterventional Surgery, Society for Vascular Medicine, and Society for Vascular Surgery. Circulation 2011;124:489–532.
13. Jahromi AS, Cina CS, Liu Y, et al. Sensitivity and specificity of color duplex ultrasound measurement in the estimation of internal carotid artery stenosis: a systematic review and meta-analysis. J Vasc Surg 2005;41:962–72.
14. Leonardo G, Crescenzi B, Cotrufo R, et al. Improvement in accuracy of diagnosis of carotid artery stenosis with duplex ultrasound scanning with combined use of linear array 7.5 MHz and convex array 3.5 MHz probes: validation versus 489 arteriographic procedures. J Vasc Surg 2003;37:1240–7.
15. Henderson RD, Steinman DA, Eliasziw M, et al. Effect of contralateral carotid artery stenosis on carotid ultrasound velocity measurements. Stroke 2000;31:2636–40.
16. Jaff MR, Goldmakher GV, Lev MH, et al. Imaging of the carotid arteries: the role of duplex ultrasonography, magnetic resonance arteriography, and computerized tomographic arteriography. Vasc Med 2008;13:281–92.
17. Koelemay MJ, Nederkoorn PJ, Reitsma JB, et al. Systematic review of computed tomographic angiography for assessment of carotid artery disease. Stroke 2004;35:2306–12.
18. Woodcock RJ Jr, Goldstein JH, Kallmes DF, et al. Angiographic correlation of CT calcification in the carotid siphon. AJNR Am J Neuroradiol 1999;20: 495–9.
19. Saba L, Sanfilippo R, Pirisi R, et al. Multidetector-row CT angiography in the study of atherosclerotic carotid arteries. Neuroradiology 2007;49:623–37.

20. Nainani N, Panesar M. Nephrogenic systemic fibrosis. Am J Nephrol 2009;29:1–9.

21. U-King-Im JM, Trivedi RA, Cross JJ, et al. Measuring carotid stenosis on contrast-enhanced magnetic resonance angiography: diagnostic performance and reproducibility of 3 different methods. Stroke 2004;35:2083–8.

22. DeMarco JK, Huston J 3rd, Bernstein MA. Evaluation of classic 2D time-of-flight MR angiography in the depiction of severe carotid stenosis. AJR Am J Roentgenol 2004;183:787–93.

23. American College of Cardiology Foundation (ACCF), American College of Radiology (ACR), American Institute of Ultrasound in Medicine (AIUM), et al. ACCF/ACR/AIUM/ASE/ASN/ICAVL/SCAI/SCCT/SIR/SVM/SVS 2012 appropriate use criteria for peripheral vascular ultrasound and physiological testing part I: arterial ultrasound and physiological testing: a report of the American College of Cardiology Foundation appropriate use criteria task force, American College of Radiology, American Institute of Ultrasound in Medicine, American Society of Echocardiography, American Society of Nephrology, Intersocietal Commission for the Accreditation of Vascular Laboratories, Society for Cardiovascular Angiography and Interventions, Society of Cardiovascular Computed Tomography, Society for Interventional Radiology, Society for Vascular Medicine, and Society for Vascular Surgery. J Am Coll Cardiol 2012;60:242–76.

24. Sfyroeras GS, Koutsiaris A, Karathanos C, et al. Clinical relevance and treatment of carotid stent fractures. J Vasc Surg 2010;51:1280–5.

25. Coppi G, Moratto R, Veronesi J, et al. Carotid artery stent fracture identification and clinical relevance. J Vasc Surg 2010;51:1397–405.

26. Lal BK, Beach KW, Roubin GS, et al. Restenosis after carotid artery stenting and endarterectomy: a secondary analysis of CREST, a randomised controlled trial. Lancet Neurol 2012;11:755–63.

27. AbuRahma AF, Abu-Halimah S, Bensenhaver J, et al. Optimal carotid duplex velocity criteria for defining the severity of carotid in-stent restenosis. J Vasc Surg 2008;48:589–94.

28. Borisch I, Hamer OW, Zorger N, et al. In vivo evaluation of the carotid wallstent on three-dimensional contrast material-enhanced MR angiography: influence of artifacts on the visibility of stent lumina. J Vasc Interv Radiol 2005;16:669–77.

29. Frolich AM, Pilgram-Pastor SM, Psychogios MN, et al. Comparing different MR angiography strategies of carotid stents in a vascular flow model: toward stent-specific recommendations in MR follow-up. Neuroradiology 2011;53:359–65.

30. Kwon BJ, Jung C, Sheen SH, et al. CT angiography of stented carotid arteries: comparison with Doppler ultrasonography. J Endovasc Ther 2007;14:489–97.

31. Romero JM, Ackerman RH, Dault NA, et al. Noninvasive evaluation of carotid artery stenosis: indications, strategies, and accuracy. Neuroimaging Clin N Am 2005;15:351–65, xi.

32. Hawkins BM, Kennedy KF, Giri J, et al. Pre-procedural risk quantification for carotid stenting using the CAS score: a report from the NCDR CARE Registry. J Am Coll Cardiol 2012;60:1617–22.

33. Bijuklic K, Wandler A, Varnakov Y, et al. Risk factors for cerebral embolization after carotid artery stenting with embolic protection: a diffusion-weighted magnetic resonance imaging study in 837 consecutive patients. Circ Cardiovasc Interv 2013;6:311–6.

34. Roubin GS, Iyer S, Halkin A, et al. Realizing the potential of carotid artery stenting: proposed paradigms for patient selection and procedural technique. Circulation 2006;113:2021–30.

Skin to Skin
Transradial Carotid Angiography and Stenting

Sasko Kedev, MD[a],*, Tift Mann, MD[b]

KEYWORDS

- Transradial approach (TRA) • Carotid artery stenting (CAS)
- Transradial carotid angiography (TRA CA) • Transfemoral approach (TFA)

KEY POINTS

- The feasibility and success of the transradial approach in carotid artery stenting has been shown.
- Radial access is particularly indicated in patients with extensive peripheral vascular disease and patients who have anatomic variations that make cannulation of the common carotid difficult from the femoral approach.
- An important benefit of the transradial approach is reduction of bleeding and vascular complications in obese patients and the older population undergoing these procedures.
- The use of the radial approach in patients with right internal carotid disease and bovine left internal carotid disease also offers the advantage of possibly reducing catheter-induced embolization from the arch because transradial catheters do not traverse this area.
- Experience in the transradial approach is important, because these are advanced techniques, and new operators should be comfortable with transradial cerebrovascular angiography before undertaking carotid stent procedures.
- With careful technique and experienced operators, the procedure can be performed with a low complication rate.

INTRODUCTION

When performed by experienced operators, carotid artery stenting (CAS) with embolic protection is a proven alternative to carotid endarterectomy in patients with significant carotid disease.[1–5] The femoral artery is the conventional access site for carotid stent procedures. However, this approach may be difficult or associated with increased risk of complications in certain patients. Thus, transradial access has been evaluated as an alternative strategy for CAS.

Access site bleeding and vascular complications are the most common adverse events after CAS from femoral access. In the Carotid Revascularization Endarterectomy versus Stenting Trial (CREST), the need for transfusion was significantly associated with a stroke. Red blood cell transfusion was needed in 12.5% of the patients having CAS who had periprocedural stroke complications versus only 1.6% of the patients having CAS who did not have stroke ($P < .0001$).[6] Elimination of these access site bleeding complications with the transradial approach (TRA) is well documented in patients undergoing coronary interventions.

Most technical failures of CAS from the transfemoral approach (TFA) are related to a complex aortic arch. The highest risk features for CAS complications are a type III aortic arch and friable aortic

Disclosures: The authors have nothing to disclose.

[a] Medical Faculty, Department of Interventional Cardiology, University Clinic of Cardiology, University of St Cyril & Methodius, Vodnjanska 17, Skopje 1000, Macedonia; [b] Department of Cardiology, Rex Heart Center, North Carolina Heart and Vascular Associates, 2800 Blue Ridge Road, Suite 550, Raleigh, NC 27607, USA
* Corresponding author.
E-mail address: skedev@gmail.com

arch atheroma.[7] The significant incidence of symptomatic strokes (14%) contralateral to the vascular territory of the treated carotid stenosis strongly suggests that catheter manipulations in the aortic arch are a cause of atheroembolic brain lesions.[6,8] An analysis of atherosclerosis distribution in different regions of the thoracic aorta showed a higher prevalence in the arch (27.6%) distal to the innominate artery and descending aorta (38.2%), especially with increasing age.[9] The use of TRA may minimize catheter contact with the arch and thereby reduce stroke risk, particularly in cases of CAS involving the right internal carotid artery (ICA) or bovine left ICA.

Previous case reports and feasibility studies have shown that, with careful technique and experienced operators, TRA CAS can be successfully performed with a low complication rate in a high percentage of patients.[10] In addition, transradial access for CAS may be useful in patients with severe peripheral vascular disease, high bleeding risk, and those with a contraindication for postprocedure bed rest.[10–26] Early patient mobilization is an important benefit of this approach.

The transradial technique for carotid stenting involves 3 different techniques for the 3 basic anatomic types of carotid disease: right ICA, bovine left ICA, and nonbovine left ICA. This article describes the preferred technical transradial strategy for CAS in various types of carotid anatomy.

TRANSRADIAL ACCESS TECHNIQUE

The wrist is hyperextended and local anesthesia (1 mL lidocaine 2%) administered. The optimal access site is 2 cm proximal to the styloid process of the radius bone along the axis with the most powerful pulsation of the radial artery (RA). A 20-G plastic cannula-over-needle (Glidesheath

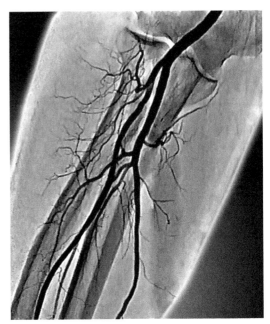

Fig. 1. Forearm arteriography with normal RA diameter.

insertion kit, Terumo, Tokyo, Japan) is inserted at a 30° to 60° angle along the vessel axis using the counterpuncture technique. When good arterial back-bleed is obtained, the 0.64-mm (0.025″) hydrophilic guidewire is advanced and the hydrophilic 5-Fr sheath (Radifocus, Terumo, Tokyo, Japan) introduced over the guidewire.

Intra-arterial vasodilator (5 mg verapamil) is injected to reduce RA spasm (RAS). Sedation may be necessary in anxious patients because circulating catecholamines can precipitate RAS. Immediately after sheath insertion, intravenous unfractionated heparin (50–70 μ/kg, up to 5000 units) or weight-based bivalirudin is administered.

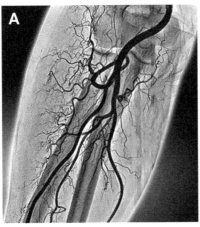 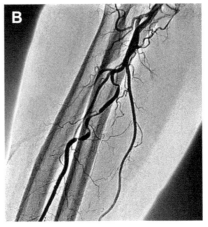

Fig. 2. Unfavorable RA anatomy. (*A*) RA with 360° loop. (*B*) Tortuous and spasmatic RA.

RA angiography is performed through the cannula or sheath, before catheter insertion (**Fig. 1**). This important step defines the RA anatomy from midforearm to brachial/axilar anastomosis and provides a roadmap for secured access. A diluted solution of 3-mL of contrast mixed with 7 mL of blood is injected briskly and recorded (see **Fig. 1**).

In cases with RAS, tortuosity, and/or radial loops and high takeoff RA, a 0.36-mm (0.014″) soft PCI guidewire can be used under fluoroscopy guidance. In most cases these anatomic variations may be negotiated for diagnostic carotid arteriography. However, patients with unfavorable RA anatomy (severe tortuosities; significant 360° RA loops; and high-takeoff, small-caliber RA) should not be considered for use of large-bore devices (**Fig. 2**).

High puncture of RA can be attempted in patients with previous RA catheterization and known RA anatomy.

TRANSRADIAL CAROTID ANGIOGRAPHY

Before the stent procedure, a complete angiographic evaluation consisting of a left anterior oblique (LAO) projection of the aortic arch as well as bilateral carotid arteriography is required. Computed tomography (CT) angiography may delineate the aortic arch and takeoff of the supra-aortic arteries. In most patients with right internal carotid disease, a right anterior oblique (RAO) angiogram of the innominate bifurcation

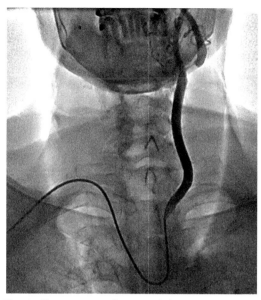

Fig. 4. Simmons 2 catheter in left common carotid artery (CCA) for diagnostic angiography.

should be evaluated. Initial angiography is performed through a 4-Fr or 5-Fr diagnostic catheter.

The specific curve of the diagnostic catheter is based on the type of arch and carotid anatomy as well as the initial configuration or orientation of the common carotid artery.

Thus, different diagnostic catheters are used for right ICA, nonbovine left ICA, and bovine left ICA.

A reversed-angle catheter, such as Simmons type 1 or 2, is primarily used for TRA carotid angiography (Cordis Corporation, Warren, NJ; Terumo, Tokyo, Japan; Merit Medical, Galway, Ireland). The

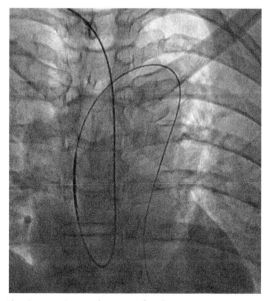

Fig. 3. Looping technique of a diagnostic Simmons 2 catheter over the hydrophilic wire in the ascending aorta.

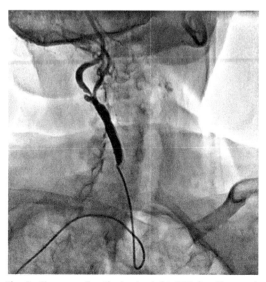

Fig. 5. Simmons 2 catheter in right CCA for diagnostic angiography.

primary curve of the catheters can be reformed using the inherent shape of the aortic arch.

There are 2 methods of reforming the natural reversed curve of the Simmons catheters within the aortic arch. The first involves passing the catheter over a hydrophilic Glidewire or J wire looped in the ascending aorta. This technique is used for a Simmons 1 or a Simmons 2 catheter in patients with a very tortuous and dilated aortic arch (**Fig. 3**).

The second method is preferred for the Simmons 2 catheter in most cases. The catheter is negotiated into the descending thoracic aorta over a standard guidewire. The curve is reformed by withdrawing the guidewire into the primary curve and prolapsing the catheter into the ascending aorta with counterclockwise rotation. With this maneuver the catheter forms a loop on itself, which often directly engages the left carotid and the catheter can also be withdrawn into the right common carotid (**Figs. 4** and **5**).[27] The Simmons 2 catheter should be used with caution in the right common carotid of women and short patients because the distal limb may reach the bifurcation. Catheters with soft reversed angle

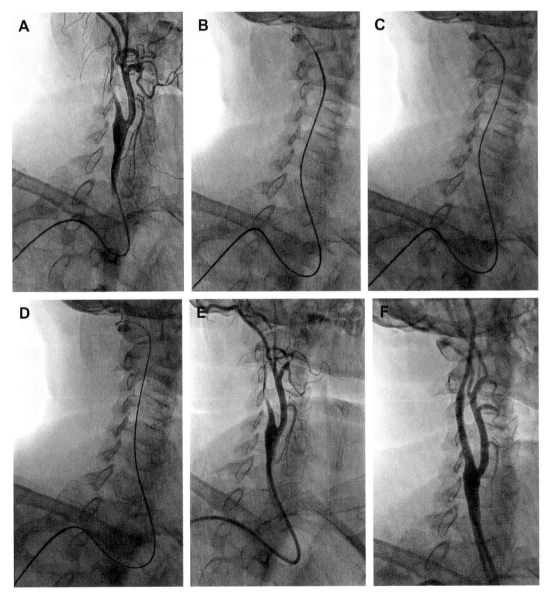

Fig. 6. Anchoring technique for right CCA cannulation. (*A*) Simmons 2 catheter in right CCA. (*B*) Simmons 2 catheter in right ECA over soft 0.89-mm (0.035″) guidewire. (*C*) Simmons 2 transfer catheter in right ECA. (*D*) Amplatz Super Stiff Guidewire in right ECA. (*E*) Shuttle sheath 6 Fr in right CCA. (*F*) Result after TRA CAS of right ICA (Precise 7.0/40 mm, Cordis Corporation, Warren, NJ).

tips are the most easy to reform and the least traumatic during diagnostic carotid angiography (Merit Medical, Galway, Ireland).

TECHNIQUES OF COMMON CAROTID ARTERY CANNULATION

TRA for CAS is usually performed through a 5-Fr or 6-Fr 90-cm Shuttle sheath (Cook, Minneapolis, MN) or Destination sheath (Terumo, Tokyo, Japan) inserted using a variation of the standard femoral technique. There are 2 different modes of common carotid artery cannulation: anchoring and telescopic.

For the anchoring technique, a diagnostic or transfer catheter positioned in the external carotid artery (ECA) is used for insertion of an exchange-length, supportive guidewire over which a guiding sheath is deployed (**Fig. 6**). In general, the diagnostic catheter initially passes into the ECA over a 0.89-mm (0.035″) Glidewire or 0.36-mm (0.014″) extrasupport coronary wire. Guidewire selection for sheath deployment is based on several factors including the specific carotid involved,

aortic arch type, and other anatomic considerations. The same technique can be used for insertion of regular guiding catheters (6 Fr to 8 Fr) or sheathless catheters (**Fig. 7**).

With the telescopic technique, a long (125 cm) wire-braided Simmons 2 catheter (Cook, Minneapolis, MN) is positioned within the Shuttle sheath and is used as the introducer. This technique is useful for sheath deployment in cases with extreme angles (**Fig. 8**).

Compatibility with the guiding sheath diameter is determined by the RA size based on preprocedural radial angiography. Repeat verapamil can be administered before insertion of the guiding sheath if RAS is anticipated. Once the sheath is in place, the technique of embolic protection device deployment and carotid stenting is the same as from the femoral artery.

Insertion of the sheath or guiding catheter from TRA necessarily involves acute angles that must be negotiated, and different strategies for sheath deployment are related to the severity of the angle between the arm and common carotid artery. In general, the different strategies vary according to

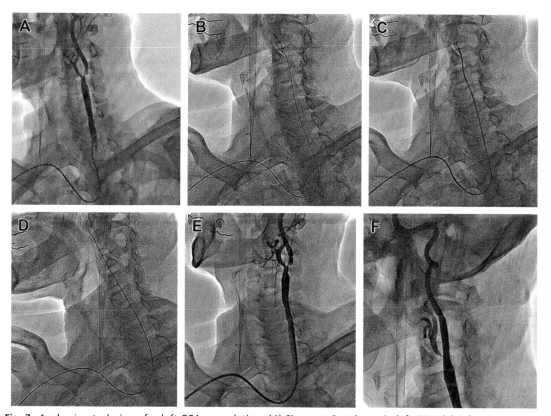

Fig. 7. Anchoring technique for left CCA cannulation. (*A*) Simmons 2 catheter in left CCA. (*B*) Advantage guidewire in left ECA. (*C*) Transfer catheter (5-Fr JR guiding catheter) in left ECA. (*D*) Amplatz Super Stiff Guidewire exchange in left ECA. (*E*) Destination 6-Fr guiding sheath in left CCA. (*F*) Result after TRA CAS of left ICA (Xact 8-6/40, Abbott Vascular, Abbott Park, IL).

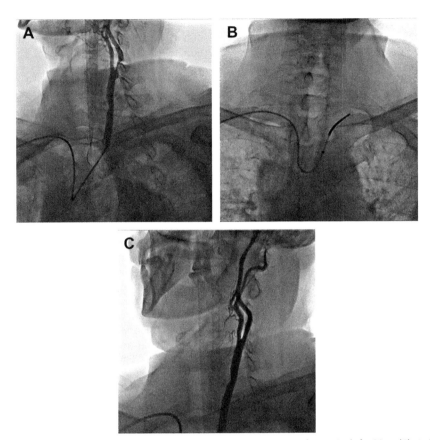

Fig. 8. Telescopic technique for left CCA cannulation. (*A*) Simmons 2 catheter in left CCA. (*B*) A 6-Fr braided Simmons 2 (125 cm) catheter into 6-Fr Shuttle sheath. (*C*) Result after TRA CAS of left ICA (Adapt 4-9/40 mm, Boston Scientific, Maple Grove, MN).

3 basic carotid artery classifications: right, bovine left, and nonbovine left.

RIGHT INTERNAL CAS

Because many procedurally related strokes originate from arch atheroembolization, the use of transradial access may minimize catheter contact with the arch, and thereby reduce stroke risk. The use of TRA in CAS of the right ICA and bovine left ICA in particular are associated with minimal catheter contact with the arch and consequently with reduced risk of atheroembolization.

An RAO arteriogram or preprocedural CT of the innominate (brachiocephalic) artery bifurcation is useful in determining the right ICA sheath insertion strategy. With less acute angles, especially when a horizontal segment of the subclavian or common carotid is present, direct cannulation with right Judkins diagnostic catheter is feasible (**Fig. 9**). The original technique of right ICA stenting involves passing the Simmons 1 or 2 catheter into the ECA over a Glidewire or extrasupport coronary

guidewire (**Fig. 10**). An exchange-length 0.89-mm (0.035″) J wire is then inserted and serves as the platform for sheath deployment. The ECA can often be directly cannulated with the hybrid 0.89-mm Advantage (distal tip hydrophilic Glidewire with stiffer nitinol core on the proximal end, Terumo; Tokyo, Japan) or the TAD II (0.89-mm exchange-length guidewire that tapers to a soft 0.46-mm [0.018″] floppy tip; Covidien, Mansfield, MA), thus omitting the step of passing the diagnostic catheter into the ECA.

When the angle of takeoff of the right common carotid is vertical or acute, a wire-braided Simmons 2 catheter positioned close to the bifurcation is used. The catheter is passed into the external over a Glidewire or extrasupport coronary wire and then exchanged for the Shuttle sheath. In this situation, an Amplatz Super Stiff Guidewire to deploy the sheath may be necessary. When the angle of takeoff of the right common carotid is particularly severe, a telescopic technique with the Shuttle sheath (90 cm) over the Simmons 2 catheter (125 cm) is used (**Fig. 11**). In general, right

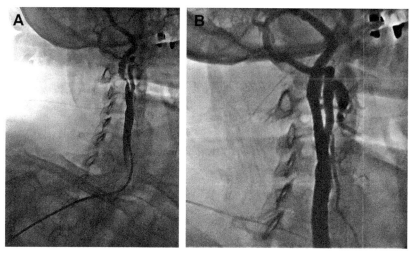

Fig. 9. (A) Direct cannulation of right CCA with Judkins right catheter. (B) Result after TRA CAS of right ICA (Xact 9-7/40, Abbott Vascular, Abbott Park, IL).

radial access provides adequate support even in acute angles of the common carotid artery with the arch of the aorta.

Patel and colleagues[12] have used the left radial approach for right internal carotid stenting. With this technique, the right common carotid artery (CCA) is selected from the left RA using a Tiger or Simmons 2 catheter. The diagnostic catheter is then passed into the ECA or high CCA and a 5-Fr or 6-Fr Shuttle sheath or 7-Fr guiding catheter

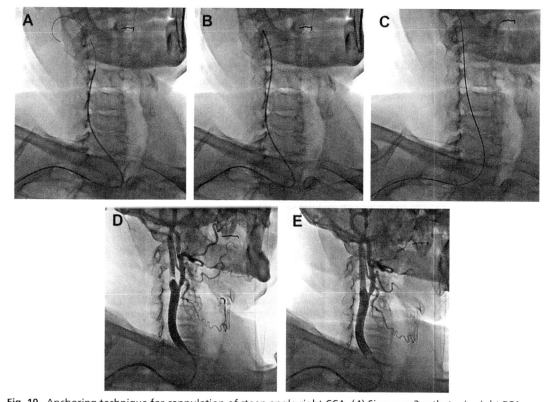

Fig. 10. Anchoring technique for cannulation of steep angle right CCA. (A) Simmons 2 catheter in right ECA over Glidewire. (B) Simmons 2 transfer catheter, deep in right ECA. (C) Amplatz Super Stiff Guidewire exchange in right ECA. (D) A 6-Fr Destination sheath in right CCA. (E) Result after TRA CAS of right ICA (Xact 8-6/30, Abbott Vascular, Abbott Park, IL).

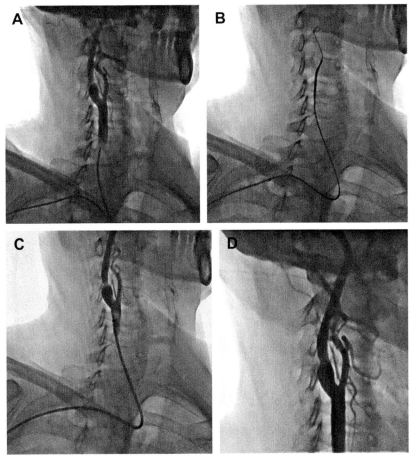

Fig. 11. Telescopic technique for right CCA cannulation. (*A*) Simmons 2 catheter in right CCA. (*B*) Simmons 2 (125 cm) catheter into 6-Fr Shuttle sheath over soft 0.89-mm (0.035″) guidewire in right ECA. (*C*) A 6-Fr Shuttle sheath in right CCA. (*D*) Result after TRA CAS of right ICA (Xact 8-6/40, Abbott Vascular, Abbott Park, IL).

is passed over a 0.89-mm (0.035″) Super Stiff Guidewire.

The telescopic technique with the 5-Fr diagnostic catheter inside the Shuttle sheath can also be used. After positioning the guiding sheath or guiding catheter beneath the bifurcation in the right CCA (**Fig. 12**A), CAS with distal embolic protection is performed in the usual fashion (see **Fig. 12**B).

BOVINE LEFT INTERNAL CAS

The bovine arch in which the right brachiocephalic and left carotid share a common trunk from the aortic arch occurs in around 13% of population.[28] Left ICA stenosis with bovine arch anatomy can easily be approached by the right arm approach (radial/brachial), and the right TRA may be the preferred strategy for carotid stenting of these lesions.

The initial takeoff of the bovine carotid is evaluated using an LAO aortic arch arteriogram. Often

no specific maneuvers are needed because wires and catheters tend to spontaneously fall into the left CCA. When the initial segment of the common carotid is horizontal, an Amplatz R2 or Judkins right diagnostic catheter is suitable (**Fig. 13**). When the initial segment is more vertical, a Simmons 1 or Simmons 2 is necessary to implement the exchange for the Shuttle sheath. Techniques similar to the right or nonbovine left internal carotid cases are used.

NONBOVINE LEFT INTERNAL CAROTID ARTERY STENTING

Transradial access for nonbovine left internal carotid disease is more challenging because of the unfavorable takeoff of the left common carotid.[10–12] The nemesis for the development of a consistent technique for nonbovine left internal carotid stenting from the right RA has been the acute angle that must be traversed for the deployment of a guiding sheath in the left

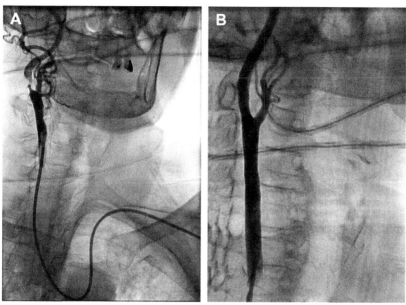

Fig. 12. Left radial access for CAS of right ICA. (*A*) A 7-Fr MP guiding catheter in right CCA. (*B*) Result after CAS of right ICA from left radial access (Wallstent 7.0/30, Boston Scientific, Maple Grove, MN).

common carotid. The angle results in poor inferior support for the catheter system with the resulting tendency for catheters to prolapse into the ascending aorta. This problem is particularly ominous should prolapse occur during stent delivery.

The use of a wire-braided Simmons 2 catheter with its long distal end provides adequate support for passing a guidewire into the ECA in most cases. A Simmons 3 catheter provides even more support and is used in cases of type II and type III arches with particularly acute angles of takeoff of the common carotid. The anchoring

technique with a stepwise exchange of Glidewire, Advantage, or TAD II wire and Amplatz Super Stiff through the diagnostic catheter in the ECA are most commonly used.

With extreme angles, a 5-Fr or 6-Fr multipurpose or Judkins R guide catheter can be used as an intermediate transfer catheter to insert an Amplatz Super Stiff Guidewire. In these extreme situations, kinking of the Shuttle sheath may occur at the acute angle and a heavily braided, semihydrophilic Destination sheath (Terumo, Tokyo, Japan) should be substituted to provide maximum support (**Figs. 14** and **15**).

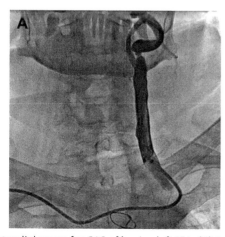
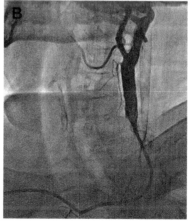

Fig. 13. Right radial access for CAS of bovine left ICA. (*A*) A 6-Fr Shuttle sheath in left bovine CCA. (*B*) Result after TRA CAS of left bovine ICA (Xact 9-7/40 mm, Abbott Vascular, Abbott Park, IL).

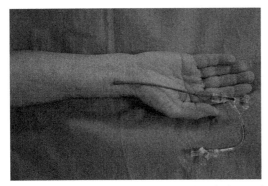

Fig. 14. A 6-Fr Destination guiding sheath (90 cm) through the right radial access.

In general, a telescopic approach with a wire-braided 125-cm long Simmons 2 diagnostic catheter within the sheath is preferred in cases of nonbovine left ICA lesions (**Fig. 16**). However, in patients with a type I arch and left internal carotid lesions, the TAD II guidewire can be passed directly into the external and usually provides sufficient support for deployment of the Shuttle sheath. This simple technique is successful only with less severe angles of takeoff of the left common carotid.

The catheter looping and retrograde engagement technique is an alternative strategy that has been described by Fang and colleagues.[13] The unique feature of this technique is the use of the right coronary cusp to provide inferior support for the system (**Fig. 17**). With this technique, a 7-Fr mutipurpose guide catheter can be used for CAS of both right ICA and left ICA with unfavorable takeoff angulations. The main disadvantage is the system instability with continuous movement of the guiding catheter and the filter. Particular attention should be made during guiding catheter removal because it could jump distally during pull-back.

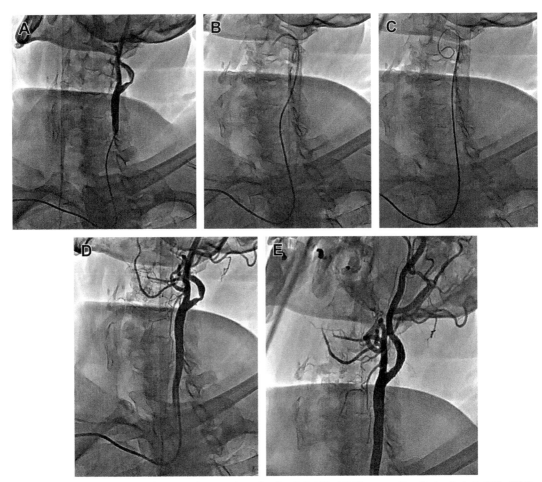

Fig. 15. Anchoring technique for cannulation of nonbovine left ICA. (*A*) Simmons 2 catheter in left CCA. (*B*) Simmons 2 transfer catheter deep in left ECA. (*C*) Amplatz Super Stiff Guidewire exchange in left ECA. (*D*) A 6-Fr Shuttle sheath in left CCA. (*E*) Result after TRA CAS of left ICA (Adapt 4-9/32 mm, Boston Scientific, Maple Grove, MN).

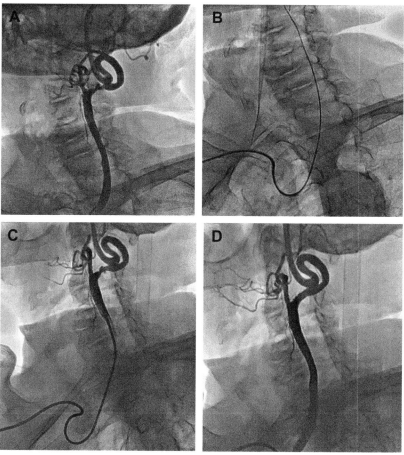

Fig. 16. Telescopic technique for CAS of nonbovine left ICA. (*A*) Simmons 1 catheter in left CCA. (*B*) A 5-Fr MP catheter (125 cm) into 7-Fr MP guiding catheter over Amplatz Super Stiff Guidewire in left ECA. (*C*) A 7-Fr MP guiding catheter in left CCA. (*D*) Result after TRA CAS of left ICA (Precise 7.0/30 mm, Cordis Corporation, Warren, NJ).

ADVANCED TRA CAS WITH MO.MA PROXIMAL PROTECTION DEVICE

The principal limitation of TRA in peripheral procedures is related to the size of the devices to be used, although feasibility of using 8-Fr sheaths in the RA has already been shown.[29] Proximal embolic protection devices (PPDs) are increasingly used during CAS because of the theoretic advantage of cerebral protection during the procedure. Two small studies suggested that PPDs are superior to distal filters for reducing surrogate end points of cerebral embolism.[30,31]

PPDs are large and cumbersome devices (8 or 9 Fr) that need specific training to become familiar with. They consist of a long sheath, with a central working lumen, connected to 2 balloons inflated to occlude the ECA and the CCA, allowing cerebral protection during all steps of CAS.

Trani and colleagues,[17] reported the first 3 cases of transradial CAS using 8-Fr proximal protection with the Mo.Ma device (Medtronic Invatec, Roncadelle, Italy). We successfully used the Mo.Ma device recently during 5 transradial CAS procedures (3 left ICA and 2 right ICA; Kedev S, MD, personal communication, 2008).

The anchoring technique is used for deployment over the 0.89-mm (0.035″) superstiff supportive guidewire positioned in the corresponding ECA. The inflated occluding balloons in ECA and in CCA, with extrasupportive 0.36-mm (0.014″) guidewire can provide additional stability of the guiding system, which is particularly important in cases with more angulated CCA takeoff (**Fig. 18**). However, CAS with Mo.Ma device by TRA should be regarded as a challenging procedure that requires significant operator experience in both radial approach and carotid interventions.

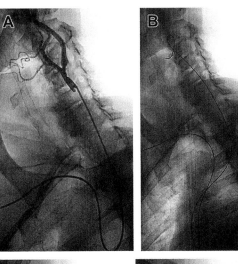

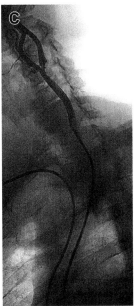
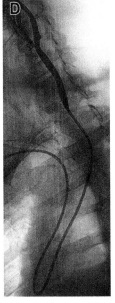

Fig. 17. Deep loop retrograde cannulation for CAS of left ICA. (*A*) Deeply looped 5-Fr MP catheter with retrograde cannulation of in left CCA below bifurcation. (*B*) Looped Advantage Glidewire in left ECA. (*C*) Looped 7-Fr MP guiding catheter with retrograde cannulation of left CCA. (*D*) Result after TRA CAS of left nonbovine ICA with deep loop retrograde cannulation technique (Wallstent 7.0/30, Boston Scientific, Maple Grove, MN).

ARTERIAL SHEATH MANAGEMENT

This incidence of RA occlusion is high and is at least in part related to the use of large-bore catheters.[32] Contemporary RA preservation techniques, especially the application of hemostasis devices using patent hemostasis, may minimize this complication.[33,34]

Radial sheath is removed immediately after the procedure and hemostasis is achieved usually by transradial band compression (Terumo, Tokyo, Japan), by inflating 15 to 18 mL of air at the puncture site. Pulse oximetry is used to confirm that hemoglobin oxygen saturation is more than 90% on the involved hand after hemostasis is obtained. Compression is applied for approximately 2 to 3-hours (depending on the sheath size) with gradual relaxation of compression after the first hour. Patients are usually discharged the following day after a careful examination by the attending physician.

ADVANTAGES OF TRA CAS

1. Alternative access in patients with extensive peripheral vascular disease.
2. Reduction of access site bleeding and vascular complications in the obese and elderly populations.
3. Alternative access in patients with anatomic variations that make cannulation of the common carotid difficult from the femoral approach.[26]
4. The preferred approach in patients with bovine left ICA disease. The use of the TRA in patients with right ICA disease and bovine left ICA disease may reduce catheter-induced embolization from the transverse aortic arch.[35–38]
5. Early patient mobilization.
6. Reduced nursing cost.

DISADVANTAGES OF TRA CAS

1. Extensive experience with both the TRA and CAS is necessary.
2. Significant learning curve for new transradial operators.
3. Sometimes longer procedures for easy TFA cases with type I aortic arch.
4. Proximal protection and larger devices cannot be used freely in all cases.
5. Postprocedure RA occlusion.

LIMITATIONS

There are several important limitations to this approach. Extensive experience with both the TRA and CAS is necessary. The transradial learning curve may limit the implementation of the described techniques. The impact of the interventionalist's learning curve on outcomes has been well established both for carotid stenting and transradial PCI; it is therefore likely that a procedure that combines these two skills may further steepen the learning curve.[3,4]

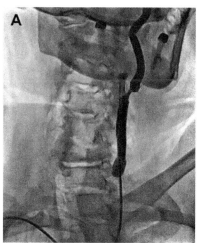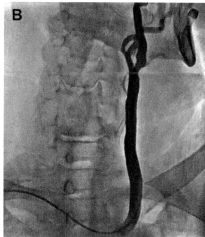

Fig. 18. Right radial access for CAS of left ICA with Mo.Ma proximal protection device. (*A*) An 8-Fr Mo.Ma proximal protection device with occlusion of left ECA and left CCA. (*B*) Result after TRA CAS of left nonbovine ICA under proximal protection with Mo.Ma 8 Fr (Crystalo Ideale 6-9/30 mm, Invatec; Medtronic, Invatec, Roncadelle, Italy).

There are some technical caveats. The potential problem of air embolization caused by the use of bulky stents in small sheaths can be eliminated with awareness and careful technique. Stents should be positioned using roadmap fluoroscopy or bony landmarks. Contrast injections are made only after careful bleed-back. Reforming 5-Fr Simmons curves may be problematic, and manipulations are minimized by using the looping technique.[27] The Simmons 2 catheter should be used with caution in the right common carotid of women and short patients because the distal limb may reach the bifurcation.

The assessment of appropriate RA size and anatomy with preliminary angiography is fundamental. Patients with unfavorable anatomy, such as significant tortuosity, loops, or other anatomic variants, should not be considered for use of large devices.

Although all commercially available stents and distal embolic protection devices can be used transradially, only the carotid Wallstent, Adapt (Boston Scientific, Maple Grove, MN), Precise (Cordis Corporation, Warren, NJ), and Crystalo Ideale (Medtronic, Invatec, Roncadelle, Italy) can be delivered though 5-Fr sheaths and through 6-Fr and 7-Fr guiding catheters.

FUTURE TECHNOLOGICAL ADVANCES

Although the feasibility and success of TRA CAS procedures with the currently available equipment has been shown, future technological advances should improve the general applicability of the technique. First, a sheath that is flexible but more supportive would be useful in patients with the most acute angles at the origin of the common carotid because lack of inferior support is the cause of most failures. Second, guiding catheters with dedicated carotid curves could facilitate common carotid cannulation. Third, the development of lower profile, more deliverable stent systems is imperative. At present, 4 carotid stents can be deployed through a 5-Fr sheath, only 2 of which are available in the United States. Smaller catheter systems would not only improve deliverability but would also reduce RA injury and occlusion.

SUMMARY

Radial access is a viable alternative approach in patients undergoing carotid stenting. It is particularly indicated in patients with extensive peripheral vascular disease and patients who have anatomic variations that make cannulation of the common carotid difficult from the femoral approach. Further, an important benefit of the TRA is reduction of bleeding and vascular complications in the obese and the elderly population undergoing these procedures. The use of the radial approach in patients with right internal carotid disease and bovine left internal carotid disease also offers the advantage of possibly reducing catheter-induced embolization from the arch because transradial catheters do not traverse this area. Experience in the TRA is important because these are advanced techniques. New operators are encouraged to become comfortable with transradial cerebrovascular angiography before undertaking carotid stent procedures.

In addition, the feasibility and success of the TRA in CAS has been shown. With careful technique and experienced operators, the procedure can be performed with a low complication rate.

REFERENCES

1. Brott TG, Hobson RW, Howard G, et al. Stenting versus endarterectomy for treatment of carotid artery stenosis. N Engl J Med 2010;363:11–23.
2. Silver FL, Mackey A, Clark WM, et al, CREST Investigators. Safety of stenting and endarterectomy by symptomatic status in the Carotid Revascularization Endarterectomy versus Stenting Trial (CREST). Stroke 2011;42:675–80.
3. Gray WA, Yadav JS, Verta P, et al, CAPTURE Trial Collaborators. The CAPTURE registry: predictors of outcomes in carotid artery stenting with embolic protection for high surgical risk patients in the early post-approval setting. Catheter Cardiovasc Interv 2007;70:1025–33.
4. Gurm HS, Yadav JS, Fayad P, et al, SAPPHIRE Investigators. Long-term results of carotid stenting versus endarterectomy in high-risk patients. N Engl J Med 2008;358:1572–9.
5. White CJ, Iyer SS, Hopkins LN, et al, BEACH Trial Investigators. Carotid stenting with distal protection in 4 high surgical risk patients: the BEACH trial 30 day results. Catheter Cardiovasc Interv 2006; 67:503–12.
6. Hill MD, Brooks W, Mackey A, et al, CREST Investigators. Stroke after carotid stenting and endarterectomy in the carotid revascularization endarterectomy versus stenting trial (CREST). Circulation 2012;126: 3054–61.
7. Macdonald S, Lee R, Williams R, et al. Delphi carotid stenting consensus panel. Towards safer carotid artery stenting: a scoring system for anatomic suitability. Stroke 2009;40:1698–703.
8. Hammer FD, Lacroix V, Duprez T, et al. Cerebral microembolization after protected carotid artery stenting in surgical high-risk patients: Results of a 2-year prospective study. J Vasc Surg 2005;42:847–53.
9. Meissner I, Whisnant JP, Khandheria BK, et al. Prevalence of potential risk factors for stroke assessed by transesophageal echocardiography and carotid ultrasonography: the SPARC study: Stroke Prevention: Assessment of Risk in a Community. Mayo Clin Proc 1999;74:862–9.
10. Etxegoien N, Rhyne D, Kedev S, et al. The transradial approach for carotid artery stenting. Catheter Cardiovasc Interv 2012;80:1081–7.
11. Folmar J, Sachar R, Mann T. Transradial approach for carotid artery stenting: a feasibility study. Catheter Cardiovasc Interv 2007;69(3):355–61.
12. Patel T, Shah S, Ranian A, et al. Contralateral transradial approach for carotid artery stenting: a feasibility study. Catheter Cardiovasc Interv 2009; 75:268–75.
13. Fang H, Chung S, Sun C, et al. Transradial and transbrachial arterial approach for simultaneous carotid angiographic examination and stenting using catheter looping and retrograde engagement technique. Ann Vasc Surg 2010;24:670–9.
14. Mendiz OA, Sampaolesi AH, Londero HF, et al. Initial experience with transradial access for carotid stenting. Vasc Endovascular Surg 2011;45:499–503.
15. Pinter L, Cagiannos C, Ruzsa Z, et al. Report on initial experience with transradial access for carotid artery stenting. J Vasc Surg 2007;45:1136–41.
16. Bakoyiannis C, Economopoulos KP, Georgopoulos S, et al. Transradial access for carotid artery stenting: a single center experience. Int Angiol 2010;29:41–6.
17. Trani C, Burzotta F, Coroleu F. Transradial carotid artery stenting with proximal embolic protection. Catheter Cardiovasc Interv 2009;74:267–72.
18. Coroleu SF, Burzotta F, Fernández-Gómez C, et al. Feasibility of complex coronary and peripheral interventions by trans-radial approach using large sheaths. Cathet Cardiovasc Diagn 2011; 79:597–600.
19. Shaw JA, Gravereaux EC, Eisenhauer AC. Carotid stenting in the bovine arch. Catheter Cardiovasc Interv 2003;60:566–9.
20. Gan HW, Bhasin A, Wu CJ. Transradial carotid stenting in a patient with bovine arch anatomy. Catheter Cardiovasc Interv 2006;75:540–3.
21. Levy EL, Kim SH, Bendok BR, et al. Transradial stenting of the cervical internal carotid artery: technical case report. Neurosurgery 2003;53: 448–51.
22. Layton KF, Kallmes DF, Cloft HJ. The radial artery access site for interventional neuroradiology procedures. AJNR Am J Neuroradiol 2006;27: 1151–4.
23. Bendok BR, Przybylo JH, Parkinson R, et al. Neuroendovascular interventions for intracranial posterior circulation disease via the transradial approach: technical case report. Neurosurgery 2005;56:626.
24. Eskioglu E, Burry MV, Mericle RA. Transradial approach for neuroendovascular surgery of intracranial vascular lesions. J Neurosurg 2004;101: 767–9.
25. Castriota F, Cremonesi A, Manetti R, et al. Carotid stenting using radial artery access. J Endovasc Surg 1999;6:385–6.
26. Yoo BS, Lee SH, Kim JY, et al. A case of transradial carotid stenting in a patient with total occlusion of distal abdominal aorta. Catheter Cardiovasc Interv 2002;56:243–5.
27. Lee D, Ahn J, Jeong S, et al. Routine transradial access for conventional cerebral angiography: a single operator's experience of its feasibility and safety. Br J Radiol 2004;77:831–8.

28. Layton KF, Kallmes DF, Cloft HJ, et al. Bovine aortic arch variant in humans: clarification of a common misnomer. AJNR Am J Neuroradiol 2006;27:1541–2.

29. Wu SS, Galani RJ, Bahro A, et al. 8 French transradial coronary interventions: clinical outcome and late effects on the radial artery and hand function. J Invasive Cardiol 2000;12:605–9.

30. Montorsi P, Caputi L, Galli S, et al. Microembolization during carotid artery stenting in patients with high-risk, lipid rich plaque: a randomized trial of proximal versus distal cerebral protection. J Am Coll Cardiol 2012;58:1656–63.

31. Bijuklic K, Wandler A, Hazizi F, et al. The PROFI study (prevention of cerebral embolization by proximal balloon occlusion compared to filter protection during carotid artery stenting): a prospective randomized trial. J Am Coll Cardiol 2012;59:1383–91.

32. Saito S, Ikei H, Hosokawa G, et al. Influence of the ratio between radial artery inner diameter and sheath outer diameter on radial artery flow after transradial coronary intervention. Catheter Cardiovasc Interv 1999;46:173–8.

33. Pancholy S, Coppola J, Patel T, et al. Prevention of radial artery occlusion–patient hemostasis evaluation trial (PROPHET study): a randomized comparison of traditional versus patency documented hemostasis after transradial catheterization. Catheter Cardiovasc Interv 2008;72:335–40.

34. Pancholy SB, Patel TM. Effect of duration of hemostatic compression on radial artery occlusion after transradial access. Catheter Cardiovasc Interv 2012;79:78–81.

35. Bendszur M, Koltzenburg M, Burger R, et al. Silent embolism in diagnostic cerebral angiography and neurointerventional procedures: a prospective study. Lancet 1999;354:1594–7.

36. El-Koussy M, Schroth G, Do DD, et al. Periprocedural embolic events related to carotid artery stenting detected by diffusion-weighted MRI: comparison between proximal and distal embolus protection devices. J Endovasc Ther 2007;14:293–303.

37. Barbato JE, Dillavou E, Horowitz MB, et al. A randomized trial of carotid artery stenting with and without cerebral protection. J Vasc Surg 2008;47:760–5.

38. Faggioli G, Ferri M, Rapezzi C, et al. Atherosclerotic aortic lesions increase the risk of cerebral embolism during carotid stenting in patients with complex aortic arch anatomy. J Vasc Surg 2009;49:80–5.

Skin to Skin
Transfemoral Carotid Angiography and Stenting

D. Christopher Metzger, MD

KEYWORDS

- Carotid artery stenting • Carotid endarterectomy • Carotid artery disease
- Transfemoral carotid angiography

KEY POINTS

- Carotid artery stenting (CAS) continues to have improving results in both standard-risk and high-risk patients with carotid artery disease.
- This successful, low-risk carotid stenting occurs when CAS is performed by experienced, appropriately trained operators who use good patient and lesion selection, sound judgment, and meticulous attention to procedural technique.
- With careful attention to these principles, CAS can be appropriately applied to help a large number of patients with carotid artery disease.

In addition to operator experience and careful case selection, meticulous attention to procedural technique is essential to successful, low-risk carotid artery stenting (CAS). This article reviews CAS procedural techniques, sharing advice and lessons learned, in the hope of providing a reference for CAS techniques. Patient preparation and the procedure from angiography through stenting are described. In addition, proximal and distal embolic protection is discussed, including advantages and nuances of technique. Also discussed are unique situations encountered, including brachiocephalic lesions, common complications of CAS, and techniques for challenging anatomy.

The author hopes that his experience of more than 1700 CAS procedures, coupled with expert opinions of many skilled CAS operators, will serve as a valuable reference for interested CAS operators.

BACKGROUND

Stroke is a devastating problem, occurring approximately 800,000 times annually in the United States and Europe.[1] A significant proportion of these strokes is due to atherosclerotic carotid artery disease. CAS has emerged as an attractive alternative to carotid endarterectomy (CEA), especially in patients at high risk for CEA. In both standard-risk and high-risk CEA patients, results of carotid stenting continue to improve, such that the last 4 major investigational exemption (IDE) trials show less than or equal to 3% stroke and death rates, even in patients at high risk for CEA (**Figs. 1 and 2**).[2–8] These improving results are likely secondary to increased operator experience, translating into better case selection and better procedural technique, as well as advances in carotid stent technology. Here the author shares his experience, hoping to provide insights into optimal techniques for CAS.

It is important to emphasize that the improving CAS results do not translate to all carotid stent operators. These results, like results in CEA procedures, are seen in centers with experienced operators. Some background considerations are critically important in relation to a description of CAS techniques. There are several important

The author has nothing to disclose.
Wellmont CVA Heart Institute, PV Dept, 2050 Meadowview Parkway, Kingsport, TN, 37660, USA
E-mail address: cmetzger@mycva.com

Intervent Cardiol Clin 3 (2014) 37–49
http://dx.doi.org/10.1016/j.iccl.2013.09.007

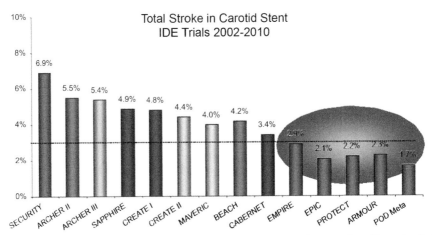

Fig. 1. Improving results in carotid artery stenting trials. IDE, investigational exemption. (*From* Bersin RM, Stabile E, Ansel GM, et al. A meta-analysis of proximal occlusion device outcomes in carotid artery stenting. Catheter Cardiovasc Interv 2012;80:1072–8; with permission.)

determinants for optimal CAS results, the first being operator experience. Before starting any independent CAS training, operators should be board certified in an interventional specialty (eg, vascular surgery, interventional radiology, neuroradiology, or interventional cardiology). Moreover, they should satisfy their society's position paper for carotid stenting, and have experience with non-CAS endovascular procedures (>50 independent endovascular procedures). Furthermore, in addition to a thorough understanding of neuroanatomy and function, an absolute minimum of 50 diagnostic

carotid angiograms and 25 hands-on proctored cases should be performed with an experienced, credentialed operator before embarking on an independent CAS career. Throughout one's CAS career, case selection cannot be overemphasized: this includes patient selection (avoiding carefully patients with decreased cerebral reserve; eg, patients with dementia; octogenarians and patients with renal insufficiency also need to be approached carefully[9,10]). Patients' lesion characteristics are also important, and cases with severe calcification, severe carotid or

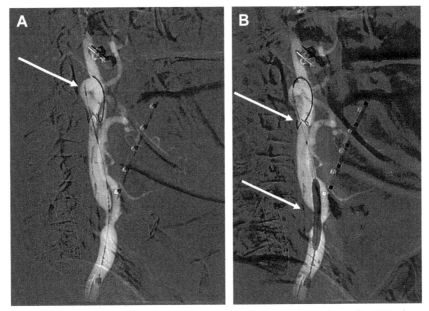

Fig. 2. (*A*) Roadmap for wiring lesion. Arrow indicates wire in place. (*B*) Roadmap for EPD placement (*higher arrow*) and predilation angioplasty (*lower arrow*).

aortic arch disease before the lesion, sharp entry or exit angles, true string signs, and so forth, should be avoided. Finally, as emphasized in this article, meticulous attention to technique is paramount to low-risk CAS. Procedures should be performed only in institutions with experience with this procedure; these patients should be placed in prospective registries where their outcomes are tracked; and they should receive pre- and post–National Institutes of Health (NIH) Stroke Scales graded by credentialed, unbiased personnel.

PREPARATION OF THE PATIENT BEFORE CAS

The author believes that it is important to personally meet each potential CAS patient in full consultation, with rare exceptions. This consultation helps the clinician to make an individual determination of the patient's candidacy for CAS, as well as to meet the patient and family and describe the risks, benefits, and alternatives to CAS. In general, a minimum for scheduling a CAS procedure would be the full clinical history in combination with a carotid duplex (CDU). The use of noninvasive imaging (magnetic resonance angiography [MRA] or computed tomographic angiography [CTA]) can be individualized. The author tends to use additional imaging in borderline cases to help guide his decision (eg, symptoms associated with borderline CDU velocities, or in octogenarian patients to help decide whether to proceed with angiography and stenting). After meeting the patient and reviewing the data, one must try to assess CAS risk as assessed in the relevant institution, and compare this CAS risk with the same patient's CEA risk and the natural history of the patient's disease with medical therapy. The author also checks whether the patient qualifies for a CAS research protocol, and performs precertification for CAS to the insurance carrier. The alternatives of CEA and medical therapy are fully disclosed and the risks of the procedures discussed, including the risk of procedural stroke. If the risk/benefit ratio appears to favor angiography and carotid stenting, both procedures are scheduled in the same setting, with performance of arch aortography and carotid angiography with CAS as appropriate after these angiograms. It is important that dual-antiplatelet therapy, usually with aspirin and clopidogrel, is instituted for at least 1 week before the therapy, with rare exceptions of loading. In most instances, patients are also asked to hold their blood pressure medicines only on the morning of their procedure, with the procedure scheduled at the convenience of the patient and family.

IN-HOSPITAL PREPARATION OF THE CAS PATIENT

In the catheter laboratory holding room, the clinician confirms that the patient has been taking aspirin and Plavix, and reassesses preadmittance laboratory data. The author personally meets with the patient and family before every procedure, regardless of the amount of time spent in the office (often there will be family from out of town not present during the initial consultation). An NIH Stroke Scale is administered as baseline for all procedures, and informed consent for research protocols is obtained. In the catheter laboratory, staff places a calibrated sticker on the target side for carotid stenting (this is a marker pigtail catheter cut, affixed to tape, and placed on the side of the carotid stent). The patient's head is placed on the carotid pillow, and a squeezable toy is placed in their contralateral hand. Detailed instructions are reviewed with the patient and reinforced early in the procedure (eg, have them squeeze their toy several times early in the procedure before CAS). In most cases no sedation is administered; we prefer to assess the patient throughout the procedure, although this can be individualized with light sedation as appropriate. Calm, reassuring demeanor is held by the physician and staff, and a nurse consistently monitors the patient.

CAS: ACCESS THROUGH ANGIOGRAMS

Femoral artery access is obtained in most CAS patients. Starting with a 6F sheath, a pigtail catheter is used to perform arch aortography. The author believes it is essential to assess the arch first in all patients. The amount of contrast used can be adjusted based on the patient's renal function (rarely if there is an MRA/CTA readily available, or prior arch aortogram was performed, these data can be used). After arch aortography, the strategy of a Shuttle sheath or guiding catheter is decided. It is the author's practice to use a 6F Shuttle sheath for more than 90% of internal carotid artery (ICA) CAS cases. 8F guiding catheters, usually a CBL modified guide, are used for challenging arches, as discussed later. The sheath or guiding catheter is placed in the descending thoracic aorta at this time. Also, based on the arch assessment, a 125-cm length neurodiagnostic catheter is used (the author considers these far preferable to coronary catheters, given the 4F and 5F diameters, hydrophilic, radiolucent tips, specialized shapes, and so forth). For type-I to -II arches, a 125-cm vertebral catheter is used. For slightly angulated arches, JB1 or H1 catheters can be used. For more difficult arches, a Vitek catheter is standard, with other possibilities being JB2 or the Simmons series.

After assessing the arch and reviewing the prior data, anticoagulation is administered early. If it is thought that there is a high likelihood to proceed with CAS, bivalirudin bolus and drip is administered to give additional protection during manipulation of catheters. Bivalirudin is used for all nonintracranial carotid stenting, as the author strongly prefers the predictable anticoagulation and lower bleeding risk of this drug, and the ability for earlier sheath removal if a closure device cannot be used. Despite its predictability, an activated clotting time (ACT) is obtained once for all CAS patients to confirm a patent intravenous line and that the patient is a responder.

After placing the sheath/guide catheter and initiating anticoagulation, the selected 125-cm neurodiagnostic catheter is first introduced into the nontarget carotid artery. Very importantly, catheters are all introduced over a 0.038 angled Glidewire. Care is taken to avoid any contact with diseased segments in the internal or distal common carotid artery, and the arch aortogram picture is placed as a reference to guide manipulations. The catheter is advanced to the mid/distal common carotid artery (CCA) and the Glidewire is removed. Importantly for every exchange, aspiration is performed through the catheter before any contrast injection or reintroduction of wires. In general, 2 angulated images are obtained of the carotid bifurcation (standard view is 40° ipsilateral and an ipsilateral straight lateral; if there is a rotated bifurcation, a contralateral 40° view is usually chosen). After the ipsilateral lateral bifurcation image is obtained, the author goes to a larger field and goes straight to the cerebral images, obtaining a straight lateral cerebral angiogram, imaging into the venous phase. Following this, an anteroposterior (AP) cranial (Towne) cerebral image is obtained. After aspiration, the Glidewire is reinserted and used as a rail to withdraw the catheter into the aorta. It is then manipulated into the target carotid artery over the angled Glidewire, again utilizing features from the arch assessment. Two diagnostic images are obtained of the target carotid artery as described earlier, followed by baseline lateral and Towne images of the target cerebral vasculature. The author considers that baseline imaging of the cerebral circulation is important for reassessment should there be a neurologic event at a later time, and that aspiration with every exchange is mandatory, as is introduction and removal of all catheters over the Glidewire.

If images of the target ICA are favorable for CAS; the best working view is selected based on the angiograms. At this point a roadmap image is obtained. If there is a clear path to the external carotid artery (ECA) on the target side, the angled Glidewire is carefully steered into the ECA. The neurodiagnostic catheter is advanced over the Glidewire into the ECA, and the previously placed sheath/guiding catheter is advanced over the Glidewire and catheter to the distal CCA (**Fig. 3**). If there is disease at the bifurcation or the ECA is occluded, a roadmap is obtained, and the Glidewire and catheter are advanced close to the bifurcation, and held tightly as the sheath/guide is advanced, taking great care to avoid any contact with the bifurcation lesion (**Figs. 4** and **5**). For most cases, there is no need to switch to a supportive wire to perform these maneuvers (the only exception being proximal protection, discussed later).

CAS: FROM GUIDE CATHETER TO COMPLETION

After the sheath/guide is placed in the distal CCA, it is attached to connecting tubing and meticulously aspirated to avoid any air in the system. A subtracted angiogram is repeated (this is important, as any tortuosity in the CCA may be transmitted northward by the larger sheath/guide, changing the angles in the ICA to be treated). An unsubtracted still frame is then placed as a reference guide shot on the right screen. The bony landmarks and neck sticker serve as important

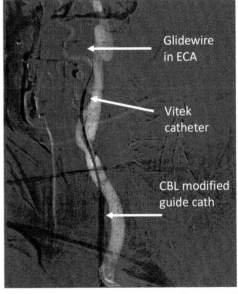

Fig. 3. Strategy for accessing difficult arches (continued). The catheter is guided into the distal CCA. CBL.

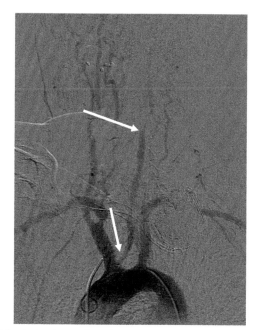

Fig. 4. Bovine arch with occluded ECA.

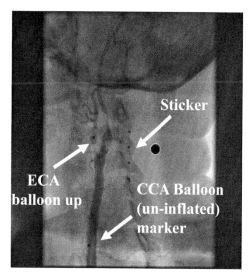

Fig. 6. Unsubtracted baseline angiogram with ECA balloon inflated. Still image with ECA, sticker, and bony landmarks.

landmarks during the CAS procedure (**Fig. 6**). After the reassessment through the guiding catheter, all equipment for the CAS procedure is selected and prepped. It is essential that all equipment is prepped in an organized fashion before beginning the CAS. Before starting the CAS procedure one may use a checklist approach, making sure that the ACT is greater than 250, the patient is relaxed and doing well, and all equipment is prepped. The staff is engaged throughout the procedure, and

confirms the administration of atropine (given in most patients before CAS, with doses individualized to the patient and their lesion). Fluid is allowed to flow at 999 mL/h during the short duration of the CAS procedure. It is confirmed that all medicines are available (the author has neosynephrine and atropine mixed for each patient, and has intravenous antihypertensive medicines available). Immediately before starting the CAS procedure, the patient is reeducated and reassured.

CAS WITH DISTAL EMBOLIC PROTECTION

After patient reeducation, CAS roadmap #1 is obtained. Using this roadmap, the lesion is wired, taking great care not to prolapse the wire. The embolic protection system (EPD) is advanced to a straight segment and deployed. Using the same roadmap, predilatation is performed in almost all cases (see **Fig. 2**). The standard balloon is a 4 × 30 noncompliant balloon. (The author is of the opinion that predilatation should be performed for all carotid stent procedures, the rationale being that there are extremely low event rates during predilatation, which facilitate atraumatic placement of the larger, self-expanding stents that will predictably expand following deployment; this takes very little time.) A balloon longer than the lesion is used; 30-mm length balloons suffice for most cases. For longer lesions a 40-mm balloon is used. This balloon is inflated briefly, usually to nominal pressures. After balloon deflation, hemodynamics and the patient are reassessed. After aspirating the system, CAS roadmap #2 is

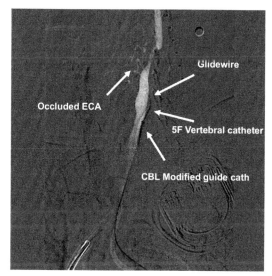

Fig. 5. Guide advancement strategy with occluded ECA. CBL.

performed. Very importantly, for stent deployment the author does not administer any contrast and tends to choose longer stents if there is any questionable circumstance; using the roadmap, bony landmarks from the guiding angiogram, sticker on the neck, and so forth, stents can be accurately placed without use of contrast (**Fig. 7**). After the stent is deployed, the roadmap is removed; reassessment with angiograms is not done yet. Fluoroscopic magnification is increased (mag up) to examine the stent. If there is any waist, it is postdilated with a balloon that has already been prepped. In most cases this is a 5 × 20 noncompliant balloon, with the balloon always at least 10 mm less than the length of the stent (for long lesions a 30-mm balloon inside the 40-mm stent is used). Balloon inflation is performed under high magnification to localize the waist and to ensure that the balloon is within the stent (**Fig. 8**); contrast is not needed for this. If there is no waist seen on increased magnification, postdilatation may not need to be performed. Inflations are of short duration. The goal is a single inflation each for predilatation and postdilatation, avoiding multiple inflations, which increase embolic events.

After postdilatation, a subtracted angiogram is obtained, which is important to ensure that there is not slow flow (discussed later) that would require aspiration thrombectomy before EPD removal. If the stent is well positioned and there is normal antegrade flow, the embolic protection system is removed with the retrieval catheter. Following EPD removal, a second oblique angiogram of the carotid bifurcation is obtained. The baseline lateral and AP Towne cerebral angiograms are then repeated. Very importantly, before sheath/guide

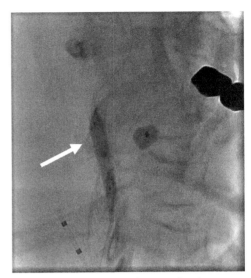

Fig. 8. Postdilatation on high magnification.

removal, a neurologic examination is performed on the table. If there are deficits, the cerebral angiograms are reevaluated, and the risk/benefit of potential neurorescue is considered. If the angiograms and neurologic checks are normal, the angled Glidewire is inserted just beyond the sheath, and the sheath removed over the wire while performing active aspiration to minimize any distal embolization.

Following the carotid stent procedure, femoral arteriograms are routinely performed to assess the suitability for closure device use. The author believes that use of a closure device use allows for earlier mobility of the patient, which may be beneficial, especially in cases of lower blood pressure often seen after CAS.

STENT SELECTION FOR CAS

Stent selection is individualized to the patient's lesion and clinical characteristics. General practice is to use longer stents as there is little penalty in terms of restenosis, and this reduces stent manipulation. The author also tends to use larger-diameter stents, using 10 × 8 tapered stents for most cases, or 10-mm stents for most nontapered stents. Although there are no pure randomized data, in the author's opinion, in patients with straight vessels with significant ulceration or calcification, and/or in symptomatic patients, closed-cell stents are preferable because of their increased scaffolding and radial strength (eg, XACT, Wallstent). For significantly tortuous vessels, a hybrid or open-cell stent (Precise stent) is preferred (others include Acculink, Protégé, and Wallstent). For almost all cases, the carotid stent

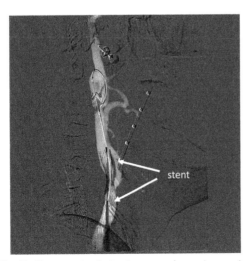

Fig. 7. Placement of stent on roadmapping, using landmarks and no contrast.

will be deployed from the internal carotid into the CCA. One must avoid leaving short segments in the CCA, as this increases difficulties with EPD removal.

MEDICATIONS DURING CAS

As discussed earlier, bivalirudin is used for essentially all CAS cases with administration of little to no sedation. Neosynephrine is given in 50- to 100-μg boluses as needed for systolic blood pressure lower than 80 mm Hg, especially if associated with symptoms. If there is sustained hypotension, patients are placed on a neosynephrine drip at 40 μg/min overnight, and weaned slowly in the morning, with the patient still discharged on post-CAS day 1. Intravenous fluid is administered throughout the procedure. For hypertension that persists after postdilatation, intravenous labetalol, apresoline, or nipride is used, depending on heart rate and blood pressure, with a lower threshold for intravenous continued infusion and a stay in the intensive care unit for persistent hypertension, especially for tighter lesions in patients with recent neurologic events, to avoid hyperperfusion syndrome (the author does not treat hypertension in patients without prior CEA before CAS, but does so immediately if the blood pressure is not lower after stent postdilatation).

PROXIMAL EMBOLIC PROTECTION FOR CAS

Proximal embolic protection likely has the best in class data for CAS results. Both American IDE trials (ARMOUR and EMPIRE) showed less than 3% stroke and death rates in patients at high risk for endarterectomy in carefully controlled trials.[6,7] Furthermore, a large meta-analysis by Bersin and colleagues[8] showed excellent stroke and death rates (<2%), with the procedure very well tolerated by patients. There are randomized data showing fewer new cerebral lesions after CAS with proximal protection compared with distal protection, both by transcranial Doppler and diffusion-weighted magnetic resonance imaging studies.[11,12] Furthermore, the benefits of proximal embolic protection appear to be consistent across the usual high-risk groups of CAS patients, including consistent excellent results in octogenarian patients and symptomatic patients.[6–8] Of importance, proximal EPD use is somewhat restricted in the United States because of lack of registry trials for patient enrollment. In the author's opinion, proximal EPD may be important in a large percentage of CAS patients, especially higher-risk patients, provided that reimbursement is available and anatomy is suitable (see later discussion).

THEORETICAL ADVANTAGES OF PROXIMAL EPD OVER DISTAL EPD

- Decreased event rates in high-risk patients seen in clinical trials[6–8]
- Fewer new cerebral lesions after CAS[11,12]
- Stable guide position with 2 balloons serving as anchors (**Figs. 9** and **10**)
- ECA balloon serves as another landmark for stent deployment (see **Figs. 6** and **10**)
- Proximal EPD protects throughout the entirety of CAS, including wiring of the lesion
- Protects against embolization of particles of essentially all sizes
- Can use with any 0.014 guide wire and any stent system
- Can be used in combination with distal EPD if appropriate
- Is well tolerated in more than 98% of patients[8]

RELATIVE REQUIREMENTS FOR PROXIMAL EPD

- Patent ipsilateral ECA vessel and no high-grade disease in the distal CCA
- Some collateral support to the treated hemisphere
- Anatomy supporting 9F catheters (the author has found that this is essentially all vessels; the device can always be advanced provided a supportive wire can be placed in the ECA, as discussed below)

The aforementioned are relative requirements, and an individualized risk/benefit evaluation is applied when considering proximal EPD.

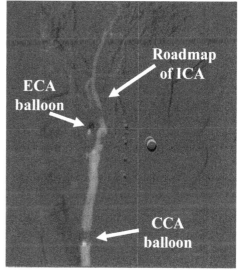

Fig. 9. Roadmap with ECA and CCA balloons inflated.

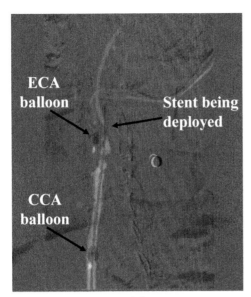

Fig. 10. Stent deployment (after percutaneous transluminal angioplasty) on roadmap, with proximal protection.

PROXIMAL EPD TECHNIQUE DURING CAS

The same principles for CAS described earlier apply, with the following modifications. A 9F long sheath is placed first (this helps with losing any of the support of the device in tortuous iliac vessels). A roadmap is used as described earlier, and an angled Glidewire is advanced into one of the terminal larger branches of the ECA. The neurodiagnostic catheter is advanced over the Glidewire and is used to exchange for a supportive wire (the author uses an exchange-length Supra-Core wire). Over the SupraCore wire, and through the 9F sheath, the MOMA system is advanced such that the ECA balloon (clearly delineated with a marker) is placed in the proximal external carotid artery (of note, the Gore flow reversal system is being taken off the market and is not discussed). It is important that the supportive wire is left in place until the ECA balloon is inflated, as the wire cannot be reinserted. After confirming a good position, the ECA balloon is inflated in the proximal external carotid artery (ideally, this will be below all branches of the ECA; however, there are instances whereby small superior thyroidal arteries are at the bifurcation, in which case it is not important to cover these branches completely and risk prolapse of the ECA balloon into the bifurcation). A nonsubtracted angiogram is obtained with the ECA balloon inflated (see **Fig. 6**) and this is used as a reference, showing the lesion, bony landmarks, and position of the ECA balloon relative to the carotid lesion (see **Figs. 6** and **9**). As

described earlier, all carotid stent equipment is then selected and prepared, after which the Supra Core wire is removed. The selected 0.014 guide wire is shaped and positioned just distal to the CCA balloon (delineated with a second marker, see **Fig. 6**). The author uses a slightly larger curve to verify that the wire moves freely distal to the CCA balloon. (There is a tract between the CCA and ECA balloons; the wire can go into this and is therefore not steerable; if this is the case, the wire is withdrawn just distal to the CCA marker and redirected. The author finds it helpful to confirm this freedom before initiating proximal protection.) With all equipment prepped and the guide wire just distal to the CCA balloon, a roadmap is obtained (see **Fig. 9**). This roadmap will stay in place until after the stent is deployed. Following roadmapping the CCA balloon is inflated, and the stump pressure is noted on arterial monitoring. After proximal protection is confirmed with a lower stump pressure, the lesion is wired. Using the same roadmap, angioplasty is performed as described earlier (usually a 4 × 30 balloon). After this, with the same roadmap, the previously prepped stent is advanced and deployed, using the roadmap, bony landmarks, and the ECA balloon position as reference for deployment (see **Fig. 10**). After stent deployment, the roadmap is removed. The same magnified views are obtained of the stent, with postdilatation performed using increased magnification as discussed earlier (see **Fig. 8**). Following postdilatation, aspiration is performed with at least three 20-mL syringes (the author finds it helpful to place approximately 2 mL of saline in the syringes, which helps to overcome the vacuum in the system). It is important to aspirate slowly to avoid neurologic intolerance. Aspiration is performed until there are 3 clean filtered 20-mL syringes (if a distal EPD is also used, three 20-mL syringes are aspirated, then the distal EPD is removed while proximal balloons are still inflated, after which an additional two 20-mL syringes are aspirated). After aspirations the ECA balloon is deflated, followed by deflation of the CCA balloon. The true systemic pressure is then reassessed with monitoring. After carefully aspirating as described, angiograms are obtained through the proximal embolic protection sheath of both the bifurcation and cerebral vessels. Of importance, the neurologic examination is performed while the MOMA balloons are still in place, as they can be reinflated if additional work is necessary. If the postprocedure angiograms and neurologic assessments are satisfactory, the MOMA device is removed. A wire cannot be reinserted (it may exit the CCA balloon and not reenter the ECA balloon, thus traumatizing the vessel).

Instead, the balloon is simply withdrawn under fluoroscopic observation while the assistant aspirates actively from the system. Closure devices are then considered, as discussed earlier.

PROXIMAL VERSUS DISTAL EPD DECISION

The decision to use proximal embolic protection versus distal embolic protection is individualized to the patient. Financial and research considerations are also important. It is the author's experience that proximal embolic protection is tolerated by most patients, and the system can be used in almost all patients provided a supportive wire can be placed in the ECA. It is his practice to use proximal embolic protection if the patient is highly symptomatic, has a lesion that appears to have a high embolic risk, is an octogenarian, or has a suboptimal landing zone for distal EPD systems, or if there are expected to be significant challenges with wiring the lesion or placing a distal EPD device across the lesion.

COMMON PROBLEMS ENCOUNTERED DURING CAS

1. *Difficulty passing the retrieval device to capture a distal EPD system.* If this occurs, it is essential to carefully watch both the distal EPD and the distal end of the guide/sheath. One should never force the retrieval catheter or pull the distal EPD system, as the EPD may become entangled in the stent, or the sheath prolapse into the aorta. Instead, slow back and forth neck rotations are performed with the nurse's assistance as the operator slowly advances and withdraws the retrieval catheter. This action will free the device from the stent tines in most (>90%–95%) cases. If this does not work after several deliberate attempts, use a bont tip retrieval device (Boston Scientific; works with all distal EPD systems), which can be directed away from the stent tines. If these maneuvers do not work, additional angioplasty can be performed at the site of resistance within the stent. Lastly, the guide/sheath can be introduced inside the stent (over a Glidewire and vertebral catheter).
2. *Slow flow after CAS with distal EPD.* It is necessary to perform one angiogram after stenting with a distal EPD. If there is slow flow, this is almost always due to a full basket. One should perform aspiration thrombectomy (regardless of the patient's symptom status) before removal of the full basket. If there is thought to be a very high debris burden, a second wire can be placed within the basket for

additional thrombectomy. After performing aspiration (to remove any suspended debris proximal to the EPD), simply remove the EPD filter slowly with the retrieval catheter, thus restoring normal flow characteristics. Careful neurologic and angiographic assessment is needed, as these patients will tend to have higher event rates despite the restoration of normal flow.

3. *Symptoms develop during CAS.* If the patient becomes symptomatic after an EPD device has been placed and angioplasty performed, in general it will be prudent to complete the CAS procedure (it is unhelpful to have a patient with a stroke and a partially treated, high-grade lesion). If they cannot squeeze a toy on several attempts, patients are not asked further. Reassess the etiology, hydrate and increase the blood pressure, and check that the ACT is adequate. After placing the carotid stent, assess for slow flow and, if present, treat as above. Obtain careful assessments of the precerebral and postcerebral angiograms, and weigh the risks/benefits of neurorescue (discussed below).

SPECIAL SITUATIONS IN CAS

1. *Difficult aortic arches.* In general, for severely difficult arches one should carefully reassess the risks and benefits of CAS in that particular patient. If there is significant calcification and/or disease in the CCA or aorta, manipulation via this will lead to an increased risk of embolic events before CAS. In significantly angulated arches (type III, bovine, and so forth), the author uses the following modifications in technique. The author is more likely to use guiding catheters (they provide additional support and steerability, and are less likely to have kinking or prolapse). Via these, use the advanced neurodiagnostic catheters (Vitek predominately; others include JB2 or Simmons catheters). In the target carotid artery, place these catheters lower in the CCA and perform a roadmap (see **Fig. 3**; **Figs. 11** and **12**). (If there is no significant disease in the CCA and there is a patent ECA, one may be confident in accessing the lesion safely in most cases.) An angled Glidewire is advanced deep into an ECA terminal branch. The catheter is slowly advanced with the support of the guiding catheter and deep ECA wire position. Often the author introduces the guiding catheter in a stepwise approach, engaging the CCA to provide additional support, then advancing the diagnostic catheter. Ultimately, the guiding catheter is advanced in

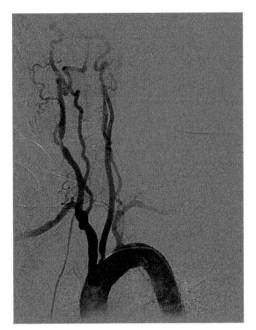

Fig. 11. Type II to III aortic arch.

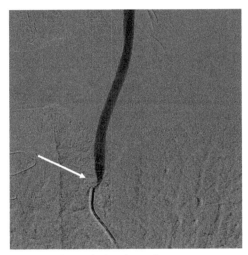

Fig. 13. Ostial CCA lesion (*arrow*).

a telescoping fashion, using the roadmap (see **Fig. 3**). Occasionally, if the Vitek catheter cannot be advanced, with the guiding catheter in the CCA one may use an exchange-length Glidewire in place of a vertebral catheter, which may be easier to advance into the ECA, and then perform the telescoping maneuver with the guiding catheter. Rarely, it is exchanged for a supportive wire in the ECA catheter. It is important to repeat a pre-CAS angiogram to re-assess the effect on ICA tortuosity after traversing the angulated arch vessels with larger guiding catheters, before proceeding with CAS. After this repeat angiogram, consideration may be given to use of proximal embolic protection, as the balloons provide sheath stability in difficult arch vessels. Extremely angulated arches or CCAs without a clear path to a patent ECA are challenging for CAS. Careful attempts can be made using roadmapping, placing a catheter and supportive wire short of the bifurcation and slowly advancing a guiding catheter (see **Figs. 4** and **5**). Great care should be taken to avoid contact with the lesion, and the procedure should be aborted if this cannot be safely performed.

2. *Ostial common carotid/innominate lesions* (**Figs. 13–18**). For ostial CCA and innominate lesions, distal EPD should be used in most cases

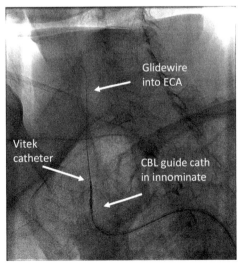

Fig. 12. Strategy for accessing a type III arch. CBL.

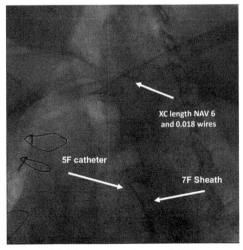

Fig. 14. Ostial CCA strategy (see text). XC.

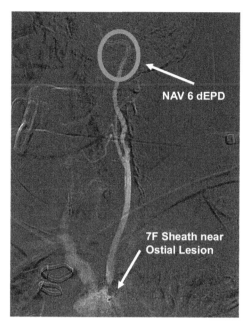

Fig. 15. Ostial CCA strategy continued. 7F Sheath and distal EPD (dEPD).

with the following modified approach. Use a 7F Shuttle sheath (to facilitate the usual 8–10 mm balloon-expandable stents needed, and to provide adequate lumens for angiograms around the stent). Very importantly, exchange-length wires are needed. Use the NAV-6 system, as this allows an exchange-length independent wire to be placed. Use also a second 0.014 or 0.018 guide wire simultaneously placed in the ECA. Both of these wires are placed through a neurodiagnostic catheter within the 7F Shuttle sheath, with a no-touch technique, whereby the

catheter is placed close to but not touching the ostial lesion, directing the wires into the ICA or ECA. After wiring, the 7F Shuttle sheath is slowly advanced to the ostial lesion over the catheter, and this catheter is removed from the Shuttle sheath over both exchange-length wires. The distal EPD is placed in the ICA over the appropriate wire. After this, predilatation is performed in the ostial CCA, usually with a 5- to 6-mm, 0.014-compatible balloon. After reassessment, a balloon-expandable, 0.035-compatible stent is chosen. Importantly this is placed over both exchange-length wires, carefully positioned, and deployed with a short inflation. Often the stent balloon is withdrawn partially in the aortic arch with a second angioplasty performed. After angiographic reassessment, the distal EPD is carefully removed. This action will often require a bent-tip retrieval device as described earlier. A modification for treatment of innominate lesions is to use right radial or brachial access to place an EPD from the right arm. This approach allows use of a 0.035 guide wire from femoral artery access to place a stent, with the protection being provided via right arm access. For the innominate artery, the author usually uses 10-mm balloon-expandable stents after predilatation.

3. *Neurorescue.* In carefully selected patients treated with CAS by experienced operators with attention to detail, neurorescue should be a rare consideration. It is the author's practice to only perform neurorescue if the patient has a major, persistent neurologic deficit and has a visible, approachable cutoff in a major cerebral vessel. Ideally, one has an excellent working relationship with a neuroradiologist or

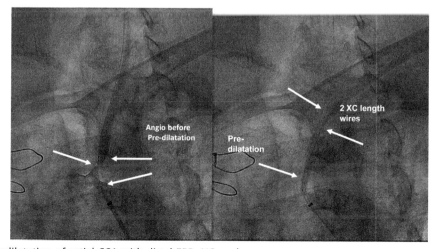

Fig. 16. Predilatation of ostial CCA with distal EPD. XC, exchange.

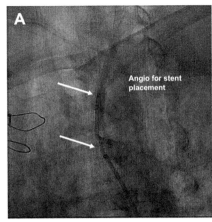
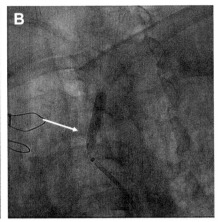

Fig. 17. Stenting of ostial CCA. (*A*) Angiography for stent placement. (*B*) Stent up.

interventional neurosurgeon at his or her facility. If this is not the case and the above criteria are met, the author proceeds with neurorescue, trying to keep it simple. In general, a neurointerventional sheath is placed higher into the petrous segment of the ICA (eg, Neuron or Envoy catheters). Via this sheath, a 0.014 wire is very carefully advanced across the lesion. Small doses of tissue plasminogen activator (eg, 1 mg at a time) can be administered locally, and angiographic and neurologic reassessment is performed. If this is unsuccessful, balloon angioplasty with a very small balloon (1.25, 1.5) can be performed, versus aspiration thrombectomy. If one is familiar with the neurorescue devices, these can be used as well. It is very important that this be done only for large neurologic deficits, and great care should be used to keep all wires within the lumen of the vessel and to avoid overdilatation, wire perforations, or dissections, which can be catastrophic. Again, with careful patient selection and procedural technique, this should be a very rare event (at the author's facility, only 1 of more than 1700 CAS cases).

SUMMARY

CAS continues to have improving results in both standard-risk and high-risk patients with carotid artery disease.[13,14] This successful, low-risk carotid stenting occurs when CAS is performed by experienced, appropriately trained operators who use good patient and lesion selection, sound judgment, and meticulous attention to procedural technique. With careful attention to these principles, CAS can be appropriately applied to help a large number of patients with carotid artery disease.

REFERENCES

1. American Heart Association: Heart disease and stroke statistics: 2004 update. Available at: http://www.americanheart.org/downloadable/heart/1079 736729696HDSStats2004Update REV3-19-04.pdf. Accessed July 1, 2004.
2. Yadav JS, Wholey MH, Kuntz RE, et al. Protected carotid artery stenting versus endarterectomy in high-risk patients. N Engl J Med 2004;351:1493–501.
3. Brott TG, Hobson RW, Roubin GS, et al, CREST Investigators. Stenting versus endarterectomy for treatment of carotid-artery stenosis. N Engl J Med 2010;363:11–23.
4. Myla S, Bacharach JM, Ansel GM, et al. Carotid artery stenting in high surgical risk patients using the FiberNet embolic protection system: the EPIC trial results. Catheter Cardiovasc Interv 2010;75:817–22.
5. The PROTECT Study, presented at 2009 International Stroke Conference at the American Heart Association 02/18/09, San Diego, CA; Chaturedi S,

Fig. 18. Final angiographic result (*arrow*) after stenting.

Gray WA, Matsumara J. Safety Outcomes for the PROTECT Carotid Artery Stenting Multicenter Study. Stroke 2009;40:2.

6. Hopkins LN. The EMPIRE trial results. Presented at TCT October 17, 2008. Washington, DC.

7. Ansel GM, Hopkins LN, Jaff MR, et al. Safety and effectiveness of the Invatec MoMa proximal cerebral protection device during carotid artery stenting: results from the ARMOUR pivotal trial. Cathet Cardiovasc Interv 2010;76:1–8.

8. Bersin RM, Stabile E, Ansel GM, et al. A meta-analysis of proximal occlusion device outcomes in carotid artery stenting. Catheter Cardiovasc Interv 2012;80:1072–8.

9. White CJ, Metzger DC, Ansel GM, et al. Safety and efficacy of carotid stenting in the very elderly. Cathet Cardiovasc Interv 2010;75(5):651–5.

10. Roubin GS, Iyer S, Halkin A, et al. Realizing the potential of carotid artery stenting proposed paradigms for patient selection and procedural technique. Circulation 2006;113:2021–30.

11. Montorsi P, Caputi L, Gali S, et al. Microembolization during carotid artery stenting in patients with high risk lipid rich plaque. A randomized trial of proximal vs. distal cerebral protection. J Am Coll Cardiol 2011;58:1656–63.

12. Birjuklic K, Wandler A, Hazizi F, et al. The PROFI Study (prevention of cerebral embolization by proximal balloon occlusion compared to filter protection during carotid artery stenting): a prospective, randomized trial. J Am Coll Cardiol 2012;59:1383–9.

13. Metzger DC, Hibbard D, Massop D, et al. Peri-procedural outcomes after carotid artery stenting in the first 15,000 patients enrolled in SAPPHIRE WW Study. JACC 2012;60(Supplement B):17.

14. Massop D, Dave R, Metzger C, et al. Stenting and angioplasty with protection in patients at high risk for Endarterectomy: SAPPHIRE World-Wide Registry in the First 2001 Patients. Cathet Cardiovasc Interv 2009;73:129–36.

Patient, Anatomic, and Procedural Characteristics That Increase the Risk of Carotid Interventions

Christopher J. White, MD

KEYWORDS

• Carotid artery stent • Angioplasty • High risk

KEY POINTS

• Carotid artery stenting (CAS) was developed as a less invasive alternative to carotid endarterectomy (CEA) in patients at increased risk of complications with conventional surgery.
• Several randomized trials have demonstrated equipoise between CAS and CEA in both high-risk and average-risk surgery patients.
• Current evidence suggests that there are identifiable patient, anatomic, and procedural characteristics that increase the incidence of carotid stenting complications.
• Such evidence reaffirms the importance of careful case selection when performing CAS.

INTRODUCTION

Carotid artery stenting (CAS) was developed as a less invasive alternative to carotid endarterectomy (CEA) in patients at increased risk of complications with conventional surgery (**Table 1**). Multiple randomized controlled trials and registry studies conducted in high surgical risk patients, average surgical risk patients, symptomatic patients, and asymptomatic patients have clearly shown equipoise for CAS versus CEA, and in some cases CAS is preferred over CEA.[1–14] CAS is a very young procedure, and as would be expected, there has been significant improvement in outcomes over the past 10 years (**Fig. 1**). These data led to Food and Drug Administration device approval for the carotid stent system (RX ACCU-LINK; Abbott Vascular, Abbott Park, Il) and to multisocietal guidelines that recommended CAS as an alternative to CEA in average and low surgical risk

symptomatic (Level I) and asymptomatic (Level II) patients who require carotid revascularization for stroke prevention.[15,16]

As high-risk patients were identified for surgery, it has also become apparent that there are patients who are at increased risk for complications with stenting. The purpose of this article was to review the evidence supporting risk stratification of patients being considered for CAS.

CAROTID STENT RISK ASSESSMENT

Presumptive high-risk features for complications of CAS include thrombus-containing lesions, heavily calcified lesions, very tortuous vessels, and near occlusions. In addition, patients have been considered to be at increased risk for complications if they have (1) contraindications to dual antiplatelet therapy (aspirin and thienopyridines), (2) a history of bleeding complications,

Disclosures: None relative to this topic.
Department of Medicine and Cardiology, Ochsner Medical Center and Ochsner Clinical School of the University of Queensland, John Ochsner Heart and Vascular Institute, Ochsner Medical Institutions, 1514 Jefferson Highway, New Orleans, LA 70121, USA
E-mail address: cwhite@ochsner.org

Intervent Cardiol Clin 3 (2014) 51–61
http://dx.doi.org/10.1016/j.iccl.2013.09.001

Table 1
Features associated with high surgical risk for carotid disease

Medical Comorbidity	Anatomic Criteria
Elderly (>75/80 y) Congestive heart failure (NYHA III/IV) Unstable angina	Surgically inaccessible lesions • At or above C2 • Below the clavicle
CAD with ≥2 vessels ≥70% stenosis	Prior neck irradiation or surgery (prior CEA)
Recent heart attack (≤30 d)	Spinal immobility of the neck
Planned open heart surgery (≤30 d)	Contralateral carotid artery occlusion
Ejection fraction ≤30%	Laryngeal palsy
COPD with FEV ≤30%	Tracheostoma

Abbreviations: C2, cervical spine vertebral body #2; CAD, coronary artery disease; CEA, carotid endarterectomy; COPD, chronic obstructive pulmonary disease; FEV, forced expiratory volume; NYHA, New York Heart Association.

and/or (3) severe peripheral arterial disease (PAD) making femoral artery vascular access difficult.

Variables that increase the risk of CAS complications can be placed into 3 categories: (1) patient characteristics, (2) anatomic or lesion features, and (3) procedural factors (**Table 2**). Some of these high-risk features have been identified empirically by expert consensus (eg, thrombus-containing lesions), whereas other criteria of CAS risk are supported by clinical trial evidence (eg, operator experience).[17]

In terms of expert consensus, a multidisciplinary Delphi Carotid Stenting Consensus Panel made recommendations regarding CAS risk factors.[18] High-risk CAS features were those that (1) prolonged catheter or guide wire manipulation in the aortic arch, (2) made crossing a carotid stenosis more difficult, (3) decreased the likelihood of successful deployment or retrieval of an embolic protection device (EPD), or (4) made stent delivery or placement more difficult. The highest-risk feature for CAS was determined to be a Type III aortic arch (**Fig. 2**) followed by friable aortic arch atheroma. The least important feature for predicting CAS complications, by expert consensus, was the severity of the carotid stenosis.

CAS patient selection criteria were proposed in 2006 by Roubin and colleagues.[19] They identified clinical features, such as older age (≥80 years) and decreased cerebral reserve (dementia, multiple prior strokes, or intracranial microangiopathy), as being associated with increased CAS risk. They also identified anatomic features, such as excessive tortuosity (more than two 90° bends within

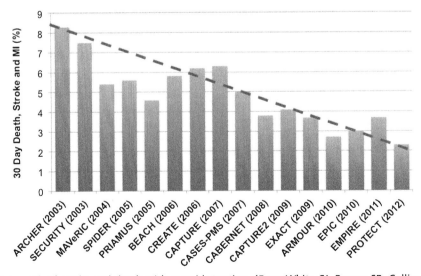

Fig. 1. Declining risk of stroke and death with carotid stenting. (*From* White CJ, Ramee SR, Collins TJ, et al. Carotid artery stenting: patient, lesion, and procedural characteristics that increase procedural complications. Catheter Cardiovasc Interv 2013. http://dx.doi.org/10.1002/ccd.24984; with permission.)

Table 2
Features that increase the risk of a carotid stent procedure

Medical Comorbidity	Anatomic Criteria	Procedural Factor
Older age (>75/80 y)	Type III aortic arch	Inexperienced operator
Symptomatic status	Vessel tortuosity	Inexperienced center
Hypercoagulable state	Heavy calcification	EPD not used
Bleeding risk	Lesion-related thrombus	Open-cell vs closed-cell stent
Chronic kidney disease	Echolucent plaque	Time delay from onset
Decreased cerebral reserve	Aortic arch atheroma	—

5 cm of the target lesion) and heavy calcification (concentric calcification ≥ 3 mm in width), with increased CAS complications.

PATIENT COMORBIDITIES THAT INCREASE CAS RISK
Patient Characteristics

Patients with severe medical comorbidities have been deemed to be at higher risk of periprocedural complications with CAS than patients who have unfavorable anatomy for surgery. Supporting evidence comes from the Boston Scientific EPI: A Carotid Stenting Trial for High-Risk Surgical Patients (BEACH) trial, which found that the 30-day periprocedural complication rates for patients enrolled

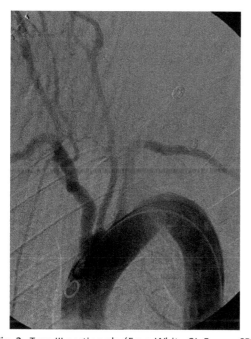

Fig. 2. Type III aortic arch. (*From* White CJ, Ramee SR, Collins TJ, et al. Carotid artery stenting: patient, lesion, and procedural characteristics that increase procedural complications. Catheter Cardiovasc Interv 2013. http://dx.doi.org/10.1002/ccd.24984; with permission.)

due to their medical comorbidities (see **Table 1**) were higher than patients enrolled for unfavorable CEA anatomy (9.1% vs 3.6%, $P = .016$).[5]

Clinical characteristics, such as hypercoagulability, increased bleeding risk, inability to take dual antiplatelet therapy, and decreased cerebral reserve, have routinely excluded patients from CAS clinical trials but have not been prospectively evaluated to assess their contribution to CAS procedure risk. A single-center European series of 624 consecutive CAS patients reported that poor glycemic control (HbA1c >7%) was the strongest independent risk predictor for a procedural complication with an adjusted odds ratio of 3.8.[20] Patients with chronic kidney disease are frequently excluded from clinical trials of CAS because of contrast risk. A post-market surveillance trial, Carotid RX Acculink/Accunet Post-Approval Trial to Uncover Unanticipated or Rare Events (CAPTURE), did not find a correlation between CAS complications and chronic kidney disease.[6]

Patients 75/80 years or older have been identified as a high-risk group for complications related to both CEA and CAS (**Table 3**).[19,21,22] Elderly patients may have a less favorable "risk-to-benefit" calculation based on their relatively shorter expected life expectancy than younger patients. In other words, if the procedure risk is fixed, then a longer life span allows a much greater benefit to accrue.

In an early study, CAS patients 80 years or older had an almost threefold higher periprocedural complication rate compared with younger patients.[23] The lead-in phase of CREST raised significant concerns in octogenarians by showing a 12.1% stroke or death rate at 30 days following CAS.[24] Increased periprocedural complications, including stroke, has been documented in elderly patients in 2 device-approval trials.[6,25] In the BEACH trial, elderly patients made up about one-third of the patients, but accounted for almost two-thirds of CAS complications.

A breakpoint for increased CAS complications has been identified at the later part of the

Table 3
Carotid artery stent risk in elderly patients

	Roubin et al,[19] [N, 1031] (%)	CREST LEAD-IN[24] [N, 532] (%)	CAPTURE[6] [N, 2217] (%)	BEACH[74] [N, 1316] (%)
<80 y	6	2.8	5.6	3.4[a]
≥80 y	16	12.1	8.1	9.1[b]
P value	<.01	<.01	<.05	<.002

Brackets are Odd Ratios and 95% confidence limits. LEAD-IN means patients treated during the qualifying period for each operator.
  Abbreviations: BEACH, Boston Scientific EPI: A Carotid Stenting Trial for High-Risk Surgical Patients; CAPTURE, Carotid RX Acculink/Accunet Post-Approval Trial to Uncover Unanticipated or Rare Events; CREST, Carotid Revascularization End-arterectomy Versus Stenting Trial.
  [a] <75 years of age.
  [b] ≥75 years of age.

sixth decade of life in both the European Stent-Protected Angioplasty versus Carotid Endarterectomy (SPACE) trial and CREST in the United States.[26,27] Advanced age is also an independent risk factor for the lesions detected by magnetic resonance imaging (MRI) or diffusion-weighted imaging (DWI) after CAS.[28]

The increased procedural risk in the elderly is multifactorial.[29,30] Octogenarian patients are more likely to have anatomic features that increase the risk for CAS, such as a type III aortic arch, decreased cerebral reserve, aortic arch vessel calcification, excessive cervical vessel tortuosity, and severe lesion calcification.[19,30–33]

Despite the potential for increased risk in the elderly, there are multiple case series documenting safety and low CAS complication rates in the very elderly.[31,34–38] It is apparent that experienced operators, working in experienced centers, are able to select patients for CAS among the very elderly and achieve excellent outcomes. Importantly, although age should certainly factor into the decision regarding risks of revascularization, there should not be an arbitrary age cutoff for eligibility of patients for CAS.

Symptomatic Versus Asymptomatic Patients

Being a symptomatic patient, defined as having a recent (<60 days) transient ischemic attack (TIA) or stroke, is an independent predictor of poor outcomes with CAS.[6,29,36,39] Symptomatic patients have demonstrated a doubling of the 30-day stroke and death risk (6.25% compared with 3.34% for elective procedures).[36] Patients with a hemispherical TIA or minor stroke had a significant increase in periprocedural risk compared with asymptomatic patients, or to those who had only retinal symptoms for CAS.[39] A large meta-analysis found that a symptomatic presentation and presenting with a cerebral event versus retinal event were both

associated with a significantly higher risk of stroke or death when treated with CAS.[29]

ANATOMIC OR LESION CHARACTERISTICS THAT INCREASE CAS RISK
Type III Aortic Arch and Aortic Arch Vessel Tortuosity

As discussed previously, the strongest predictor of adverse outcomes related to CAS by expert consensus was a type III aortic arch (see **Fig. 2**).[18] The Sienna Risk Score for CAS complications found a 2.5-fold increase in periprocedural strokes with Type III aortic arches.[36] Other investigators have confirmed a threefold to fourfold increased risk for periprocedural complications for complex aortic arch anatomy.[40] Higher death and stroke rates were associated with more complex atherosclerotic aortic arch anatomy in an analysis of a 3388-patient subset of the Carotid RX Acculink/Accunet Post-Approval Trial to Uncover Rare Events (CAPTURE-2).[17]

Complex aortic arch anatomy correlates with finding DWI-MRI abnormalities following diagnostic cerebral angiography.[41] Although patients with complex aortic arch morphologies are frequently excluded from clinical trials, the volume of embolic brain lesions is significantly greater with a Type III aortic arch and these lesions are more likely to affect the contralateral hemisphere.[42] In another analysis, aortic arch angulation and proximal common carotid artery tortuosity significantly contributed to both technical failure and neurologic complications of CAS, whereas tortuosity of the distal internal carotid artery was not a significant factor.[43]

Contralateral Carotid Stenosis or Occlusion

Although contralateral carotid occlusion is a recognized risk for CEA (see **Table 1**), multiple trials have failed to demonstrate any correlation for CAS complications.[6,28,36,44] In the BEACH trial (n = 747 high surgical risk patients), there was no difference in the periprocedural complications for CAS patients with unilateral or bilateral carotid disease.[5]

Aortic Arch Atheroma

Large (>5 mm or mobile debris) aortic arch atheroma found on transesophageal echocardiography (TEE) correlate with the number and volume of cerebral lesions found on brain DWI-MRI imaging after CAS. An association exists between the presence of protruding or mobile atherosclerotic plaques of the aortic arch and the risk of contralateral periprocedural embolization.[42] Increasing complexity of the aortic arch and increasing patient age both correlate with increasing amounts of aortic arch calcification.[32] Additionally, the presence of arch calcification is associated with threefold to fourfold increased risk of periprocedural stroke after CAS.[36]

Carotid Lesion Characteristics

DWI-MRI brain lesions are surrogates for cerebral embolization. The clinical importance of new DWI-MRI lesions is uncertain at the present time. New DWI-MRI lesions were seen in 51% of CAS patients. Lesion features independently associated with new DWI-MRI defects included an ulcerated stenosis or a lesion longer than 1 cm (**Fig. 3**).[44–46] Consistent with the increased periprocedural stroke risk with longer lesions is the association of increased complications with longer carotid stent lengths or the need for multiple stents.[6,47,48] Ulcerated lesions and lesions with irregular borders are also associated with an increased risk of CAS clinical complications.[20,36,48]

Heavily Calcified Plaque

Heavily calcified lesions or those with circumferential calcium are often excluded from CAS trials because of presumptive high carotid stent risk. A major concern with dense calcification is difficult balloon expansion and the potential risk of carotid artery rupture in nonexpandable lesions. Unfortunately, without an objective way to identify and classify calcified lesions, it is difficult to know which specific lesions pose a greater procedural risk.

Calcified lesions, defined as being radiographically opaque, were related to stroke risk in 2 large series of CAS.[20,36] Two other reports disagreed. In a series of 231 patients with one-third of the lesions graded as calcified, there was no association with CAS complications.[44] The CAPTURE registry (n = 3500) found no relationship between lesion calcification and increased procedural

stroke risk.[6] Major confounders in these trials include a lack of a uniform definition of lesion calcification, the subjective nature of lesion selection, and variable techniques used to perform CAS.

Echolucent Plaque

There have been indications that low plaque echogenicity (echolucent plaque) is associated with an increased number of emboli after CEA and CAS.[49] An ultrasound-based parameter of plaque echogenicity, the gray scale median (GSM), is an independent predictor of periprocedural stroke after CAS.[50] The Carotid Angioplasty and Risk of Stroke (ICAROS) registry included 418 cases of CAS collected from 11 international centers and found that 7.1% (11/155) with GSM of 25 or less had a periprocedural stroke, whereas only 1.5% (4/263) of patients with GSM greater than 25 had a stroke (P = .005).

MRI data characterizing atherosclerotic carotid artery plaque have recently been used to predict

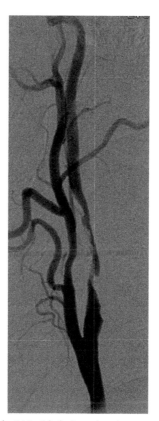

Fig. 3. High CAS risk lesion due to excessive lesion length. (*From* White CJ, Ramee SR, Collins TJ, et al. Carotid artery stenting: patient, lesion, and procedural characteristics that increase procedural complications. Catheter Cardiovasc Interv 2013. http://dx.doi.org/10.1002/ccd.24984; with permission.)

cerebral embolism related to CAS. MRI indicators of vulnerable plaque (signal intensity ratio [SIR] and plaque volume) correlate with new cerebral lesions following carotid stenting.[51] The ability to noninvasively identify subsets of patients at increased risk for cerebral embolism will be an important tool to guide treatment selection, perhaps affecting the choice of stent used or the method of embolic protection used.

PROCEDURAL FACTORS THAT INCREASE CAS RISK
Inexperienced Operator and Center

Administrative databases and clinical trial results both support the inverse relationship for complications of CAS and operator and site volume.[52] Analysis of the Sienna CAS Score[36] demonstrated a threshold with an operator with more than 100 CAS cases had better outcomes compared with an operator with fewer than 50 CAS cases. In the CAPTURE-2 postmarket study,[17] there was an inverse correlation between operator and institutional volume for CAS complications. From this dataset of several thousand patients, a threshold of 72 CAS cases was needed to achieve a complication rate of less than 3%. Not only volume, but also provider specialty may affect CAS outcomes. For the lead-in phase of CREST, there was a statistically higher complication rate noted for vascular surgeons compared with interventional cardiologists and neuroradiologists (**Fig. 4**).[53] This was attributed to a lack of focused catheter-based training among the surgeons.

Failure to Use an Embolic Protection Device

The efficacy of a variety of embolic protection devices (EPDs) to reduce the risk of cerebral emboli has been accepted relatively broadly without comparative evidence to support a clinical benefit. The Food and Drug Administration rarely accepts surrogate evidence of "safe and effective" for device approval, but did in the case of carotid EPDs, accepting the argument that prevention of embolic debris was justified by the low risk of complications associated with their use.[54] Furthermore, the Centers for Medicare and Medicaid Services has required the use of an EPD with CAS for reimbursement, without any comparative evidence to support the criteria of "reasonable and necessary."

CAS patients were randomized to a filter-type EPD or to no EPD in 2 small trials and found no difference in the rate of DWI-MRI lesions.[55,56] However, in a review of 134 published reports, including 24 studies that included data on both protected and unprotected CAS, the relative risk (RR) for stroke reduction was 0.59 (95% confidence interval [CI] 0.47–0.73) in favor of protected CAS ($P<.001$).[57] These data have been confirmed in a meta-analysis that found a lower risk for stroke or death when an EPD was used.[29] The benefit for protected CAS was evident in both symptomatic and asymptomatic patients ($P<.05$).[58]

In the SPACE trial, 25% of the CAS procedures used EPDs and 75% were unprotected. The incidence of ipsilateral stroke or ipsilateral stroke and death within 30 days was numerically lower in the unprotected group (6.2%, 26/418 patients) compared with the protected group (8.3%, 12/145 patients, $P = .40$).[59] In both of these trials, the operators were inexperienced, with some being tutored in how to perform CAS.[60] In the International Carotid Stenting Study (ICSS) trial, two-thirds (6 of 9) of operators were very inexperienced, having performed fewer than 50 CAS procedures, which may explain why the added procedural complexity with an EPD led to more complications than expected.[61]

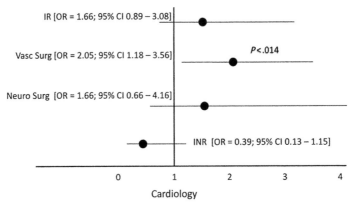

CREST Lead-In Specialty Outcomes

IR [OR = 1.66; 95% CI 0.89 – 3.08]

Vasc Surg [OR = 2.05; 95% CI 1.18 – 3.56] $P<.014$

Neuro Surg [OR = 1.66; 95% CI 0.66 – 4.16]

INR [OR = 0.39; 95% CI 0.13 – 1.15]

0   1   2   3   4

Cardiology

Fig. 4. Differences in CAS outcomes stratified by operator subspecialty in the CREST lead-in trial. (*From* White CJ. Carotid artery stent placement. JACC Cardiovasc Interv 2010;3:469; with permission.)

Despite the use of EPDs, there is evidence of periprocedural embolic events occurring. Emboli may occur before lesion crossing with catheter manipulation in the aortic arch or when placing the guide catheter or sheath into the common carotid artery. Filter EPDs may allow embolic debris smaller than the filter pores to pass through to the brain. The filter device may release plaque debris when advanced across the carotid stenosis. Finally, if the filter is not completely apposed to the wall of the carotid artery, some emboli may pass outside of the filter.

A meta-analysis of 2397 patients undergoing CAS with proximal protection demonstrated a stroke risk of less than 2%. The only independent predictors of risk were older age and diabetes mellitus. Gender, symptom status, and other baseline characteristics were not risk predictors for stroke complications with proximal protection.[62] Two smaller studies have suggested that proximal occlusion devices are superior to distal filters for reducing surrogate end points of cerebral embolism.[63,64]

Stent Design

The self-expanding stents used for CAS come in a variety of designs (open or closed cell, tapered and nontapered) and materials (nitinol or stainless steel). Performance characteristics ascribed to stent design characteristics, for example trackability and conformability, are often superior in tortuous arteries with open cell designs. The argument has also been made that smaller space between cells (free cell area) of closed-cell stents may reduce embolization. Unfortunately, there are few comparative data regarding stent designs. One randomized trial of 40 patients did not demonstrate any difference in DWI-MRI outcomes based on stent type.[65]

It has been suggested that closed-cell stents are associated with a lower risk of periprocedural complications than open cell stents, particularly in symptomatic patients.[66] In a secondary analysis of symptomatic SPACE trial patients, those treated with a closed-cell stent had a lower risk of periprocedural complications (5.6% [95% CI 3.7%–8.2%]) compared with those treated with an open-cell stent (11.0%, 95% CI 6.2%–17.8%; P = .029).[59]

Significant confounders make evaluating stent designs difficult. For example, data may be biased by operators selecting flexible, deliverable open-cell stents in tortuous carotid lesions, which are independently associated with higher complication rates. In a more rigorous analysis of a multicenter, consecutive series of 1684 CAS patients,

there was no difference between closed-cell versus open-cell (P = .77) stents.[67]

Lack of Femoral Artery Access

A major contraindication to CAS in all premarket and postmarket surveillance trials was severe peripheral arterial disease, preventing common femoral artery access. Recently, several investigators have demonstrated comparable procedural outcomes for CAS from radial artery access.[68,69] A reason to explore transradial access is that in CREST the need for transfusion was associated with a stroke.[48] Red blood cell transfusion was needed in 12.5% of the CAS patients with a periprocedural stroke complication versus only 1.6% of the CAS patients who did not have stroke (P<.0001). Transradial access for CAS would virtually eliminate access site bleeding.

Time to Procedure

Although symptomatic lesions are associated with higher periprocedural CAS complications, data regarding whether the timing ($\leq$14 days) of the intervention adds additional risk are conflicting. CAPTURE found significantly higher rates of periprocedural complications for symptomatic patients receiving CAS within 14 days of symptom onset.[6] In 2124 CAS procedures, 78.9% of the patients experiencing a complication were recently symptomatic, suggesting an association for periprocedural CAS complications and recent onset of symptoms.[36]

In contrast, a smaller multicenter European registry reported that the time from symptom onset to intervention (<14 days) made no difference for CAS outcome.[70] There was no difference in the 30-day stroke and death rates in 142 patients treated for fewer than 14 days (7%) and 178 patients treated for 14 days or more (9.6%; P = .54) from symptom onset. A meta-analysis of CAS data has confirmed the lack of risk associated early intervention after symptom onset finding no relationship between CAS risk and timing of the intervention.[29] Although this issue remains unsettled, in light of the known benefit of early CEA in symptomatic patients, it appears that CAS should emulate that strategy until proven otherwise.[71–73]

SUMMARY

CAS has been one of the most studied cardiovascular procedures of all time, with tens of thousands of patients enrolled in clinical trials. Several randomized trials have been demonstrated equipoise between CAS and CEA in both high-risk and average-risk surgery patients.

Current evidence suggests that there are identifiable patient, anatomic, and procedural characteristics that increase the incidence of carotid stenting complications. Such evidence reaffirms the importance of careful case selection when performing CAS.

REFERENCES

1. Yadav JS, Wholey MH, Kuntz RE, et al. Protected carotid-artery stenting versus endarterectomy in high-risk patients. N Engl J Med 2004;351:1493–501.

2. Gurm HS, Yadav JS, Fayad P, et al. Long-term results of carotid stenting versus endarterectomy in high-risk patients. N Engl J Med 2008;358:1572–9.

3. Hopkins LN, Myla S, Grube E, et al. Carotid artery revascularization in high surgical risk patients with the NexStent and the Filterwire EX/EZ: 1-year results in the CABERNET trial. Catheter Cardiovasc Interv 2008;71:950–60.

4. Higashida RT, Popma JJ, Apruzzese P, et al, on behalf of the MAVErIC I and II Investigators. Evaluation of the Medtronic Exponent Self-Expanding Carotid Stent System with the Medtronic Guardwire Temporary Occlusion and Aspiration System in the treatment of carotid stenosis: combined from the MAVErIC (Medtronic AVE Self-expanding CaRotid Stent System with distal protection In the treatment of Carotid stenosis) I and MAVErIC II Trials. Stroke 2010;41:e102–9.

5. White CJ, Iyer SS, Hopkins LN, et al. Carotid stenting with distal protection in high surgical risk patients: the BEACH trial 30 day results. Catheter Cardiovasc Interv 2006;67:503–12.

6. Gray WA, Yadav JS, Verta P, et al, Capture Trial Collaborators. The CAPTURE registry: Predictors of outcomes in carotid artery stenting with embolic protection for high surgical risk patients in the early post-approval setting. Catheter Cardiovasc Interv 2007;70:1025–33.

7. Safian RD, Bresnahan JF, Jaff MR, et al. Protected carotid stenting in high-risk patients with severe carotid artery stenosis. J Am Coll Cardiol 2006;47:2384–9.

8. Gray WA, Hopkins LN, Yadav S, et al. Protected carotid stenting in high-surgical-risk patients: the ARCHeR results. J Vasc Surg 2006;44:258–68.

9. Massop D, Dave R, Metzger C, et al. Stenting and angioplasty with protection in patients at high-risk for endarterectomy: SAPPHIRE Worldwide Registry first 2,001 patients. Catheter Cardiovasc Interv 2009;73:129–36.

10. Gray WA, Chaturvedi S, Verta P. Thirty-day outcomes for carotid artery stenting in 6320 patients from 2 prospective, multicenter, high-surgical-risk registries. Circ Cardiovasc Interv 2009;2:159–66.

11. Myla S, Bacharach JM, Ansel GM, et al. Carotid artery stenting in high surgical risk patients using the FiberNet embolic protection system: The EPIC trial results. Catheter Cardiovasc Interv 2010;75:817–22.

12. Ansel GM, Hopkins LN, Jaff MR, et al. Safety and effectiveness of the INVATEC MO.MA proximal cerebral protection device during carotid artery stenting: results from the ARMOUR pivotal trial. Catheter Cardiovasc Interv 2010;76:1–8.

13. Brott TG, Hobson RW 2nd, Howard G, et al. Stenting versus endarterectomy for treatment of carotid-artery stenosis. N Engl J Med 2010;363:11–23.

14. Silver FL, Mackey A, Clark WM, et al. Safety of stenting and endarterectomy by symptomatic status in the Carotid Revascularization Endarterectomy Versus Stenting Trial (CREST). Stroke 2011;42:675–80.

15. Furie KL, Kasner SE, Adams RJ, et al. Guidelines for the prevention of stroke in patients with stroke or transient ischemic attack: a guideline for healthcare professionals from the American Heart Association/American Stroke Association. Stroke 2011;42:227–76.

16. Brott TG, Halperin JL, Abbara S, et al. 2011 ASA/ACCF/AHA/AANN/AANS/ACR/ASNR/CNS/SAIP/SCAI/SIR/SNIS/SVM/SVS guideline on the management of patients with extracranial carotid and vertebral artery disease: executive summary: a report of the American College of Cardiology Foundation/American Heart Association Task Force on Practice Guidelines, and the American Stroke Association, American Association of Neuroscience Nurses, American Association of Neurological Surgeons, American College of Radiology, American Society of Neuroradiology, Congress of Neurological Surgeons, Society of Atherosclerosis Imaging and Prevention, Society for Cardiovascular Angiography and Interventions, Society of Interventional Radiology, Society of NeuroInterventional Surgery, Society for Vascular Medicine, and Society for Vascular Surgery Developed in Collaboration With the American Academy of Neurology and Society of Cardiovascular Computed Tomography. J Am Coll Cardiol 2011;57:1002–44.

17. Gray WA, Rosenfield KA, Jaff MR, et al. Influence of site and operator characteristics on carotid artery stent outcomes: analysis of the CAPTURE 2 (Carotid ACCULINK/ACCUNET Post Approval Trial to Uncover Rare Events) clinical study. JACC Cardiovasc Interv 2011;4:235–46.

18. Macdonald S, Lee R, Williams R, et al, on behalf of the Delphi Carotid Stenting Consensus Panel. Towards safer carotid artery stenting: a scoring system for anatomic suitability. Stroke 2009;40:1698–703.

19. Roubin GS, Iyer S, Halkin A, et al. Realizing the potential of carotid artery stenting: proposed paradigms for patient selection and procedural technique. Circulation 2006;113:2021–30.

20. Hofmann R, Niessner A, Kypta A, et al. Risk score for peri-interventional complications of carotid artery stenting. Stroke 2006;37:2557–61.

21. Kazmers A, Perkins AJ, Huber TS. Carotid surgery in octogenarians in Veterans Affairs medical centers. J Surg Res 1999;81:87–90.

22. Wennberg D, Lucas F, Birkmeyer J, et al. Variation in carotid endarterectomy mortality in the Medicare population. JAMA 1998;279:1278–81.

23. Roubin GS, New G, Iyer SS, et al. Immediate and late clinical outcomes of carotid artery stenting in patients with symptomatic and asymptomatic carotid artery stenosis: a 5-year prospective analysis. Circulation 2001;103:532–7.

24. Hobson RW 2nd, Howard VJ, Roubin GS, et al. Carotid artery stenting is associated with increased complications in octogenarians: 30-day stroke and death rates in the CREST lead-in phase. J Vasc Surg 2004;40:1106–11.

25. Iyer SS, White CJ, Hopkins LN, et al. Carotid artery revascularization in high-surgical-risk patients using the Carotid WALLSTENT and FilterWire EX/EZ: 1-year outcomes in the BEACH Pivotal Group. J Am Coll Cardiol 2008;51:427–34.

26. Eckstein HH, Ringleb P, Allenberg JR, et al. Results of the Stent-Protected Angioplasty versus Carotid Endarterectomy (SPACE) study to treat symptomatic stenoses at 2 years: a multinational, prospective, randomised trial. Lancet Neurol 2008;7:893–902.

27. Voeks JH, Howard G, Roubin GS, et al. Age and outcomes after carotid stenting and endarterectomy: the carotid revascularization endarterectomy versus stenting trial. Stroke 2011;42:3484–90.

28. Groschel K, Ernemann U, Schnaudigel S, et al. A risk score to predict ischemic lesions after protected carotid artery stenting. J Neurol Sci 2008; 273:112–5.

29. Touze E, Trinquart L, Chatellier G. Systematic review of the perioperative risks of stroke or death after carotid angioplasty and stenting. Stroke 2009; 40:e683–93.

30. Lam RC, Lin SC, DeRubertis B, et al. The impact of increasing age on anatomic factors affecting carotid angioplasty and stenting. J Vasc Surg 2007; 45:875–80.

31. Setacci C, de Donato G, Chisci E, et al. Is carotid artery stenting in octogenarians really dangerous? J Endovasc Ther 2006;13:302–9.

32. Bazan HA, Pradhan S, Mojibian H, et al. Increased aortic arch calcification in patients older than 75 years: implications for carotid artery stenting in elderly patients. J Vasc Surg 2007;46:841–5.

33. Bates ER, Babb JD, Casey DE Jr, et al. ACCF/SCAI/SVMB/SIR/ASITN 2007 Clinical Expert Consensus Document on carotid stenting. Vasc Med 2007;12:35–83.

34. Zahn R, Ischinger T, Hochadel M, et al. Carotid artery stenting in octogenarians: results from the ALKK Carotid Artery Stent (CAS) Registry. Eur Heart J 2007;28:370–5.

35. Velez CA, White CJ, Reilly JP, et al. Carotid artery stent placement is safe in the very elderly (> or =80 years). Catheter Cardiovasc Interv 2008; 72:303–8.

36. Setacci C, Chisci E, Setacci F, et al. Siena carotid artery stenting score: a risk modelling study for individual patients. Stroke 2010;41:1259–65.

37. Grant A, White C, Ansel G, et al. Safety and efficacy of carotid stenting in the very elderly. Catheter Cardiovasc Interv 2010;75:651–5.

38. Alvarez B, Matas M, Ribo M, et al. Transcervical carotid stenting with flow reversal is a safe technique for high-risk patients older than 70 years. J Vasc Surg 2012;55:978–84.

39. Kastrup A, Groschel K, Schulz JB, et al. Clinical predictors of transient ischemic attack, stroke, or death within 30 days of carotid angioplasty and stenting. Stroke 2005;36:787–91.

40. Faggioli GL, Ferri M, Freyrie A, et al. Aortic arch anomalies are associated with increased risk of neurological events in carotid stent procedures. Eur J Vasc Endovasc Surg 2007;33:436–41.

41. Bendszus M, Koltzenburg M, Burger R, et al. Silent embolism in diagnostic cerebral angiography and neurointerventional procedures: a prospective study. Lancet 1999;354:1594–7.

42. Faggioli G, Ferri M, Rapezzi C, et al. Atherosclerotic aortic lesions increase the risk of cerebral embolism during carotid stenting in patients with complex aortic arch anatomy. J Vasc Surg 2009; 49:80–5.

43. Faggioli G, Ferri M, Gargiulo M, et al. Measurement and impact of proximal and distal tortuosity in carotid stenting procedures. J Vasc Surg 2007;46: 1119–24.

44. Mathur A, Roubin GS, Iyer SS, et al. Predictors of stroke complicating carotid artery stenting. Circulation 1998;97:1239–45.

45. Sayeed S, Stanziale SF, Wholey MH, et al. Angiographic lesion characteristics can predict adverse outcomes after carotid artery stenting. J Vasc Surg 2008;47:81–7.

46. Krapf H, Nagele T, Kastrup A, et al. Risk factors for periprocedural complications in carotid artery stenting without filter protection: a serial diffusion-weighted MRI study. J Neurol 2006; 253:364–71.

47. Groschel K, Schnaudigel S, Ernemann U, et al. Size matters! Stent-length is associated with

thrombembolic complications after carotid artery stenting. Stroke 2008;39:e131–2 [author reply: e133].

48. Hill MD, Brooks W, Mackey A, et al. Stroke after carotid stenting and endarterectomy in the Carotid Revascularization Endarterectomy Versus Stenting Trial (CREST). Circulation 2012;126: 3054–61.

49. Tegos TJ, Sabetai MM, Nicolaides AN, et al. Correlates of embolic events detected by means of transcranial Doppler in patients with carotid atheroma. J Vasc Surg 2001;33:131–8.

50. Biasi GM, Froio A, Diethrich EB, et al. Carotid plaque echolucency increases the risk of stroke in carotid stenting: the Imaging in Carotid Angioplasty and Risk of Stroke (ICAROS) Study. Circulation 2004;110:756–62.

51. Tanemura H, Maeda M, Ichikawa N, et al. High-risk plaque for carotid artery stenting evaluated with 3-dimensional T1-weighted gradient echo sequence. Stroke 2013;44:105–10.

52. Nallamothu BK, Gurm HS, Ting HH, et al. Operator experience and carotid stenting outcomes in Medicare beneficiaries. JAMA 2011;306:1338–43.

53. Hopkins LN, Roubin GS, Chakhtoura EY, et al. The carotid revascularization endarterectomy versus stenting trial: credentialing of interventionalists and final results of lead-in phase. J Stroke Cerebrovasc Dis 2010;19:153–62.

54. Cremonesi A, Manetti R, Setacci F, et al. Protected carotid stenting: clinical advantages and complications of embolic protection devices in 442 consecutive patients. Stroke 2003;34:1936–41.

55. Macdonald S, Evans DH, Griffiths PD, et al. Filter-protected versus unprotected carotid artery stenting: a randomised trial. Cerebrovasc Dis 2010;29: 282–9.

56. Barbato JE, Dillavou E, Horowitz MB, et al. A randomized trial of carotid artery stenting with and without cerebral protection. J Vasc Surg 2008;47:760–5.

57. Kastrup A, Nagele T, Groschel K, et al. Incidence of new brain lesions after carotid stenting with and without cerebral protection. Stroke 2006;37: 2312–6.

58. Garg N, Karagiorgos N, Pisimisis GT, et al. Cerebral protection devices reduce periprocedural strokes during carotid angioplasty and stenting: a systematic review of the current literature. J Endovasc Ther 2009;16:412–27.

59. Jansen O, Fiehler J, Hartmann M, et al. Protection or nonprotection in carotid stent angioplasty: the influence of interventional techniques on outcome data from the SPACE Trial. Stroke 2009;40:841–6.

60. Roffi M, Sievert H, Gray WA, et al. Carotid artery stenting versus surgery: adequate comparisons? Lancet Neurol 2010;9:339–41.

61. Gensicke H, Zumbrunn T, Jongen LM, et al. Characteristics of ischemic brain lesions after stenting or endarterectomy for symptomatic carotid artery stenosis: results from the International Carotid Stenting Study-Magnetic Resonance Imaging Substudy. Stroke 2013;44:80–6.

62. Bersin RM, Stabile E, Ansel GM, et al. A meta-analysis of proximal occlusion device outcomes in carotid artery stenting. Catheter Cardiovasc Interv 2012;80:1072–8.

63. Montorsi P, Caputi L, Galli S, et al. Microembolization during carotid artery stenting in patients with high-risk, lipid-rich plaque a randomized trial of proximal versus distal cerebral protection. J Am Coll Cardiol 2011;58:1656–63.

64. Bijuklic K, Wandler A, Hazizi F, et al. The PROFI study (Prevention of Cerebral Embolization by Proximal Balloon Occlusion Compared to Filter Protection During Carotid Artery Stenting): a prospective randomized trial. J Am Coll Cardiol 2012;59: 1383–9.

65. Timaran CH, Rosero EB, Higuera A, et al. Randomized clinical trial of open-cell vs closed-cell stents for carotid stenting and effects of stent design on cerebral embolization. J Vasc Surg 2011;54: 1310–6.e1 [discussion: 1316].

66. Bosiers M, de Donato G, Deloose K, et al. Does free cell area influence the outcome in carotid artery stenting? Eur J Vasc Endovasc Surg 2007; 33:135–41 [discussion: 142–33].

67. Schillinger M, Gschwendtner M, Reimers B, et al. Does carotid stent cell design matter? Stroke 2008;39:905–9.

68. Patel T, Shah S, Malhotra H, et al. Transradial approach for stenting of vertebrobasilar stenosis: a feasibility study. Catheter Cardiovasc Interv 2009;74:925–31.

69. Fang HY, Chung SY, Sun CK, et al. Transradial and transbrachial arterial approach for simultaneous carotid angiographic examination and stenting using catheter looping and retrograde engagement technique. Ann Vasc Surg 2010;24:670–9.

70. Groschel K, Knauth M, Ernemann U, et al. Early treatment after a symptomatic event is not associated with an increased risk of stroke in patients undergoing carotid stenting. Eur J Neurol 2008;15:2–5.

71. Sacco RL, Adams R, Albers G, et al. Guidelines for prevention of stroke in patients with ischemic stroke or transient ischemic attack: a statement for healthcare professionals from the American Heart Association/American Stroke Association Council on Stroke: Co-sponsored by the Council on Cardiovascular Radiology and Intervention: The American Academy of Neurology affirms the value of this guideline. Stroke 2006;37:577–617.

72. White CJ, Ramee SR, Collins TJ, et al. Carotid artery stenting: Patient, lesion, and procedural

characteristics that increase procedural complications. Catheter Cardiovasc Interv 2013. http://dx.doi.org/10.1002/ccd.24984.

73. White CJ. Carotid artery stent placement. JACC Cardiovasc Interv 2010;3:467–74.

74. White CJ, for the Beach Investigators. BEACH Trial: 30 day outcomes of carotid wallstent and filterwire EX/EZ distal protection system placement for treatment of high surgical risk patients. J Am Coll Cardiol 2005;45:28A.

Carotid Artery Stenting Versus Carotid Endarterectomy for Treatment of Asymptomatic Carotid Disease

R. Kevin Rogers, MD, MSc[a], Sanjay Gandhi, MD[b],
Kenneth Rosenfield, MD, MHCDS[c],*

KEYWORDS

- Asymptomatic carotid artery stenosis • Stroke • Carotid artery stent • Carotid endarterectomy

KEY POINTS

- Patients with asymptomatic carotid artery stenosis are at increased risk for stroke, which carries significant morbidity and mortality.
- Carotid artery revascularization with carotid endarterectomy has been shown in randomized trials that enrolled from 1983 to 2003 to reduce the risk for stroke in asymptomatic patients compared with medical therapy alone.
- There are limited level I data comparing carotid artery stent with carotid endarterectomy in asymptomatic patients with carotid artery stenosis.
- Based on current limited randomized and observational data, carotid artery stenting is noninferior to endarterectomy in clinical outcomes in patients at standard and high surgical risk with asymptomatic carotid artery stenosis.
- Operator volume and experience with patient selection play an important role in outcomes for carotid stenting; similarly, emerging techniques such as proximal embolic protection may also reduce adverse periprocedural events.
- Decision of revascularization strategy for a patient should be individualized based on the patient's clinical and anatomic lesion characteristics, the local operator experience, and patient preference.

INTRODUCTION

Revascularization of stenoses caused by atherosclerotic plaque that is not causing symptoms is generally not indicated for most vascular territories. However, disease of the carotid artery bifurcation is one of the few exceptions in which revascularization may be appropriate, even in the absence of symptoms. Two decades ago, landmark trials comparing carotid endarterectomy (CEA) with medical therapy showed a clear benefit of stroke reduction in patients treated with surgery.[1–3] In 2000, carotid artery stenting (CAS) emerged as an available technical alternative to CEA for carotid revascularization. At present, 87% of carotid

Disclosures: R.K. Rogers is a site Principle Investigator for the SAPPHIRE registry. S. Gandhi has no disclosures. K. Rosenfield is the National Co-PI for the ACT I study. He also receives compensation as member of Scientific Advisory Board for Abbott Vascular, the Medicines Company, and Vortex-Angiodynamics. He receives delayed royalty payments from Angioguard. His insitution receives research funding from Cordis, Abbott Vascular, Bard-Lutonix, Silk Road, and Medtronic.
[a] Section of Vascular Medicine and Intervention, Division of Cardiology, University of Colorado, 12401 E 17th Avenue, Aurora, CO 80045, USA; [b] Heart and Vascular Center, MetroHealth Campus, Case Western Reserve University, 2500 MetroHealth Drive, Cleveland, OH 44122, USA; [c] Section of Vascular Medicine and Intervention, Division of Cardiology, Massachusetts General Hospital, 55 Fruit Street, Boston, MA 02114, USA
* Corresponding author.
E-mail address: krosenfield@fastmail.us

Intervent Cardiol Clin 3 (2014) 63–72
http://dx.doi.org/10.1016/j.iccl.2013.09.009

revascularization procedures are performed for asymptomatic disease.[4]

Trials of CEA versus CAS have been the subject of much criticism and debate and, in particular, have highlighted the importance of case selection and operator experience for CAS. Most of these trials(CEA versus medical therapy and CEA versus CAS) have included patients who are of standard surgical risk, limiting the ability to generalize the evidence base to high-surgical-risk patients.[1–3,5–8] The ability to generalize trials comparing CEA and CAS is further limited by pooling both symptomatic and asymptomatic patients, subgroups with clearly different event rates.[5–9] This article summarizes the evidence base and related controversies regarding CEA versus CAS for the revascularization of carotid disease in asymptomatic patients.

INDICATIONS FOR REVASCULARIZATION OF ASYMPTOMATIC CAROTID STENOSIS

The indications for revascularization of asymptomatic carotid disease are based largely on the seminal trials of CEA versus medical therapy. These trials are summarized in **Table 1**. Each trial showed a substantial benefit of carotid endarterectomy compared with medical therapy for patients with greater than 60% to 70% asymptomatic carotid stenosis.[1–3] Several observations merit mention: (1) these trials enrolled primarily in the 1980s to 1990s and, as such, contemporary medical therapy was not available to many study participants. (2) Patients with medical comorbidities and/or anatomic high-risk features (eg, prior CEA or inaccessible lesion) were excluded. Additional selection biases may also have affected outcomes. (3) Life expectancy for participants was at least ~3 years, so that operative risks could be offset by longevity for overall benefit in stroke risk reduction. Although some argue that medical therapy has caught up to CEA, multisocietal guidelines indicate that CEA is appropriate for patients with low surgical risk and asymptomatic carotid stenoses greater than 70%.[10]

RANDOMIZED TRIAL EVIDENCE COMPARING CEA AND CAS IN STANDARD-SURGICAL-RISK PATIENTS

There are 4 large randomized trials comparing CAS with embolic protection with CEA in standard-surgical-risk patients and, of these,[5–8] only 1 trial has included asymptomatic patients.[8] In the Carotid Revascularization Endarterectomy versus Stenting (CREST) trial, standard-surgical-risk patients were randomized to CEA or CAS with distal embolic protection. Of 2502 randomized patients,

47% were asymptomatic. The primary outcome was not powered to enable comparison between therapies by symptomatic status. At 30 days, compared with the CEA group, there were trends for less myocardial infarction (MI) but more strokes in the CAS group; however, these differences were not statistically significant (**Table 2**). There were no deaths at 30 days for asymptomatic patients in either the CAS or CEA groups.

RANDOMIZED TRIAL EVIDENCE COMPARING CEA AND CAS IN HIGH-SURGICAL-RISK PATIENTS

Several clinical and anatomic features are generally accepted as conferring high-risk status to patients for CEA (**Box 1**). These variables have largely served as exclusion criteria in most carotid revascularization trials. Only 1 carotid revascularization trial has included solely high-surgical-risk patients.[9]

In the Stenting and Angioplasty with Protection in Patients at High Risk for Endarterectomy (SAPPHIRE) trial, 334 patients at high risk for CEA were randomized to CAS with distal embolic protection or CEA (**Table 3**). Approximately 70% of the study population was asymptomatic, but the trial was not powered to be analyzed by symptomatic status. The primary outcome was a composite of death, stroke, or MI within 30 days after revascularization and death or ipsilateral stroke between day 31 and 1 year. At 30 days, death, MI, and stroke occurred in 5.4% of asymptomatic patients having CAS and in 10.2% of the asymptomatic patients having CEA ($P = .20$). At 1 year in the asymptomatic subgroup, the primary outcome occurred in 9.9% of patients in the CAS arm and in 21.5% of patients in the CEA arm ($P = .02$ for comparison, $P = .55$ for test for interaction).[9] At 3 years, strokes occurred in 10.3% of the asymptomatic patients having CAS and in 9.2% of asymptomatic participants with CEA.[11] Overall, based on this sample size and design, this finding should be interpreted as indicating that CAS is not inferior to CEA in asymptomatic patients at high risk for endarterectomy.

LIMITATIONS OF RANDOMIZED CONTROLLED TRIAL EVIDENCE COMPARING CEA WITH CAS IN ASYMPTOMATIC PATIENTS

A primary limitation of randomized trial evidence comparing CEA with CAS in asymptomatic patients is the paucity of level I data. Across the 4 trials of carotid stenting versus CEA in standard-surgical-risk patients, only 1175 of 5940 (20%) patients were asymptomatic.[5–8] In the only trial of high-surgical-risk patients, 233 patients were asymptomatic.[9]

Table 1
Trials of CEA versus medical therapy in asymptomatic patients

Trial	N	Years Enrolled	Medical Therapy	Inclusion	Pertinent Exclusion	Mean Follow-up (y)	Results
ACST[1]	3120	1993–2003	At last year of follow-up, 90% were on antiplatelet, 80% on antihypertensive, and 70% on lipid-lowering medications	60% asymptomatic carotid stenosis by duplex	Prior ipsilateral CEA Poor surgical risk cardioembolic source Major life-threatening condition	3.4	6.4% vs 11.8% for all strokes and perioperative deaths
VA study[2]	445	1983–1991	84% aspirin	50% asymptomatic carotid stenosis by angiography	Prior stroke Prior ipsilateral CEA Life expectancy <5 y High surgical risk caused by medical illness Anatomically inaccessible lesion	4	14.7% vs 24.5% all strokes and perioperative deaths
ACAS[3]	1662	1987–1993	All received aspirin 325 mg daily	Asymptomatic 60% stenosis by angiography or duplex	Symptomatic lesion Disorder that could seriously complicate surgery Life expectancy <5 y	2.7	5.1% vs 11.0% for all strokes and perioperative deaths

Abbreviations: ACAS, Asymptomatic Carotid Atherosclerosis Study; ACST, Asymptomatic Carotid Surgery Trial; VA study, Veteran Affairs Cooperative Study Group.

Table 2
Results from CREST in asymptomatic patients

Stroke (%)			MI (%)			Death (%)		
CAS	CEA	P Value	CAS	CEA	P Value	CAS	CEA	P Value
2.5	1.4	.15	1.2	2.2	.2	0	0	NA

Data from Brott TG, Hobson RW 2nd, Howard G, et al. Stenting versus endarterectomy for treatment of carotid artery stenosis. N Engl J Med 2010;363(1):11–23.

This lack of data hinders the validity of any conclusions regarding a dominant revascularization strategy for asymptomatic carotid disease. Furthermore, to the extent that the asymptomatic subgroups in these trials were not specifically randomized, results in the asymptomatic patients may be subject to unmeasured confounding.

A major limitation of randomized controlled trial evidence comparing CEA with CAS in asymptomatic patients is the poor ability to generalize. Randomized trials of CEA versus CAS to date have pooled symptomatic and asymptomatic patients. Extrapolating results from the trials as a whole to asymptomatic patients is not possible. The distinction between symptomatic and asymptomatic

Box 1
High-risk features for carotid endarterectomy

Clinical

Age greater than 75 to 80 years

Severe heart failure (class III/IV)

Left ventricular ejection fraction less than 30% to 35%

Acute coronary syndrome

Severe pulmonary disease[a]

Contralateral cranial nerve injury

End-stage renal disease

Anatomic

Previous CEA with recurrent stenosis

Surgically inaccessible lesion

Lesion at or above C2

Below the clavicle

Contralateral carotid occlusion

History of radiation therapy to neck

Prior radical neck surgery

Severe tandem lesions

Spinal immobility of the neck

[a] Defined as need for home oxygen, Po_2 less than 60 mm Hg on room air, forced expiratory volume in 1 second less than 30% to 50% of predicted.

patients is important, because these two subgroups have distinct natural histories. For example, in the medical therapy group in the North American Symptomatic Carotid Endarterectomy Trial, the stroke and death rate for patients with symptomatic 70% to 99% carotid stenoses was 32%, and the stroke rate for patients with symptomatic 50% to 69% stenoses was 22% at 5 years.[12] In contrast, in the medical therapy group of the Asymptomatic Carotid Surgery Trial (ACST), freedom from stroke and perioperative death up to 5 years was 11.8%.[1] Thus, any generalization of results of carotid stenting versus CEA trials to asymptomatic patients should be done with caution.

Asymptomatic Carotid Trial I is a randomized controlled trial that will provide additional level I evidence comparing CEA with CAS in asymptomatic standard-surgical-risk patients. This trial was recently completed (terminated early) and results are expected to be reported early in 2014.

OBSERVATIONAL EVIDENCE OF CAS IN ASYMPTOMATIC PATIENTS

Given the paucity of data from randomized trials on CAS in asymptomatic patients, results from observational studies are important to provide additional insight into outcomes and techniques for CAS in this patient population. The most reliable studies are Investigational Device Exemption (IDE) or Postmarket Approval (PMA) registries

Table 3
Death, MI, and stroke rates in SAPPHIRE

Follow-up Period	CAS (%), n = 117	CEA (%), n = 120	P Value
30 d	5.4	10.2	.20
1 y[a]	9.9	21.5	.02[b]
3 y	21.4	29.2	NS

[a] Outcome reported was for composite of death, stroke, or MI within 30 days after revascularization and death or ipsilateral stroke between day 31 and 1 year.
[b] $P = .55$ for test for interaction.
Data from Yadav JS, Wholey MH, Kuntz RE, et al. Protected carotid-artery stenting versus endarterectomy in high-risk patients. N Engl J Med 2004;351(15):1493–501.

of patients at high risk for CEA with either symptomatic stenoses greater than 50% or asymptomatic lesions greater than 70% to 80%. Approximately 75% of patients in these studies were asymptomatic.[13–18]

Two of the largest and most recent observational studies of CAS were the EXACT (Emboshield and Xact Post Approval Carotid Stent Trial, n = 2145) and CAPTURE 2 (Carotid RX ACCULINK/RX ACCUNET Post-Approval Trial to Uncover Unanticipated or Rare Events, n = 5297) studies.[13] In both, there was independent adjudication of neurologic outcomes. In EXACT, 90.1% of patients were asymptomatic. At 30 days, the rate of death was 0.9% and the rate of all strokes was 3.6%. Of the first 3500 patients enrolled in CAPTURE 2, 3018 (86%) were asymptomatic. In these asymptomatic, high-risk patients, the 30-day stroke rate was 4.1%.

CONTROVERSIES IN 2013

The primary controversies regarding carotid revascularization in asymptomatic patients are whether revascularization, either by CEA or CAS, has a role in this era of improved contemporary medical therapy, whether carotid stenting is equivalent to CEA and should be offered to asymptomatic patients, and whether intervention is of benefit rather than medical therapy alone in high-surgical-risk patients who have either anatomic or comorbid conditions that confer a higher risk of revascularization. These controversies are fueled by the potential impact on decisions for reimbursement by the Centers for Medicare and Medicaid Services (CMS), and concerns that inappropriate procedures might be undertaken without supportive data or oversight.

CMS Reimbursement

In 2005, 1 year after the US Food and Drug Administration (FDA) approved the first carotid stent, CMS issued a national coverage determination (NCD) for reimbursement for carotid stenting.[19] That NCD persists currently and provides coverage for CAS using FDA-approved carotid platforms in CMS-certified institutions for (1) patients with symptomatic carotid stenoses greater than 50% at high risk for CEA or (2) patients with symptomatic carotid stenoses greater than 50% or asymptomatic carotid stenoses greater than 80% at high risk for CEA if enrolled in an IDE or PMA study.[20] The result of the NCD has been restriction of carotid stenting to certain patients at particular institutions. For example, in 2007, among United States hospitals equipped to provide invasive cardiovascular procedures, only

59% offered carotid stenting. In contrast, 96% of such hospitals offered carotid endarterectomy, 90% offered coronary PCI with drug-eluting stents, 85% offered implantable cardiac defibrillators, and 75% offered coronary artery bypass grafting.[19] Also, the NCD restricts technology for carotid stenting. For example, because there are no ongoing registries for flow stasis or reversal devices, these embolic protection devices are not an option for patients with carotid disease unless symptomatic with greater than 70% stenosis and high risk for CEA (~7% of carotid revascularization procedures). The IDE and PMA registry restrictions prohibit tailoring the most appropriate technology for a specific patient when performing CAS. Furthermore, the number of IDE trials has been limited and, as of this writing, only a single postmarket surveillance study remains active; it allows use of a single, first-generation stent and embolic protection device.

Natural History of Asymptomatic Carotid Disease with Optimal Contemporary Medical Therapy

The natural history of asymptomatic, severe carotid disease in the setting of contemporary medical therapy is unknown. As mentioned earlier, the annual total stroke rate (total number strokes/average follow-up in years) in the control arm of CEA versus medical therapy trials was 3% to 4%.[1–3] These trials enrolled from 1983 to 2003. During that time frame, the FDA approved the first 3-hydroxy-3-methyl-glutaryl (HMG) coreductase inhibitor (lovastatin, 1987), and multiple other medications in this class, as well as powerful new antihypertensive agents, have become available.[21] These advances in medical therapy are occurring in the setting of reduced smoking prevalence and recognition of the effectiveness of antiplatelet therapy. As such, it is expected that the stroke rates for patients with asymptomatic carotid disease on contemporary medical therapy is improved compared with the control arms in the CEA versus medical therapy trials.

However, is the natural history now sufficiently favorable such that revascularization is no longer warranted? That is, is the stroke rate for severe asymptomatic disease less than that seen in the CEA arms of the CEA versus medical therapy trials? A single-author systematic review and meta-analysis attempted to address this important issue.[22] In this analysis, data from 11 studies were pooled to ascertain annual stroke rates for asymptomatic patients with carotid stenoses greater than 50%. Logistic regression was used to estimate the contemporary yearly stroke rate.

This estimated yearly stroke rate exceeded the 1.1% annual rate observed in the largest, most contemporary CEA versus medical therapy trial, ACST. The difference between medical therapy and CEA in this comparison would likely be more pronounced had the meta-analysis included only patients with stenoses greater than 70%, the threshold at which most multisocietal guidelines recommend revascularization for asymptomatic patients.[10] Nonetheless, the ideal future trial of carotid revascularization in asymptomatic patients would include a comparison arm of optimal contemporary medical therapy.

Impact of Proximal Embolic Protection on CAS Outcomes

It is generally agreed that CAS is safer with embolic protection than without it. Although there is no randomized evidence for the use of distal embolic protection during CAS, a meta-analysis of 4747 patients undergoing CAS showed a strong association between filter use and decreased stroke rates (relative risk, 0.59; 95% confidence interval, 0.47–0.73).[23] More recently, low periprocedural strokes rates were seen with the use of proximal embolic protection devices.[24–28]

The initial concept of a proximal occlusion device with flow reversal during CAS was shown to be safe by Parodi and colleagues.[29] Two commercially available proximal occlusion devices have included a flow reversal system and a flow stasis system, although manufacture of the flow reversal system is currently suspended. The general premise is that, in the internal carotid being treated, flow is arrested or reversed, such that embolic debris does not travel distally to the brain. Cerebral perfusion is maintained by the circle of Willis. One main advantage of this approach is neuroprotection during the initial guidewire and device traversal of the lesion. In contrast, for distal embolic protection devices, there is no cerebral protection in place while advancing a guidewire or filter device across a stenosis. Proximal embolic protection devices are also useful for cases in which tortuosity or disease distal to the carotid bifurcation lesion precludes the delivery of a filter device.

Data with proximal embolic protection devices are more limited than for distal embolic protection devices, but are emerging (**Table 4**). A meta-analysis of 4 studies (N = 2397) was published in 2012 and included standard-surgical-risk and high-surgical-risk patients as well as symptomatic and asymptomatic patients (69% asymptomatic).[24] There was independent neurologic assessment in each study. The pooled 30-day stroke rate for all patients was 1.7%. Device intolerance caused by global cerebral ischemia during flow stasis/reversal was only 0.63%. A small randomized trial examining the incidence of magnetic resonance imaging–diffusion-weighted imaging defects has also shown that, although a significant effect on clinical outcome has yet to be shown, there is less distal embolization with proximal than with distal embolic protection devices.[30] These results suggest that proximal embolic protection devices provide excellent neuroprotection during CAS, and may expand the safety margin as well as the pool of patients eligible for CAS.

Influence of Operator Volume

Higher institutional and operator volumes of carotid revascularization procedures are associated with improved outcomes for both CEA and CAS.[31,32] For example, in CAPTURE 2, a prospective, multicenter, observational study of carotid stenting in high-risk patients, operator outcomes were assessed in asymptomatic patients less than 80 years old. Thirty-day stroke and death

Table 4
Studies of CAS with proximal embolic protection devices

Study	Device	Number of Patients	Asymptomatic (%)	30-d Death/Stroke (%)
Meta-analysis[24]	Flow reversal and stasis	2397	69.3	2.25[a]
Single center registry[25]	Flow stasis	1300	72.2	1.4
ARMOUR[26]	Flow stasis	262	84.9	2.3[a]
Nikas et al,[27]	Flow reversal	122	72	1.6
EMPiRE[28]	Flow reversal	245	68	2.9
PRIAMUS[38]	Flow stasis	416	36.5	4.6

Abbreviations: ARMOUR, Proximal Protection with the MO.MA Device During Carotid Stenting; EMPiRE, The Embolic Protection with Reverse Flow Clinical Study; PRIAMUS, Proximal Flow Blockage Cerebral Protection During Carotid Stenting.
  [a] Death/MI/stroke.

rates decreased as operator caseload increased. Logistic regression predicted that 72 cases were the threshold for operators in this study to have death and stroke rates less than 3%. This operator volume is significantly higher than that reported in all CEA versus CAS trials, except for SAPPHIRE (**Table 5**).[5–9] It is clear that inexperienced operators should not perform carotid stenting. Ensuring adequate operator experience for quality care in the current era of restricted availability of carotid stenting is a major challenge for this treatment modality. An appropriate training pathway needs to be developed, both for initial certification and for recertification.

Revascularization of Asymptomatic Disease in the Elderly

Several aspects of carotid revascularization for asymptomatic disease in the elderly are controversial. First, offering carotid revascularization to octogenarians can be unattractive because of concerns about sufficient life expectancy to offset procedural risk. Second, there have been mixed signals in the evidence regarding the overall benefit of carotid revascularization, including by CEA, for the elderly. ACST was the only trial of CEA versus medical therapy to include patients more than 75 years old.[1] There was a treatment effect for less benefit in this subgroup compared with younger patients. Although there was a trend for overall benefit in the CEA group in patients

Table 5 Operator requirements for the clinical trials	
Trial	**Operator CAS Experience**
CAVATAS[39]	Training in PTA but not necessarily in carotid artery
EVA 3S[6]	5 CAS procedures
SPACE[5]	25 angioplasty, any bed
ICSS[7]	10 carotid procedures
CREST[8]	Median 30 CAS procedures to be considered for trial. Lead-in phase with mean 9 CAS cases
SAPPHIRE[9]	64 median CAS
CAPTURE 2[32]	Optimal threshold 72 CAS to achieve <3% stroke/death

Abbreviations: CAPTURE 2, Carotid ACCULINK/ACCUNET Post Approval Trial to Uncover Rare Events; CAVATAS, Carotid and Vertebral Artery Transluminal Angioplasty Study; EVA 3S, Endarterectomy Versus Angioplasty in Patients with Symptomatic Severe Carotid Stenosis; ICSS, International Carotid Stenting Study; PTA, percutaneous transluminal angioplasty; SPACE, Stent-Protected Angioplasty versus Carotid Endarterectomy.

more than 75 years old, it did not reach statistical significance. There was a stronger signal for increased periprocedural stroke rates for elderly patients receiving CAS versus CEA in CREST.[8] Of the 2502 patients in CREST, 686 (27%) were more than 75 years old, and 43% of these patients were asymptomatic. It is important to recognize that randomization in CREST was not stratified by age; nonetheless, there were no obvious or statistically significant differences between the patients having CEA and CAS more than 75 years old. The periprocedural stroke and ipsilateral postprocedure strokes rates for patients more than 75 years old in this trial were 6.9% ± 1.4% for the CAS group and 3.1% ± 0.9% for the CEA group ($P = .035$). The primary outcome in this subgroup was 9.0% ± 1.6% for the CAS arm versus 5.9% ± 1.3% for the CEA arm ($P = .16$). Symptomatic status did not statistically alter this treatment effect.[33]

In an observational study published from 4 high-volume centers in the United States, adverse outcomes for elderly patients undergoing CAS were low.[34] In this study, data were provided on 389 patients 80 years of age or older who underwent carotid stenting. Of the study population, 270 patients (69%) were asymptomatic. Most procedures were done in a registry or trial, and independent neurologic assessment was routine. The 30-day stroke and death rate was only 1.5%. Similar results have been published from high-volume centers in Europe in elderly populations.[35]

The mixed results of carotid stenting in elderly patients may reflect not only differences in operator volume but also the experience to select appropriate patients for CAS and the freedom to do so in a real-world setting as opposed to a trial. Factors associated with advanced age increase the risk of carotid revascularization. For CAS, these variables are predominantly anatomic and likely include increased tortuosity of the aorta and great vessels, increased calcification, increased burden of atherosclerosis, and reduced cerebrovascular reserve.[34] For CEA, pertinent issues likely include comorbidities, complications related to anesthesia, frailty, and cardiovascular/cerebrovascular reserve. These and related risk factors, as well as age, should be considered when managing patients with asymptomatic carotid disease.

Importance of Periprocedural Stroke versus MI

The inclusion of MI as an outcome in CREST and SAPPHIRE has sparked much controversy.[8,9] The relative importance of these two end points have been subjectively debated but also objectively studied with quality-of-life measures and impact on mortality.

Health-related quality of life (HRQOL) was assessed in all CREST participants at baseline, 2 weeks following revascularization, 1 month, and 1 year. Overall, HRQOL favored CAS at 2 weeks but there was no difference in HRQOL between CAS and CEA at 1 year. In particular, MI was not associated with poorer HRQOL, but periprocedural stroke did predict poorer HRQOL at 1 year.[36]

Another analysis from CREST evaluated the impact of periprocedural MI on mortality.[37] MI in CREST was defined as increased biomarkers and either chest pain or electrocardiographic evidence of ischemia. Compared with patients without periprocedural MI, patients with MI associated with either CEA or CAS (n = 42) had a hazard ratio of 3.40 (1.67–6.92) for death over 4 years. This association remained significant after adjustment for confounding.

Neither periprocedural MI or stroke is desirable. These outcomes should be considered when selecting a treatment strategy for the individual patient.

DECIDING THERAPY FOR THE INDIVIDUAL PATIENT

Managing asymptomatic, severe carotid disease can be challenging for providers in light of sparse data, biases, and conflicting opinions and literature interpretation. Correctly informing patients of their options can be difficult for the same reasons.

The first issue is whether revascularization should be offered to an asymptomatic patient with a severe carotid stenosis. It is reasonable that the threshold for revascularization should increase as the natural history for stroke improves because of advances in medical therapy. As such, perhaps medical therapy is most appropriate for a patient with life expectancy of only 3 years and carotid stenosis no more than 70% in severity, particularly if there are risk factors for revascularization. As an alternative, a patient with a life expectancy of much more than 5 years and an asymptomatic stenosis of greater than 90% would likely opt for revascularization unless there were prohibitive associated risks.

High-risk features for CEA have been well described but are less well known for CAS, particularly in asymptomatic patients. It is generally accepted that more complicated aortic arch types, increased tortuosity, heavy calcification, and higher burden of atherosclerosis (for all of which, age is a surrogate) confer additional risk for CAS. The presence of these CAS risk factors may lead to pursuing CEA, as would lack of institutional and operator experience in CAS. In contrast, CAS should be considered for patients with risk factors for CEA (see **Box 1**), which would be supported by the results from SAPPHIRE.[9] Experienced operators and the use of proximal embolic protection devices are associated with excellent outcomes from carotid stenting; access to centers with this expertise would make CAS a more attractive alternative.[24] In addition, patient preference and shared decision making should have a large role and be based on accurate information of MI, stroke, and cranial palsy risks; other procedural characteristics, such as length of stay and recovery times; and long-term outcomes and durability.

SUMMARY

Carotid endarterectomy, CAS, and optimal medical therapy should be thought of as complementary, rather than competing, treatment options for patients with severe, asymptomatic carotid disease. The management for asymptomatic carotid disease should involve an educated assessment of individual patient risk factors for revascularization, informed patient preferences, particular institutional strengths, and certain operators' skill sets. However, nihilistic, emotional, and unilateral stances favoring a single treatment modality for this disease are prevalent. Moving beyond this obstacle, forming multidisciplinary approaches to caring for patients with carotid disease and lifting the restrictions on reimbursement for carotid stenting (which limit patient choice and reduce both operator experience and further technological improvement for CAS devices) would improve the available care for patients with asymptomatic carotid disease. Furthermore, thoughtful evaluation, with level I randomized trials examining outcomes of optimal medical therapy alone versus medical therapy with associated revascularization, are required to address the question of which patients will benefit from revascularization in the current era. For patients in whom revascularization is deemed appropriate, it is likely that a portion will be better served with CEA, and another group with CAS. For the remaining patients, equipoise will exist between CEA and CAS, and selection of therapy must be individualized based on the preferences of an informed patient who is sharing in the decision.

REFERENCES

1. Halliday A, Mansfield A, Marro J, et al. Prevention of disabling and fatal strokes by successful carotid endarterectomy in patients without recent neurological

symptoms: randomised controlled trial. Lancet 2004; 363(9420):1491–502.

2. Hobson RW 2nd, Weiss DG, Fields WS, et al. Efficacy of carotid endarterectomy for asymptomatic carotid stenosis. The Veterans Affairs Cooperative Study Group. N Engl J Med 1993; 328(4):221–7.

3. Endarterectomy for asymptomatic carotid artery stenosis. Executive Committee for the Asymptomatic Carotid Atherosclerosis Study. JAMA 1995;273(18): 1421–8.

4. Naylor AR. What is the current status of angioplasty vs endarterectomy in patients with asymptomatic carotid artery disease? J Cardiovasc Surg (Torino) 2007;48(2):161–80.

5. Ringleb PA, Allenberg J, Bruckmann H, et al. 30 day results from the SPACE trial of stent-protected angioplasty versus carotid endarterectomy in symptomatic patients: a randomised non-inferiority trial. Lancet 2006;368(9543):1239–47.

6. Mas JL, Chatellier G, Beyssen B, et al. Endarterectomy versus stenting in patients with symptomatic severe carotid stenosis. N Engl J Med 2006; 355(16):1660–71.

7. International Carotid Stenting Study, Ederle J, Dobson J, Featherstone RL, et al. Carotid artery stenting compared with endarterectomy in patients with symptomatic carotid stenosis (International Carotid Stenting Study): an interim analysis of a randomised controlled trial. Lancet 2010; 375(9719):985–97.

8. Brott TG, Hobson RW 2nd, Howard G, et al. Stenting versus endarterectomy for treatment of carotid-artery stenosis. N Engl J Med 2010;363(1):11–23.

9. Yadav JS, Wholey MH, Kuntz RE, et al. Protected carotid-artery stenting versus endarterectomy in high-risk patients. N Engl J Med 2004;351(15): 1493–501.

10. American College of Cardiology Foundation/American Heart Association Task F, American Stroke A, American Association of Neuroscience N, American Association of Neurological S, American College of R, American Society of N, Brott TG, Halperin JL, Abbara S, et al. 2011 ASA/ACCF/AHA/AANN/AANS/ACR/ASNR/CNS/SAIP/SCAI/SIR/SNIS/SVM/SVS guideline on the management of patients with extracranial carotid and vertebral artery disease: executive summary. J Neurointerv Surg 2011;3(2):100–30.

11. Gurm HS, Yadav JS, Fayad P, et al. Long-term results of carotid stenting versus endarterectomy in high-risk patients. N Engl J Med 2008;358(15): 1572–9.

12. Barnett HJ, Taylor DW, Eliasziw M, et al. Benefit of carotid endarterectomy in patients with symptomatic moderate or severe stenosis. North American Symptomatic Carotid Endarterectomy Trial Collaborators. N Engl J Med 1998;339(20):1415–25.

13. Gray WA, Chaturvedi S, Verta P. Thirty-day outcomes for carotid artery stenting in 6320 patients from 2 prospective, multicenter, high-surgical-risk registries. Circ Cardiovasc Interv 2009;2(3):159–66.

14. Gray WA, Hopkins LN, Yadav S, et al. Protected carotid stenting in high-surgical-risk patients: the ARCHeR results. J Vasc Surg 2006;44(2):258–68.

15. Higashida RT, Popma JJ, Apruzzese P, et al. Evaluation of the Medtronic exponent self-expanding carotid stent system with the Medtronic Guardwire temporary occlusion and aspiration system in the treatment of carotid stenosis: combined from the MAVErIC (Medtronic AVE Self-expanding CaRotid Stent System with distal protection In the treatment of Carotid stenosis) I and MAVErIC II trials. Stroke 2010;41(2):e102–9.

16. Hopkins LN, Myla S, Grube E, et al. Carotid artery revascularization in high surgical risk patients with the NexStent and the Filterwire EX/EZ: 1-year results in the CABERNET trial. Catheter Cardiovasc Interv 2008;71(7):950–60.

17. Safian RD, Bresnahan JF, Jaff MR, et al. Protected carotid stenting in high-risk patients with severe carotid artery stenosis. J Am Coll Cardiol 2006;47(12): 2384–9.

18. White CJ, Iyer SS, Hopkins LN, et al. Carotid stenting with distal protection in high surgical risk patients: the BEACH trial 30 day results. Catheter Cardiovasc Interv 2006;67(4):503–12.

19. Groeneveld PW, Epstein AJ, Yang F. Medicare's policy on carotid stents limited use to hospitals meeting quality guidelines yet did not hurt disadvantaged. Health Aff (Millwood) 2010;30(2):312–21.

20. Safian RD. Carotid artery stenting: payment, politics, and equipose. J Am Coll Cardiol 2012; 59(15):1390–1.

21. Endo A. The discovery and development of HMG-CoA reductase inhibitors. J Lipid Res 1992;33(11): 1569–82.

22. Abbott AL. Medical (nonsurgical) intervention alone is now best for prevention of stroke associated with asymptomatic severe carotid stenosis: results of a systematic review and analysis. Stroke 2009; 40(10):e573–83.

23. Garg N, Karagiorgos N, Pisimisis GT, et al. Cerebral protection devices reduce periprocedural strokes during carotid angioplasty and stenting: a systematic review of the current literature. J Endovasc Ther 2009;16(4):412–27.

24. Bersin RM, Stabile E, Ansel GM, et al. A meta-analysis of proximal occlusion device outcomes in carotid artery stenting. Catheter Cardiovasc Interv 2012;80(7):1072–8.

25. Stabile E, Salemme L, Sorropago G, et al. Proximal endovascular occlusion for carotid artery stenting: results from a prospective registry of 1,300 patients. J Am Coll Cardiol 2010;55(16):1661–7.

26. Ansel GM, Hopkins LN, Jaff MR, et al. Safety and effectiveness of the INVATEC MO.MA proximal cerebral protection device during carotid artery stenting: results from the ARMOUR pivotal trial. Catheter Cardiovasc Interv 2010;76(1):1–8.

27. Nikas D, Reith W, Schmidt A, et al. Prospective, multicenter European study of the GORE flow reversal system for providing neuroprotection during carotid artery stenting. Catheter Cardiovasc Interv 2012;80(7):1060–8.

28. Clair DG, Hopkins LN, Mehta M, et al. Neuroprotection during carotid artery stenting using the GORE flow reversal system: 30-day outcomes in the EMPiRE Clinical Study. Catheter Cardiovasc Interv 2011;77(3):420–9.

29. Parodi JC, La Mura R, Ferreira LM, et al. Initial evaluation of carotid angioplasty and stenting with three different cerebral protection devices. J Vasc Surg 2000;32(6):1127–36.

30. Bijuklic K, Wandler A, Hazizi F, et al. The PROFI study (Prevention of Cerebral Embolization by Proximal Balloon Occlusion Compared to Filter Protection During Carotid Artery Stenting): a prospective randomized trial. J Am Coll Cardiol 2012;59(15):1383–9.

31. Holt PJ, Poloniecki JD, Loftus IM, et al. Meta-analysis and systematic review of the relationship between hospital volume and outcome following carotid endarterectomy. Eur J Vasc Endovasc Surg 2007;33(6):645–51.

32. Gray WA, Rosenfield KA, Jaff MR, et al. Influence of site and operator characteristics on carotid artery stent outcomes: analysis of the CAPTURE 2 (Carotid ACCULINK/ACCUNET Post Approval Trial to Uncover Rare Events) clinical study. JACC Cardiovasc Interv 2011;4(2):235–46.

33. Voeks JH, Howard G, Roubin GS, et al. Age and outcomes after carotid stenting and endarterectomy: the Carotid Revascularization Endarterectomy versus Stenting trial. Stroke 2011;42(12):3484–90.

34. Grant A, White C, Ansel G, et al. Safety and efficacy of carotid stenting in the very elderly. Catheter Cardiovasc Interv 2010;75(5):651–5.

35. Setacci C, de Donato G, Chisci E, et al. Is carotid artery stenting in octogenarians really dangerous? J Endovasc Ther 2006;13(3):302–9.

36. Cohen DJ, Stolker JM, Wang K, et al. Health-related quality of life after carotid stenting versus carotid endarterectomy: results from CREST (Carotid Revascularization Endarterectomy Versus Stenting Trial). J Am Coll Cardiol 2011;58(15):1557–65.

37. Blackshear JL, Cutlip DE, Roubin GS, et al. Myocardial infarction after carotid stenting and endarterectomy: results from the carotid revascularization endarterectomy versus stenting trial. Circulation 2011;123(22):2571–8.

38. Coppi G, Moratto R, Silingardi R, et al. PRIAMUS–proximal flow blockage cerebral protection during carotid stenting: results from a multicenter Italian registry. J Cardiovasc Surg (Torino) 2005;46(3):219–27.

39. Endovascular versus surgical treatment in patients with carotid stenosis in the Carotid and Vertebral Artery Transluminal Angioplasty Study (CAVATAS): a randomised trial. Lancet 2001;357(9270):1729–37.

Surgery Versus Stenting in Symptomatic Patients

Jun Li, MD[a,b], Rahul Sakhuja, MD, MPP, MSc, FACC[c],
Sahil A. Parikh, MD, FACC, FSCAI[a,b],*

KEYWORDS

- Symptomatic carotid artery stenosis • Carotid artery stenting • Carotid endarterectomy • Stroke

KEY POINTS

- Carotid artery stenosis is an important cause of ischemic stroke, which carries significant social and economic burden.
- Revascularization with carotid endarterectomy (CEA) decreases the incidence of recurrent stroke in patients with symptomatic carotid stenosis.
- The technique of carotid artery stenting (CAS) has evolved over the past several decades with improvement in patient selection, adjunctive medical therapy, stent design, and embolic protection devices.
- CAS has been demonstrated to be equivalent to CEA in randomized, controlled, prospective clinical trials when considering the composite endpoint of death, myocardial infarction, and ipsilateral stroke in both standard-risk and high-risk patients.
- The choice of revascularization modality (CEA vs CAS) should be an individualized, patient-specific decision based on comorbidities, target vessel and plaque characteristics, and patient preference.

INTRODUCTION

Stroke is the fourth leading cause of death in the United States. It is estimated to account for close to 130,000 deaths per year with a case fatality rate of approximately 16%.[1,2] Moreover, stroke continues to be associated with significant morbidity and economic costs. From the Framingham Heart Study population, it is estimated that 16% of stroke patients are subsequently institutionalized; 20% are dependent for mobility, and 31% are dependent for self-care.[3] In the United States, stroke is associated with an annual economic burden of 312.6 billion dollars in combined direct (eg, medical) and indirect (eg, lost productivity) costs.[2]

It is estimated that more than 80% of strokes are ischemic, and of these, approximately 15% to 20% are thought to be the direct result of carotid atherosclerosis.[4–6] The dominant mechanism for symptomatic carotid artery–related stroke is artery-to-artery embolization from atherosclerotic disease in the carotid bifurcation, although embolization from the intracranial carotid artery, proximal vertebral artery, and the aortic arch are also common.[6] Other mechanisms, such as carotid artery dissection and multivessel occlusive plaque, are uncommon causes of symptomatic carotid

Disclosures: Drs Li and Sakhuja report no disclosures. Dr Parikh serves as a consultant for Abbott Vascular, Boston Scientific, and Medtronic and receives research support from Boston Scientific and Medtronic.
[a] Department of Medicine, Case Western Reserve University School of Medicine, 11100 Euclid Avenue, Cleveland, OH 44106, USA; [b] Division of Cardiovascular Medicine, Harrington Heart and Vascular Institute, University Hospitals Case Medical Center, 11100 Euclid Avenue, Cleveland, OH 44106, USA; [c] Department of Medicine, Division of Cardiology, Wellmont CVA Heart Institute, 2050 Meadowview Pkwy, Kingsport, TN 37660, USA
* Corresponding author. Department of Medicine, Case Western Reserve University School of Medicine, 11100 Euclid Avenue, Cleveland, OH 44106.
E-mail address: Sahil.Parikh@UHhospitals.org

Intervent Cardiol Clin 3 (2014) 73–90
http://dx.doi.org/10.1016/j.iccl.2013.09.006
2211-7458/14/$ – see front matter © 2014 Elsevier Inc. All rights reserved.

interventional.theclinics.com

disease. With the tremendous societal and personal burden of stroke, carotid stenosis is an important disease to combat.

Revascularization remains the mainstay of therapy for patients with symptomatic carotid stenosis. Carotid endarterectomy (CEA) has traditionally been the strategy for surgical revascularization, with significant reduction in the recurrence of stroke compared with medical therapy alone. In the past 3 decades, the advent of endovascular techniques and carotid artery stenting (CAS) have led to the current paradigm of revascularization with either CEA or CAS, in conjunction with aggressive medical management for the treatment of patients with symptomatic disease. Candidates for revascularization should have a predicted periprocedural stroke or death rate of less than 6%, a benchmark set by early CEA trialists for which surgical benefits outweigh risks.[7–10]

PATIENT EVALUATION

Screening for carotid stenosis is typically triggered by the presence of symptoms or signs on physical examination (eg, abnormal palpation of carotid pulse, presence of a carotid bruit). Symptoms of carotid stenosis include transient ischemic attack (TIA) and stroke. Although an imperfect correlation, severity of stenosis and symptomatic disease remain the most important clinical indicators for embolic potential of carotid atherosclerosis.[7,11]

In symptomatic patients, the association between disease severity and stroke risk are closely related. With greater degrees of stenosis, the risk of recurrent stroke increases substantially. Specifically, data from the North American Symptomatic Carotid Endarterectomy Trial (NASCET) illustrate that patients with greater than 70% stenosis had a stroke rate of 24% at 18 months, versus patients with 50% to 69% stenosis with a stroke rate of 22% at more than 5 years.[12] In addition, the greatest risk of recurrence exists soon after the index event, estimated to be 10% to 25% within the first month.[6,7,13] Thus, timely determination of the degree of carotid stenosis is essential in symptomatic patients. A proposed algorithm for the assessment of patients with symptomatic carotid stenosis is outlined in **Fig. 1**.

There are a variety of modalities for estimating severity of stenosis. Although the gold standard for assessment of the presence and degree of carotid stenosis has been catheter-based digital subtraction angiography, advances in noninvasive imaging techniques have led to their widespread use as the first-line screening test.[14–17] **Table 1** shows the different imaging modalities commonly used, the technique of quantifying degree of

stenosis, and their respective strengths and weaknesses. There are 2 methods of measuring the degree of stenosis on angiography, modeled after the NASCET and the European Carotid Surgery Trial (ECST) studies (**Fig. 2**).[7,8,11,12,18] The most commonly used technique in clinical trials and practice has traditionally been the NASCET approach; 70% stenosis by NASCET correlates well with approximately 85% stenosis by the ECST approach.[7,12]

The optimal imaging modality depends on patient-related and practice-related factors. Patient-related factors include age, renal function, prior surgical interventions affecting the imaging field, and importantly, patient ability to comply with necessary testing. Practice-related factors derive primarily from the available expertise in a health care system. For example, if a center has technologists skilled in carotid duplex ultrasound (CDUS) and physicians trained in the nuanced interpretation of carotid duplex, this may be the best imaging modality at that facility.

CDUS is often a simple, sensitive, and inexpensive initial study to evaluate stenosis severity. Patients with severe stenosis and high-risk features for CEA, as shown in **Table 2**, are considered for carotid angiography and CAS as indicated.[19] Patient characteristics that portend a need for further anatomic study before carotid angiography—either with computed tomography (CT) or magnetic resonance (MR)—are listed in **Table 3**.

Imaging in the setting of acute stroke differs, as CT and MR are fundamental to the evaluation of an acute stroke. CT is less time-consuming and more sensitive than MR for the detection of intracranial hemorrhage. However, diffusion-weighted MR is much more sensitive for the detection of infarction in the setting of recent cerebrovascular occlusion.

MEDICAL TREATMENT

The immediate management of a patient with acute ischemic stroke is composed of thrombolytic therapy if deemed appropriate and supportive care to minimize intracranial hypoxemia and hypotension to reduce parenchymal injury.[11,17] Following a first stroke or TIA, modifiable risk factors to treat aggressively include hypertension, tobacco use, diabetes, dyslipidemia, physical inactivity, and dietary choices.[20,21] The role of interventional therapies for restoration of cerebral perfusion remain actively under investigation.

The foundation for secondary prevention of stroke is based on lowering of blood pressure and cholesterol, as well as the use of antiplatelet therapy.[21] The amount of benefit derived from

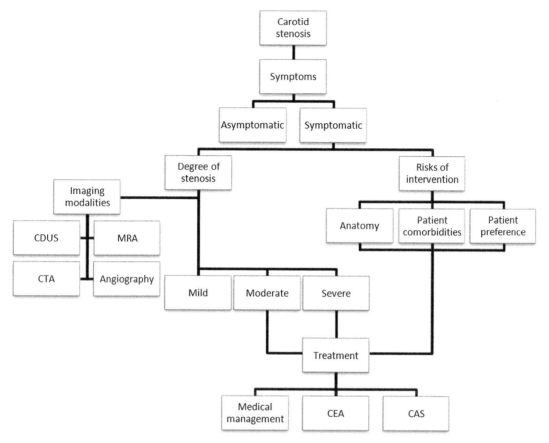

Fig. 1. This schematic illustration depicts the components that are taken into account in the evaluation of a patient with carotid stenosis, as well as potential treatment modalities. CTA, computed tomography angiography; MRA, magnetic resonance angiography.

antihypertensives is reported to be directly related to the degree of blood pressure lowering, regardless of the choice of agent.[21,22] Likewise, benefits of statins in stroke prevention are most evident in those with the greatest amount of low-density lipoprotein reduction.[21,23] Antiplatelet therapy with aspirin alone, clopidogrel alone, or aspirin plus dipyridamole has been shown to have comparable efficacy in secondary prevention, while balancing the risk of bleeding.[21,24–26] The recommendations for the secondary prevention of stroke are applicable regardless of patient candidacy for reperfusion therapy or revascularization.[7]

There is continued debate over optimal medical management versus revascularization for asymptomatic carotid stenosis. Anticipated trials including the Transatlantic Asymptomatic Carotid Intervention Trial (TACIT), the Carotid Revascularization Endarterectomy versus Stenting Trial 2 (CREST-2), and the Asymptomatic Carotid Surgery Trial 2 (ACST-2) have been proposed. Conversely, with stroke rates as high as 15% to 26% in the control groups of randomized CEA

trials, revascularization—via either endarterectomy or endovascular stenting—remains the cornerstone of therapy for managing symptomatic carotid stenosis.[8,9] A detailed review of management of asymptomatic carotid stenosis and primary stroke prevention can be found in the sections entitled "Surgery versus Stenting in Asymptomatic Patients" and "Primary Stroke Prevention: Medical Therapy versus Revascularization," respectively elsewhere in this issue.

SURGICAL INTERVENTION

Surgical techniques for CEA were initially described in 1953 by Dr Michael DeBakey. As the techniques were refined, there was a dramatic 7-fold increase in the number of CEAs performed, from 15,000 in 1971 to 107,000 in 1985.[18] Although there was an associated decline in the overall number of strokes, this was independent of significant geographic variation in rates of CEA, drawing into question the benefit of CEA versus concurrent improvements in medical therapy.[18]

Table 1
Different imaging modalities to determine the degree of carotid stenosis

	Measurement	Sensitivity	Specificity	Strengths	Weaknesses
Digital subtraction angiography (DSA)	• NASCET method: comparing diameter in the area of stenosis to that of the internal carotid distally • ECST method: comparing diameter of the stenotic lumen to probable original diameter	• Gold standard	• Gold standard	• Can be diagnostic and therapeutic if able to perform stenting at the time of catheterization	• Invasive nature with associated morbidity and mortality, including stroke risk • Cost
Carotid duplex ultrasound (CDUS)	• Peak systolic velocity in ICA • Carotid index calculated as ratio of peak systolic velocity in ICA/CCA	• 70%–99% stenosis: 91%	• 70%–99% stenosis: 87%	• Noninvasive • Correlates well with angiographic stenosis	• Difficult to determine subtotal vs total occlusion • Cutoff between <70% and >70% stenosis may be arbitrary given nondirect measurement • Image quality is operator dependent
Magnetic resonance angiography (MRA)	• Majority of studies used NASCET method	• 70%–99% stenosis: TOF 91.2%, CE 94.6% • Total occlusion: TOF 94.5%, CE 99.4%	• 70%–99% stenosis: TOF 88.3%, CE 91.9% • Total occlusion: TOF 99.3%, CE 99.6%	• Noninvasive • 3-dimensional rendering • Safe for use in renal failure when contrast excluded (ie, TOF)	• Difficult to determine subtotal vs total occlusion • TOF can be limited due to overlying neck anatomy • Cost
Computed tomography angiography (CTA)	• Majority of studies used NASCET method	• 70%–99% stenosis: 85% • Total occlusion: 97%	• 70%–99% stenosis: 93% • Total occlusion: 99%	• Noninvasive • 3-dimensional rendering • Fast compared to CDUS and MRA	• Radiation exposure • Calcified plaques and metallic implants or clips obscure image • Iodinated contrast

Abbreviations: CE, contrast enhanced; TOF, time-of-flight, using the principle of blood flow to characterize arterial architecture.
Data from Refs.[14–17]

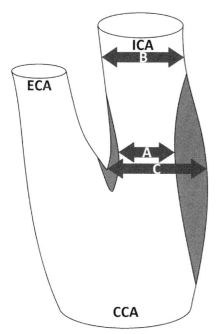

Fig. 2. Degree of stenosis as measured in NASCET and ECST. NASCET calculates stenosis as the residual lumen size (A) compared to normal distal ICA (B), where percentage stenosis is $[(B - A)/B] \times 100$.[7] ECST calculates it based on residual lumen (A) to estimated diameter of carotid bulb (C), where percent stenosis is $[(C - A)/C] \times 100$.[7] ECA, external carotid artery. (*Data from* Refs.[7,8,11,18])

Table 2	
High-risk patients for CEA	
Anatomic	**Clinical**
Contralateral carotid occlusion	Heart failure NYHA class III or IV and/or LVEF <30%
Previous CEA with recurrent stenosis	Recent MI >24 h but <4 wk
Severe tandem lesions	Unstable angina CCS class III or IV
Surgical inaccessibility High cervical ICA CCA lesions below the clavicle	Coexistent severe cardiac disease Left main disease or ≥2 vessel coronary disease Need for urgent CT surgery Abnormal stress test
Prior neck radiation or surgery	Severe pulmonary disease
Tracheostomy	Severe renal disease
Severe immobility of neck	Age >80

Adapted from Massop D, Dave R, Metzger C, et al. Stenting and angioplasty with protection in patients at high-risk for endarterectomy: SAPPHIRE Worldwide Registry first 2,001 patients. Catheter Cardiovasc Interv 2009;73(2):129–36; with permission.

Operative Technique

The choice of general versus local anesthesia is based on patient and practitioner preference. General anesthesia has the advantage of increased patient comfort, improved airway and ventilation management, and increased cerebral blood flow coupled with decreased cerebral metabolic demand. However, there is an increased frequency of the use of internal shunting to preserve continuous perfusion of the ischemic penumbra and to prevent exacerbation of neurologic deficits.[11,27] Internal shunting is not without risk, including introduction of air or thrombotic emboli, disruption of distal intima resulting in arterial dissection, and limiting complete visualization of the surgical field.[11]

Local anesthesia carries the advantage of performing neurologic evaluations during the surgery, as well as the ability to assess for adequate collateral circulation during trial clamping of the common, external, and internal carotid arteries to prevent unnecessary use of internal shunting.[11] In patients undergoing CEA with local anesthesia, it is estimated that 10% to 15% of patients will require shunting due to inadequate collateral

flow.[11] However, study data to date have not shown a definite benefit in the outcome of patients stratified for general versus local anesthesia.[27,28]

Patients are positioned supine with neck extension to expose the surgical site. Incision is either vertical along the anterior border of the sternocleidomastoid muscle or obliquely along a skin crease. The carotid sheath is incised, with retraction of the internal jugular vein and vagus nerve. The facial vein approximates the carotid bifurcation; it is suture ligated and divided to expose the underlying carotid artery. Cranial nerve XII is typically mobilized to prevent intraoperative injury.

Following isolation of the carotid artery, trial clamping and potential shunting are performed. Dissection is made at the level of the internal elastic lamina, separating the diseased intima from the media. After removal of the atheromatous intima, careful examination is performed to ensure all debris is extracted. Suturing of the carotid can then be performed with or without a patch. If an internal shunt is used, it is removed before complete suturing of the artery. Verification of the surgical result can be performed intraoperatively with

Table 3
Patient factors that may benefit from additional imaging to determine course of therapy[a]

Imaging Characteristics	Patient Characteristics Associated with High-Risk CAS
Borderline[b] or inconclusive[c] findings on CDUS	Elderly and women[d]
Discrepant findings between examination and imaging[e]	Presence of diabetes, chronic kidney disease[f]
Total occlusion on CDUS requiring confirmation	Calcified aortic arch or unfavorable arch anatomy

[a] These particular patient characteristics may confer an increased risk during catheter angiography.
[b] Peak systolic velocity on CDUS correlating with borderline stenosis of 50%–69%; because velocities are an indirect measure of stenosis, true luminal narrowing may be underestimated.
[c] Shadowing from calcific plaques may limit the full assessment of carotid velocities.
[d] Elderly and female patients have an increased likelihood of complex arches, as well as tortuous "entry" and "exit" angles with regards to lesion.
[e] For example, late-peaking, loud systolic bruit on examination but minimal stenosis on CDUS.
[f] Diabetic or renal patients with increased propensity for atherosclerotic burden. Those who are suitable candidates for CT or MR angiography must have acceptable risk for multiple contrasted studies.

either direct angiography or ultrasound and waveform analysis.

Clinical Trials of Endarterectomy

Large randomized trials, such as NASCET and ECST, have established the superiority of CEA over medical therapy in patients with symptomatic carotid stenosis. In contrast to the medical armamentarium available today, the best medical therapy serving as control in the NASCET era consisted of aspirin up to 1300 mg daily, and blood pressure and cholesterol management at the practicing clinician's discretion.[18]

In pooled analysis of the large randomized controlled trials of symptomatic patients—including NASCET, ECST, and the Veterans Affairs Trial 309—the incidence of stroke at 30 days was 7.1% in the surgical group.[29] At 5 years, there was marginal benefit to CEA in patients with moderate 50% to 69% stenosis by NASCET criteria (absolute risk reduction 4.6%), but significant benefit in those with greater than 70% stenosis (absolute risk reduction 16.0%).[29] These large, early clinical trials established CEA as the standard of care for symptomatic, severe carotid stenosis.[30,31]

Limitations of Existing Literature

In clinical practice, each patient should be assessed for suitability for surgical intervention based on their individualized surgical risk and the predicted complication rates of the operating surgeon. In these large trials, only very experienced surgeons were included. For example, in NASCET, all trial surgeons had a preceding perioperative complication rate of less than 6%.[10] The results of this selective group of operators resulted in an overall 30-day perioperative death and stroke rate of 6.5% in all patients and 5.8% in patients with severe stenosis.[10] In addition, many of the patients included in these trials were low-risk surgical patients. **Table 4** shows a summary of the perioperative wound and cranial nerve injuries that were reported in the NASCET study population.[10] However, the rates of adverse events and mortality are

Table 4
Non-MI, nonstroke complications of CEA

	Mild	Moderate	Severe	Total
Wound hematoma	55 (3.9%)	42 (3.0%)	4 (0.3%)	101 (7.1%)
Wound infection	19 (1.3%)	10 (0.7%)	—	29 (2.0%)
Facial nerve injury	28 (2.0%)	3 (0.2%)	—	31 (2.2%)
Vagus nerve injury	31 (2.2%)	5 (0.4%)	—	36 (2.5%)
Spinal accessory nerve injury	3 (0.2%)	—	—	3 (0.2%)
Hypoglossal nerve injury	50 (3.5%)	2 (0.2%)	—	52 (3.7%)

Mild complication resulted in no delay in discharge or return to operating room; moderate complication resulted in a delay in discharge, return to operating room, readmission, or—in the event of a nerve injury—documented deficit that never recovered; severe complication resulted in permanent functional disability or death.

Data from Ferguson GG, Eliasziw M, Barr HWK, et al. The North American Symptomatic Carotid Endarterectomy Trial: surgical results in 1415 patients. Stroke 1999;30(9):1751–8.

higher in patients with high-risk clinical or anatomic features previously noted (see **Table 2**). In fact, when CEA was performed in community hospitals, the 30-day mortality rate was 2-fold to 4-fold higher than that seen in these randomized trials (**Fig. 3**).[32] Finally, none of the early landmark surgical trials used specialists to adjudicate stroke via a standardized scoring system, such as the current National Institutes of Health Stroke Scale (NIHSS). As such, there does exist a possible reporting bias that underestimates the true incidence of stroke in the earlier clinical trials.

ENDOVASCULAR INTERVENTION

The first endovascular carotid artery balloon angioplasty was initially described by Dr CW Kerber in 1980. Since its development, numerous advances have been made in the technique, mirroring the evolution of other endovascular fields such as interventional cardiology. The concept of CAS was introduced in the mid-1990s and the use of embolic protection devices (EPD) to decrease showering of emboli was conceived in the early 2000s. Current interventional techniques incorporate many innovations from the past 3 decades into practice.

Interventional Techniques

An important predictor of CAS procedural success is patient selection. Preprocedural assessment may entail noninvasive evaluation of the extracranial vasculature so as to properly assess the lesion and develop a list of tools needed for any individual procedure. Aortic arch anatomy, internal carotid artery (ICA) tortuosity, the presence of proximal common carotid lesions, and collateral circulation are factors that should be considered before

CAS. Some examples of anatomy that favors CAS—as opposed to CEA—are outlined in **Fig. 4**.

Femoral arterial access is the preferred approach, although radial or brachial access is a feasible alternative. Baseline angiography may depend on preprocedural noninvasive imaging. Arch aortography can help understand anatomy and select equipment. After establishing an activated clotting time of 225 to 300, the ipsilateral common carotid artery (CCA) is often accessed using a 5-Fr diagnostic catheter and 0.038″ hydrophilic wire. Imaging of the ipsilateral CCA, bifurcation, ICA, and ipsilateral anterior intracranial circulation is essential. After diagnostic angiography, an interventional 6-Fr sheath or 8-Fr guide catheter are advanced into the CCA. In difficult arches (eg, type III) or those with tortuous access, a supportive 0.035″ wire may be advanced into the external carotid artery for additional support in advancing interventional equipment.

The target lesion should be subjected to as little manipulation as possible to prevent distal embolization. It has been shown that during unprotected CAS, most microembolic events occur during stenting, followed by predilation and postdilation.[33] EPDs are intended to prevent distal embolization and potential associated neurologic deficits and should be placed before target intervention. Following EPD placement, the target lesion is then predilated with an undersized balloon (3–4 mm diameter × 15–40 mm in length). Often, pretreatment with atropine and a fluid bolus can blunt anticipated bradycardia and hypotension during manipulation of the carotid bulb. Given that 90% of stenoses involve the cervical portion of the distal CCA or proximal ICA, self-expanding stents are preferred. Stent lengths of 30 to 40 mm are most commonly chosen and deployed

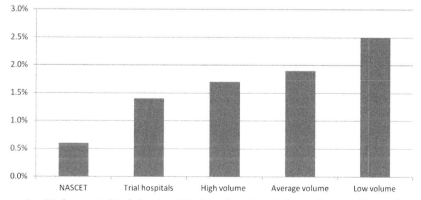

30 day CEA mortality rates by hospital experience

Fig. 3. Perioperative 30-day mortality following CEA based on hospital experience, with NASCET data as reference. (*Data from* Wennberg DE, Lucas FL, Birkmeyer JD, et al. Variation in carotid endarterectomy mortality in the Medicare population: trial hospitals, volume, and patient characteristics. JAMA 1998;279(16):1278–81.)

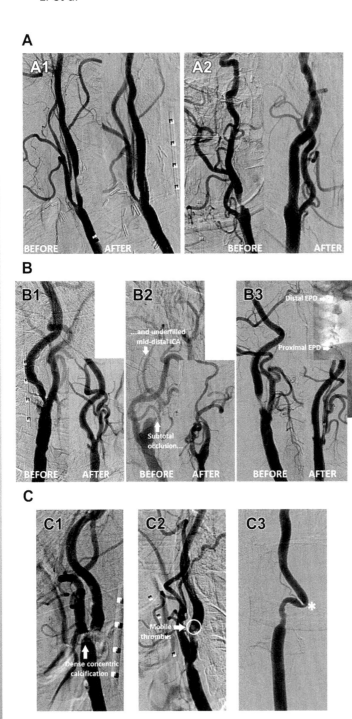

Fig. 4. Angiographic features of low-risk, intermediate-risk, and high-risk patients for carotid artery stenting. (*A*) Examples of "type A" lesions for carotid stenting (*A1* and *A2*). Angiographically, these are often lower risk for CAS. These include focal stenosis with straight landing zone rendering it easier to deliver distal EPD. (*B*) Examples of "type B" lesions for carotid stenting, which are angiographically intermediate risk, but the risk-benefit ratio may favor CAS. These include (*B1*) moderately calcified, nonconcentric lesions without other high-risk features, (*B2*) focal subtotal occlusions with "string sign" present (particularly with proximal EPD, if external carotid patent), or (*B3*) haziness, which may suggest underlying thrombus which could require special attention to embolic protection (eg, seen here with "double protection" using distal and proximal EPD in a highly symptomatic patient). (*C*) Examples of "type C" lesions, which are high risk for CAS. These include (*C1*) dense concentric calcification, (*C2*) mobile thrombus with high embolic potential, and (*C3*) tortuous "kinks" in the vessel (denoted by *asterisk*), which may be transmitted downstream by stent straightening and are unlikely to cause artery-to-artery embolization (ie, not disease, just tortuosity).

across the CCA bifurcation, "jailing" the external carotid. A residual stenosis of less than 30% is often acceptable, as there is increased risk without added benefit when aiming for a lesser residual stenosis. In fact, some operators avoid postdilation and instead rely on the stent's outward radial force to expand the lumen further. Completion angiography should evaluate the treatment zone, the EPD landing zone, and the ipsilateral anterior intracranial circulation.

Special Topics in Carotid Stenting

Stent design

Currently marketed carotid stents are composed of either nickel-titanium alloy or stainless steel.

Carotid stent designs account for the fact that the plaque is trapped behind stent struts after deployment with the attendant risk of extrusion of plaque debris between stent struts resulting in distal embolization. It is thought that adequate vessel scaffolding prevents debris from embolization.[34] Closed-cell design stents, which have more connections between adjacent ring segments compared to open-cell designs, are thought to decrease potential for embolization via improved scaffolding.[34] However, this improved scaffolding is balanced by reduced flexibility of closed-cell designs, resulting in decreased conformity to tortuous vessels. More recently, optical coherence tomography imaging corroborates greater stent malapposition with closed-cell stents with less vessel scaffolding with open-cell stents.[35] To date, clinical data reflecting reduction in emboli and improvement in clinical outcomes when using closed- versus open-cell stents are lacking.[36,37]

In addition to embolic risk, stent patency rate can be influenced by stent design. The radial force of stents has been theorized to contribute to restenosis rate. In vitro testing of multiple stent designs shows that closed-cell stents tend to have lower radial force than open-cell stents, although there are notable differences in radial force even among open-cell stents, suggesting that these may be independent qualities.[38] Increased length of stenosis has been found to be associated with decreased radial forces.[38] Finally, a number of patient-dependent factors, such as female sex, diabetes, and dyslipidemia, have been found to be independent predictors of stent patency.[39] The choice of stent should be an individualized decision based on plaque and vessel characteristics, to achieve the ideal balance between the degree of scaffolding and amount of radial force necessary. Independent of stent design, clinically important restenosis remains uncommon in CAS.

Neuroprotection

Neuroprotection involves not only the use of EPDs, but also minimizing periprocedural hemodynamic shifts to avoid hypoperfusion. As noted previously, atropine and volume resuscitation before balloon angioplasty can mitigate hypotension. Rapid recognition of hypotension is essential and can often be managed with ongoing volume resuscitation and early initiation of vasopressors (eg, phenylephrine or dopamine), which can often be weaned rapidly.

Most neurologic complications in CAS are due to intracerebral embolization. **Table 5** shows patient baseline characteristics associated with increased risk for periprocedural stroke or death. EPDs have become standard of care in carotid

Table 5
Patient characteristics that predict an increased risk of stroke or death at 30 days after CAS

Risk Factor	Odds Ratio
Age (per 10 y)	1.52[a]–1.76[b]
MI within prior 4 wk	2.79[a]
Preceding cerebrovascular event	
Stroke	2.03[b]–2.08[a]
TIA	1.71[a]
Symptomatic ipsilateral lesion within prior 6 mo	1.55[b]
Proximity to other surgical procedure	
Concomitant cardiac surgery	2.16[a]
Impending major surgery	2.20[b]
Atrial fibrillation or flutter	1.41[b]
Dialysis	2.68[a]
Angiographic characteristics	
Lesion length (per 10 mm)	1.20[a]
Type II or III aortic arch	1.24[a]
Two 90° bends	1.59[a]

[a] Data from Wimmer et al[72] extrapolated from Stenting and Angioplasty with Protection in Patients at High Risk for Endarterectomy (SAPPHIRE) population of high-risk surgical candidates.
[b] Data from Hawkins BM, Kennedy KF, Giri J, et al. Preprocedural risk quantification for carotid stenting using the CAS score: a report from the NCDR CARE Registry. J Am Coll Cardiol 2012;60(17):1617–22.

stenting to minimize the embolic risks of these interventions. There are 2 main types of EPD: "distal" and "proximal." Distal EPDs require first crossing the lesion with a guidewire, followed by deployment of a filter-type device distal to the target lesion. After the intervention, the filter is captured and removed along with the embolic debris therein. Limitations of distal filter EPDs include pore sizes resulting in nonclinically significant microemboli of less than 100 μm, a large crossing profile needed to traverse the stenotic lesion before intervention, and a possibility of poor apposition against the vessel wall.[11,40] The capture efficiency of each filter system varies based on individual characteristics including porosity (ratio of porous surface area to total surface area), pore density (ratio of total number of pores to total surface area), resistance across filter, and design eccentricity.[41]

Proximal protection devices have been developed to address these limitations. Currently available proximal EPDs deploy a balloon in the external carotid artery and CCA to stagnate flow in the ICA to prevent distal embolization. These devices provide a theoretical advantage of embolic protection before crossing with any equipment, including the guidewire. The main difficulty encountered with flow stagnation is intolerance in the setting of poor collateral flow.[40] Despite these limitations, 2 recent randomized trials have demonstrated superiority of proximal protection devices compared with distal filter in decreasing the microembolic burden.[42–44] Specifically, the PROFI study randomized 62 patients to proximal balloon occlusion versus distal filter protection, using the MoMa (Medtronic, Minneapolis, MN, USA) and Nav6 (Abbott Vascular, Santa Clara, CA, USA) devices, respectively. Diffusion-weighted MR imaging at 12 to 24 hours revealed fewer ischemic lesions in size and number with proximal EPDs.[42] An international meta-analysis of 2397 patients recapitulated these findings, with a stroke rate of 1.7%.[45] These data suggest that proximal EPDs could play an integral role in carotid stenting. A more detailed review of EPDs can be found in the section entitled "Embolic Protection for Carotid Stenting" elsewhere in this issue.

Clinical Trials of Carotid Stenting

With ongoing advances and improvements in technique, there exists inherent difficulty in studying the efficacy of endovascular carotid interventions. CEA had matured by the time of NASCET and ECST and had already undergone at least 40 years of evolution. By comparison, at the time of the first large-scale study to investigate endovascular carotid intervention, the technique had only been available for a relatively short period of time. The heterogeneities in CAS studies include the following:

1. High-risk versus standard-risk surgical patients
2. Symptomatic patients only versus inclusion of both symptomatic and asymptomatic patients
3. Use of stents not universal in all studies
4. Use of EPD not universal in all studies
5. Requirement of expertise in endovascular operators, particularly in comparison to the robust experience of surgeons used in each trial, as well as those in NASCET and ECST
6. No standardized protocol for the assessment of stroke (ie, with use of National Institutes of Health Stroke Scale)
7. Disparities in primary endpoint, including the incidence of periprocedural myocardial infarction (MI).

With the evolving technology and continued improvements in technical expertise of operators, the comparisons among endovascular interventions over time are intrinsically different and must be interpreted with caution. The large, randomized, controlled trials investigating carotid artery endovascular intervention versus endarterectomy in primarily patients with symptomatic carotid artery stenosis are summarized in this section and in **Tables 6–8**.[46–56]

The endovascular studies can be divided into investigation of high-risk and standard-risk patients. The most notable, large-scale study examining the high-risk surgical patients is the Stenting and Angioplasty with Protection in Patients at High Risk for Endarterectomy (SAPPHIRE) noninferiority study investigating the risk of perioperative stroke, MI, or death at 30 days and long-term death or ipsilateral stroke in patients undergoing CAS or CEA. The combined incidence for symptomatic and asymptomatic, high-risk patients noted noninferiority of CAS compared to CEA.[48,49]

Amongst standard-risk patients, the initial studies Carotid and Vertebral Artery Transluminal Angioplasty Study (CAVATAS), Endarterectomy versus Angioplasty in Patients with Symptomatic Severe Carotid Stenosis (EVA-3S), Stent-Supported Percutaneous Angioplasty of the Carotid Artery versus Endarterectomy (SPACE), and International Carotid Stenting Study (ICSS) have a high degree of variability in the use of stenting, EPD, and operator expertise, as noted in **Table 7**. The short-term and long-term outcomes for CAS versus CEA studies, as well as NASCET and ECST, are detailed in **Table 8**. In general, the incidence of perioperative stroke tends to occur more often in the CAS group; nonetheless, the long-term incidence of stroke and death are essentially the same between the endovascular and surgical groups.

The largest trial published in the symptomatic, standard-risk population takes into the account the above shortcomings. CREST used stents and EPDs universally as standard of care. Furthermore, an intensive lead-in phase built into the study protocol allowed for proper credentialing of interventionalists to ensure satisfactory expertise before participation in the trial.[56] There was no difference in CAS versus CEA in the primary endpoint of periprocedural stroke, MI, or death from any cause or ipsilateral stroke within 4 years.[55] Like SAPPHIRE, the primary outcome in CREST also included the incidence of periprocedural MI. Although the finding of increased periprocedural stroke in CAS persists in CREST, there is a significantly lower incidence of periprocedural MI in CAS.

Some critics have argued that periprocedural MI is not a direct measure of treatment efficacy for stroke prevention and thus serves as a diversion

Table 6
Characteristics of study populations and duration of recruitment for trials of CAS versus CEA

| | Years Conducted | Number of Patients | | Degree of Stenosis | High-Risk Surgery Patients |
		Intervention Arm	Control Arm		
CAVATAS	1992–1997	251	253	• Most are symptomatic • Variable degrees of stenosis	No
SAPPHIRE	2000–2002	167 (50 symptomatic)	167 (46 symptomatic)	• Symptomatic >50% • Asymptomatic >80%	Yes
EVA-3S	2000–2005	265	262	• Symptomatic ≥60%	No
SPACE	2001–2006	599	584	• Symptomatic ≥70% CDUS (≥50% by NASCET)	No
ICSS	2001–2008	853	857	• Symptomatic ≥50% or noninvasive equivalent	No
CREST	2000–2008	1262 (668 symptomatic)	1240 (653 symptomatic)	• Symptomatic ≥50% or ≥70% by noninvasive • Asymptomatic ≥60% or ≥70% CDUS or ≥80% MRA/CTA	No

Data from Refs.[46,48,50,52,54,55]

from the true assessment of benefit.[57] However, it has previously been shown that vascular surgeries and endovascular procedures complicated by periprocedural MI heralds worsened long-term morbidity and mortality and must be considered as an integral component in the overall benefit versus harm analysis of each respective procedure.[48,58–60] Patient characteristics that render one to be more susceptible to perioperative MI include age greater than 70 years old, diabetes, angina, ST and T wave abnormalities on resting electrocardiogram, and heart failure; these patient-specific factors should be included in the heuristic for determination of revascularization strategy, as noted in **Fig. 1**.[60]

An additional individualized patient factor that may be pertinent in revascularization success is patient age. In both SPACE and CREST there were reported differences in adverse event rates between younger and older patients, with patients less than the age of 70 with a tendency to fare better with CAS, and those over the age of 70 with improved outcomes with CEA.[53,55,61] It is speculated that the elderly cohort may have increased vascular tortuosity, atherosclerosis burden in the arch, and plaque instability accounting for the age-dependent gradation in response.[61] Although CAS may be more favorable among younger

patients, the role of age is still not entirely understood. Preprocedural imaging can play an important role in patient selection for CAS versus CEA.

LONG-TERM OUTCOMES

As with all modes of revascularization, restenosis remains a vexing problem with CEA and CAS. The cause of restenosis is thought to be secondary to neointimal hyperplasia when occurring within 2 years of an intervention, and recurrent atherosclerosis if occurring after 2 years.[62] The restenosis rates following both modes of intervention were investigated in CAVATAS and EVA-3S. Ultrasound velocities were used to establish severe or moderate restenosis, defined as ≥70% or 50% to 69%, respectively, by NASCET criteria.[62] However, the validity of CDUS for severity of stenosis has not been validated for grading in-stent restenosis compared to native disease; thus, interobserver comparisons can be difficult. Nevertheless, at the 5-year follow-up for CAVATAS patients who had undergone endovascular treatment, regardless of stenting status, had a significantly increased risk of moderate or severe restenosis compared to CEA; this risk was partially mitigated by the use of stents, which produced a significantly lower risk of restenosis compared with angioplasty alone

Table 7
Endovascular requirements for stents and/or embolic protection devices and criteria for expertise in operators for participation in trials of CAS versus CEA

	Use of Stents	Use of EPD	Operator Expertise	
			Interventionalists	Surgeons
CAVATAS	• Optional after 1994 • Used in 55 (26%) of patients	• None	• Training in neuroradiology and techniques of angioplasty • Not necessarily in the carotid artery	• Vascular surgeon or neurosurgeon • Expertise in CEA
SAPPHIRE	• Yes	• Yes	• Experience equal to or superior to the published results of carotid stenting • Median lifetime experience of 64 carotid interventions, range 20–700	• Must meet the criteria of the AHA for acceptable rates of complication during and after CEA • Annual median volume of 30 CEAs, range 15–100
EVA-3S	• Yes	• Systematic in 2003 • Used in 227 (88%) of patients	• Performed $\geq$12 carotid stenting procedures or $\geq$35 stenting procedures in the supra-aortic trunks, of which $\geq$5 were in the carotid • Centers fulfilling all other requirements except those with regard to the interventionalist can join study with supervision of CAS under experienced tutor, until deemed sufficient by tutor • 101 (39%) of procedures were performed under supervision	• $\geq$25 CEAs in the year before enrollment
SPACE	• Yes	• Optional • Used in 151 (27%) of patients	• $\geq$25 successful consecutive percutaneous carotid transluminal angioplasty or stent	• $\geq$25 consecutive CEAs, must provide mortality and morbidity rates
ICSS	• Yes	• Recommended, not mandatory • Used in 593 (72%) of patients	• $\geq$50 stenting procedures, with $\geq$10 carotid cases • Centers can join as supervised site • Supervised centers can be promoted if $\geq$20 trial cases performed with acceptable results • 102 (12%) of procedures performed in supervised centers	• $\geq$50 carotid operations, with $\geq$10 cases per year
CREST	• Yes	• Yes	• Interventionalists with >30 carotid stenting cases and low event rates, previous experience with CREST study devices were exempt from lead in phase • Lead in phase for operators with <30 carotid stent experience • Ability to participate based on evaluation of performance during lead in phase	• Validated selection process, documentation of $\geq$12 procedures per year • Rates of complications and death $\leq$3% in asymptomatic patients and $\leq$5% in symptomatic patients

Data from Refs. 46,48,50,52,54–56

Table 8
Rate of occurrence of composites, stroke, death, and MI in perioperative and follow-up periods

	30 d Composite		Perioperative Stroke		Perioperative Death		Perioperative MI		Follow-Up Composite		Follow-Up Stroke		Follow-Up Death	
	CAS (%)	CEA (%)	CAS (%)	CEA (%)	CAS (%)	CEA (%)	CAS (%)	CEA (%)	CAS (%)	CEA (%)	CAS (%)	CEA (%)	CAS (%)	CEA (%)
NASCET[a]	—	5.8	—	5.5	—	0.6	—	0.9	—	15.8	—	12.6	—	4.6
ECST[b]	—	7.0	—	6.6	—	1.2	—	—	—	37.0	—	17.4	—	27.6
CAVATAS[c]	10.0 (6.4)	9.9 (5.9)	7.2	8.3	2.8	1.6	0	1.2	45.2	50.4	21.1	15.4	48.4	43.0
SAPPHIRE[d]	4.8 (2.1)	9.8 (9.3)	3.6	3.1	1.2	2.5	2.4	6.1	24.6 (32.0)	26.9 (21.7)	9.0	9.0	18.6	21.0
EVA-3S[e]	9.6	3.9	8.8	2.7	0.8	1.2	0.4	0.8	26.9	21.6	14.2 (4.5)	9.1 (4.9)	16.1	16.0
SPACE[f]	6.8 (7.7)	6.3 (6.5)	6.7 (7.5)	6.0 (6.2)	0.7	0.9	0	0	9.5	8.8	10.9 (2.2)	10.1 (1.9)	6.3	5.0
ICSS[g]	8.5	5.2	7.7	4.1	2.3	0.8	0.4	0.5	—	—	—	—	—	—
CREST[h]	5.2 (6.7)	4.5 (5.4)	4.1 (5.5)	2.3 (3.2)	0.7	0.3	1.1 (1.0)	2.3 (2.3)	7.2 (8.6)	6.8 (8.4)	6.2 (7.6)	4.7 (6.4)	11.3	12.6

[a] Results obtained from study group with severe, symptomatic disease. Thirty-day primary composite here is of any stroke or death; follow-up composite is at 2 years, any stroke (ipsilateral or otherwise), or death.

[b] Results of all patients with any degree of stenosis. Thirty-day composite is of all stroke (with symptoms lasting more than 7 days) or death; follow-up composite is at 3 years of any major stroke or death.

[c] Results of all patients with any degree of stenosis. Thirty-day composite is of all stroke (disabling, defined as requiring help from another person for everyday activities for more than 30 days, and nondisabling) and death. Parentheses show only disabling stroke combined with death. MI is nonfatal MI; fatal MI not separately reported. Follow-up composite is at 8 years of disabling stroke or death; stroke at follow-up analysis is nonperioperative stroke.

[d] Results of all patients, both symptomatic and asymptomatic; data for symptomatic population only is shown in parentheses. Thirty-day composite is of stroke, MI, or death. Individual event rates at 30 days are not reported separately for symptomatic and asymptomatic populations. Long-term composite is stroke, MI, or death within 30 days, or ipsilateral stroke or death between days 31 and 3 years.

[e] Thirty-day composite is of any stroke or death. Cumulative follow-up at 4 years is of any stroke or death. Parentheses show rate of 4-year nonprocedural stroke. Follow-up death is secondary to nonprocedural death.

[f] Thirty-day composite is of ipsilateral stroke or death, with any stroke or death in parentheses. Two-year follow-up composite is of ipsilateral stroke plus periprocedural stroke or death. Follow-up stroke is any stroke between randomization and 3 years; parentheses show nonprocedural stroke.

[g] Short-term composite is at 120 days, of stroke, death, or procedural MI. Long-term follow-up data are pending publication.

[h] Thirty-day composite is any periprocedural stroke, MI, or death or postprocedural ipsilateral stroke. Parentheses show data for subgroup of symptomatic patients; $P = .30$ for the 30-day composite in the symptomatic group. Follow-up composite at 4 years is periprocedural stroke, MI, or death or postprocedural ipsilateral stroke. Follow-up stroke is composed of both periprocedural stroke and postprocedural ipsilateral stroke.

Data from Refs.[46–56]

in the CAVATAS population (36.2% in balloon angioplasty alone, 16.6% in CAS, and 10.5% in CEA).[62] In EVA-3S at 3-year follow-up, a significant difference was noted between CAS and CEA for restenosis ≥50% (12.5% in CAS vs 5% in CEA), but no difference in the patients with severe restenosis ≥70% (3.3% CAS vs 2.8% in CEA).[63]

Despite the well-accepted association between stroke and high-grade stenosis in a procedure-naïve vessel, neither study found a difference in the risk of ipsilateral stroke with restenosis.[62,63] The increased rate of post-CAS restenosis without a reciprocal increase in prevalence of recurrent stroke may be reflective of a difference in composition of restenosed vessels with less atherothrombotic debris resulting in fewer artery-to-artery embolic events, resulting in a lower incidence of clinical events. A lower incidence of clinical events calls for more rigorous investigation into the criteria used to diagnose clinically significant restenotic lesions and to introduce the potential use of novel intravascular imaging techniques–such as optical coherence tomography—to characterize apparently severe stenotic lesions further.[53,64]

With continuing improvements in CAS and increasing experience of operators, the number of adverse events in the periprocedural period for CAS is on the decline. Overall, in the symptomatic population, the CREST patients carried lower rates of stroke or death in CAS compared to SPACE, EVA-3S, and ICSS.[55] In Protected Carotid Artery Stenting in Patients at High Risk for Carotid Endarterectomy (PROTECT), a multicenter trial to assess outcomes of CAS with EPD for patients deemed high risk for CEA, investigators noted a composite of perioperative rate of death, stroke, and MI of 3.4%—a rate that is lower than all of the previously discussed endovascular studies.[65]

The progressively improving outcomes in CAS clinical trials in recent years may reflect more stringent credentialing of interventionalists, the advent of new technologies used in stenting and EPD, and the evolution of medical management. In clinical practice, there is a push for standardized care with a focus on improving quality of endovascular interventions, as patients in clinical trials have fewer complications.[66] This has resulted in multiple registries to monitor outcomes assessment and quality of care with real-world implementation of CAS, including the Carotid Artery Revascularization and Endarterectomy (CARE) Registry within the National Cardiovascular Data Registry (NCDR) and the Society for Vascular Surgery Vascular Registry (SVSVR).[67–69] The former registry was initiated by multidisciplinary societies within cardiology, vascular surgery, neurovascular diseases, and radiology, with a goal of providing benchmarks for best practices in carotid interventions by monitoring clinical practice, patient outcomes, and quality of administered care.[67]

Some investigators have compared the efficacy of CAS versus CEA using the SVSVR data to argue that CAS continues to be an inferior choice of carotid intervention.[68,70] However, the nonrandomized nature of patient assignment to treatment modality in a real-world setting renders the 2 populations fundamentally different.[70] An analysis of the clinical referral patterns to CAS versus CEA using the CARE Registry found that patients who have a higher propensity for CAS referral had an increased risk of mortality, suggesting that this population of patients is at an inherently increased risk of periprocedural adverse events.[71] Conclusions drawn from these types of comparisons, plagued by uncontrolled bias, should be carefully scrutinized.[70,71]

SUMMARY

In the present day, revascularization remains the standard of care for patients with symptomatic carotid disease. Although CEA has been historically established as the gold standard for revascularization in patients with symptomatic carotid stenosis, CAS has emerged as an alternative treatment option with long-term results similar to CEA. Operator expertise, patient characteristics—such as anatomy and associated comorbidities—and patient preference are factored into the consideration for modality of revascularization. CAS is undoubtedly an important modality for patients at high risk for operative revascularization. However, the mounting evidence conveyed by CAS trials suggests that it is a viable option in the standard-risk patient as well. The evidence and multispecialty guidelines consider CAS and CEA equivalent in selected patients for the management of symptomatic carotid stenosis.

The carotid artery is one of the few vascular beds in which surgery remains the dominant mode of revascularization despite strong data supportive of the use of less invasive strategies. However, the strength of recent data portend a paradigm shift in which patients referred for CAS will no longer be those who are poor candidates for surgery. Rather, some may consider CEA as an alternative to CAS for those patients who are not suitable for CAS. In this sense, patients should be deemed "poor CAS" candidate, as opposed to the current mentality of a "poor CEA" candidate.

The American Heart Association, the American Association of Neurological Surgeons, and the

Society for Vascular Surgery issued a joint recommendation in 2011 endorsing the use of either CEA or CAS for the treatment of severe, symptomatic carotid artery stenosis.[7] Furthermore, the Food and Drug Administration issued the approval of CAS for use in occlusive disease in 2004.[69] Nonetheless, the procedure is not reimbursed outside of clinical trials for large segments of the population in whom high-quality data support CAS as comparable to CEA. This concern over reimbursement has bridled enthusiasm within the field, limiting the potential for continued improvements of CAS technologies and techniques. With the recent clarification of the clinical role of CAS and the emerging transformation of health economics, one hopes that CAS will assume its proper position among therapies for the treatment of symptomatic carotid stenosis in the eyes of patients, providers, and payers alike.

REFERENCES

1. Hoyert DL, Xu JQ. Deaths: preliminary data for 2011. Hyattsville (MD): National Center for Health Statistics; 2012.

2. Go AS, Mozaffarian D, Roger VL, et al. Executive summary: heart disease and stroke statistics–2013 update: a report from the American Heart Association. Circulation 2013;127(1):143–52.

3. Gresham GE, Fitzpatrick TE, Wolf PA, et al. Residual disability in survivors of stroke — The Framingham Study. N Engl J Med 1975;293(19):954–6.

4. Adams HP, Bendixen BH, Kappelle LJ, et al. Classification of subtype of acute ischemic stroke. Definitions for use in a multicenter clinical trial. TOAST. Trial of Org 10172 in Acute Stroke Treatment. Stroke 1993;24(1):35–41.

5. Cutlip DE, Pinto DS. Extracranial carotid disease revascularization. Circulation 2012;126(22): 2636 11.

6. Rasmussen TE, Clouse WD, Tonnessen BH, et al. Handbook of patient care in vascular diseases. 5th edition. Philadelphia: Wolters Kluwer Health/Lippincott Williams & Wilkins; 2008.

7. Brott TG, Halperin JL, Abbara S, et al. 2011 ASA/ACCF/AHA/AANN/AANS/ACR/ASNR/CNS/SAIP/SCAI/SIR/SNIS/SVM/SVS guideline on the management of patients with extracranial carotid and vertebral artery disease: executive summary: a report of the American College of Cardiology Foundation/American Heart Association Task Force on Practice Guidelines, and the American Stroke Association, American Association of Neuroscience Nurses, American Association of Neurological Surgeons, American College of Radiology, American Society of Neuroradiology, Congress of Neurological Surgeons, Society of Atherosclerosis Imaging and Prevention, Society for Cardiovascular Angiography and Interventions, Society of Interventional Radiology, Society of NeuroInterventional Surgery, Society for Vascular Medicine, and Society for Vascular Surgery. Developed in collaboration with the American Academy of Neurology and Society of Cardiovascular Computed Tomography. Catheter Cardiovasc Interv 2013;81(1): E76–123.

8. Randomised trial of endarterectomy for recently symptomatic carotid stenosis: final results of the MRC European Carotid Surgery Trial (ECST). Lancet 1998;351(9113):1379–87.

9. North American Symptomatic Carotid Endarterectomy Trial Collaborators. Beneficial effect of carotid endarterectomy in symptomatic patients with high-grade carotid stenosis. N Engl J Med 1991;325(7): 445–53.

10. Ferguson GG, Eliasziw M, Barr HW, et al. The North American symptomatic carotid endarterectomy trial: surgical results in 1415 patients. Stroke 1999;30(9):1751–8.

11. Rutherford RB. Vascular surgery. 6th edition. Philadelphia: Saunders; 2005.

12. Barnett HJ, Taylor DW, Eliasziw M, et al. Benefit of carotid endarterectomy in patients with symptomatic moderate or severe stenosis. N Engl J Med 1998;339(20):1415–25.

13. Rothwell PM. Prediction and prevention of stroke in patients with symptomatic carotid stenosis: the high-risk period and the high-risk patient. Eur J Vasc Endovasc Surg 2008;35(3):255–63.

14. Moneta GL, Edwards JM, Chitwood RW, et al. Correlation of North American Symptomatic Carotid Endarterectomy Trial (NASCET) angiographic definition of 70% to 99% internal carotid artery stenosis with duplex scanning. J Vasc Surg 1993;17(1):152–9.

15. Koelemay MJ, Nederkoorn PJ, Reitsma JB, et al. Systematic review of computed tomographic angiography for assessment of carotid artery disease. Stroke 2004;35(10):2306–12.

16. Debrey SM, Yu H, Lynch JK, et al. Diagnostic accuracy of magnetic resonance angiography for internal carotid artery disease: a systematic review and meta-analysis. Stroke 2008;39(8):2237–48.

17. Jauch EC, Saver JL, Adams HP Jr, et al. Guidelines for the early management of patients with acute ischemic stroke: a guideline for healthcare professionals from the American Heart Association/American Stroke Association. Stroke 2013;44(3):870–947.

18. North American symptomatic carotid endarterectomy trial. Methods, patient characteristics, and progress. Stroke 1991;22(6):711–20.

19. Massop D, Dave R, Metzger C, et al. Stenting and angioplasty with protection in patients at high-risk for endarterectomy: SAPPHIRE Worldwide Registry

first 2,001 patients. Catheter Cardiovasc Interv 2009;73(2):129–36.

20. Goldstein LB. Primary prevention of ischemic stroke: a guideline from the American Heart Association/American Stroke Association Stroke Council: cosponsored by the Atherosclerotic Peripheral Vascular Disease Interdisciplinary Working Group; Cardiovascular Nursing Council; Clinical Cardiology Council; Nutrition, Physical Activity, and Metabolism Council; and the Quality of Care and Outcomes Research Interdisciplinary Working Group: The American Academy of Neurology affirms the value of this guideline. Circulation 2006; 113(24):e873–923.

21. Davis SM, Donnan GA. Clinical practice. Secondary prevention after ischemic stroke or transient ischemic attack. N Engl J Med 2012;366(20):1914–22.

22. Group PC. Randomised trial of a perindopril-based blood-pressure-lowering regimen among 6,105 individuals with previous stroke or transient ischaemic attack. Lancet 2001;358(9287):1033–41.

23. Amarenco P, Goldstein LB, Szarek M, et al. Effects of intense low-density lipoprotein cholesterol reduction in patients with stroke or transient ischemic attack: the Stroke Prevention by Aggressive Reduction in Cholesterol Levels (SPARCL) trial. Stroke 2007;38(12):3198–204.

24. Antithrombotic Trialists' Collaboration. Collaborative meta-analysis of randomised trials of antiplatelet therapy for prevention of death, myocardial infarction, and stroke in high risk patients. BMJ 2002;324(7329):71–86.

25. CAPRIE Steering Committee. A randomised, blinded, trial of clopidogrel versus aspirin in patients at risk of ischaemic events (CAPRIE). CAPRIE Steering Committee. Lancet 1996;348(9038): 1329–39.

26. Diener HC, Cunha L, Forbes C, et al. European Stroke Prevention Study. 2. Dipyridamole and acetylsalicylic acid in the secondary prevention of stroke. J Neurol Sci 1996;143(1–2):1–13.

27. Group GT, Lewis SC, Warlow CP, et al. General anaesthesia versus local anaesthesia for carotid surgery (GALA): a multicentre, randomised controlled trial. Lancet 2008;372(9656):2132–42.

28. Rerkasem K, Rothwell PM. Local versus general anaesthesia for carotid endarterectomy. Cochrane Database Syst Rev 2008;(4):CD000126.

29. Rothwell PM, Eliasziw M, Gutnikov SA, et al. Analysis of pooled data from the randomised controlled trials of endarterectomy for symptomatic carotid stenosis. Lancet 2003;361(9352):107–16.

30. Biller J, Feinberg WM, Castaldo JE, et al. Guidelines for carotid endarterectomy: a statement for healthcare professionals from a Special Writing Group of the Stroke Council, American Heart Association. Circulation 1998;97(5):501–9.

31. Sacco RL, Adams R, Albers G, et al. Guidelines for prevention of stroke in patients with ischemic stroke or transient ischemic attack: a statement for healthcare professionals from the American Heart Association/American Stroke Association Council on Stroke: co-sponsored by the Council on Cardiovascular Radiology and Intervention: the American Academy of Neurology affirms the value of this guideline. Stroke 2006;37(2):577–617.

32. Wennberg DE, Lucas FL, Birkmeyer JD, et al. Variation in carotid endarterectomy mortality in the medicare population: trial hospitals, volume, and patient characteristics. JAMA 1998;279(16):1278–81.

33. Al-Mubarak N, Roubin GS, Vitek JJ, et al. Effect of the distal-balloon protection system on microembolization during carotid stenting. Circulation 2001;104(17):1999–2002.

34. Bosiers M, Deloose K, Verbist J, et al. The impact of embolic protection device and stent design on the outcome of CAS. Perspect Vasc Surg Endovasc Ther 2008;20(3):272–9.

35. de Donato G, Setacci F, Sirignano P, et al. Optical coherence tomography after carotid stenting: rate of stent malapposition, plaque prolapse and fibrous cap rupture according to stent design. Eur J Vasc Endovasc Surg 2013;45(6):579–87.

36. Timaran CH, Rosero EB, Higuera A, et al. Randomized clinical trial of open-cell vs closed-cell stents for carotid stenting and effects of stent design on cerebral embolization. J Vasc Surg 2011;54(5): 1310–6.e1 [discussion: 1316].

37. Grunwald IQ, Reith W, Karp K, et al. Comparison of stent free cell area and cerebral lesions after unprotected carotid artery stent placement. Eur J Vasc Endovasc Surg 2012;43(1):10–4.

38. Voute MT, Hendriks JM, van Laanen JH, et al. Radial force measurements in carotid stents: influence of stent design and length of the lesion. J Vasc Interv Radiol 2011;22(5):661–6.

39. Lal BK, Beach KW, Roubin GS, et al. Restenosis after carotid artery stenting and endarterectomy: a secondary analysis of CREST, a randomised controlled trial. Lancet Neurol 2012;11(9):755–63.

40. Mousa AY, Campbell JE, Aburahma AF, et al. Current update of cerebral embolic protection devices. J Vasc Surg 2012;56(5):1429–37.

41. Loghmanpour NA, Siewiorek GM, Wanamaker KM, et al. Assessing the impact of distal protection filter design characteristics on 30-day outcomes of carotid artery stenting procedures. J Vasc Surg 2013;57(2):309–17.e2.

42. Bijuklic K, Wandler A, Hazizi F, et al. The PROFI study (Prevention of Cerebral Embolization by Proximal Balloon Occlusion Compared to Filter Protection During Carotid Artery Stenting): a prospective randomized trial. J Am Coll Cardiol 2012; 59(15):1383–9.

43. Ansel GM, Hopkins LN, Jaff MR, et al. Safety and effectiveness of the INVATEC MO.MA proximal cerebral protection device during carotid artery stenting: results from the ARMOUR pivotal trial. Catheter Cardiovasc Interv 2010;76(1):1–8.

44. Montorsi P, Caputi L, Galli S, et al. Microembolization during carotid artery stenting in patients with high-risk, lipid-rich plaque. A randomized trial of proximal versus distal cerebral protection. J Am Coll Cardiol 2011;58(16):1656–63.

45. Bersin RM, Stabile E, Ansel GM, et al. A meta-analysis of proximal occlusion device outcomes in carotid artery stenting. Catheter Cardiovasc Interv 2012;80(7):1072–8.

46. Endovascular versus surgical treatment in patients with carotid stenosis in the Carotid and Vertebral Artery Transluminal Angioplasty Study (CAVATAS): a randomised trial. Lancet 2001; 357(9270):1729–37.

47. Ederle J, Bonati LH, Dobson J, et al. Endovascular treatment with angioplasty or stenting versus endarterectomy in patients with carotid artery stenosis in the Carotid And Vertebral Artery Transluminal Angioplasty Study (CAVATAS): long-term follow-up of a randomised trial. Lancet Neurol 2009;8(10): 898–907.

48. Yadav JS, Wholey MH, Kuntz RE, et al. Protected carotid-artery stenting versus endarterectomy in high-risk patients. N Engl J Med 2004;351(15): 1493–501.

49. Gurm HS, Yadav JS, Fayad P, et al. Long-term results of carotid stenting versus endarterectomy in high-risk patients. N Engl J Med 2008;358(15): 1572–9.

50. Mas JL, Chatellier G, Beyssen B, et al. Endarterectomy versus stenting in patients with symptomatic severe carotid stenosis. N Engl J Med 2006; 355(16):1660–71.

51. Mas JL, Trinquart L, Leys D, et al. Endarterectomy Versus Angioplasty in Patients with Symptomatic Severe Carotid Stenosis (EVA 3S) trial: results up to 4 years from a randomised, multicentre trial. Lancet Neurol 2008;7(10):885–92.

52. SPACE Collaborative Group, Ringleb PA, Allenberg J, Brückmann H, et al. 30 day results from the SPACE trial of stent-protected angioplasty versus carotid endarterectomy in symptomatic patients: a randomised non-inferiority trial. Lancet 2006;368(9543):1239–47.

53. Eckstein HH, Ringleb P, Allenberg JR, et al. Results of the Stent-Protected Angioplasty versus Carotid Endarterectomy (SPACE) study to treat symptomatic stenoses at 2 years: a multinational, prospective, randomised trial. Lancet Neurol 2008;7(10): 893–902.

54. International Carotid Stenting Study Investigators, Ederle J, Dobson J, Featherstone RL, et al. Carotid artery stenting compared with endarterectomy in patients with symptomatic carotid stenosis (International Carotid Stenting Study): an interim analysis of a randomised controlled trial. Lancet 2010; 375(9719):985–97.

55. Brott TG, Hobson RW, Howard G, et al. Stenting versus endarterectomy for treatment of carotid-artery stenosis. N Engl J Med 2010;363(1):11–23.

56. Hopkins LN, Roubin GS, Chakhtoura EY, et al. The carotid revascularization endarterectomy versus stenting trial: credentialing of interventionalists and final results of lead-in phase. J Stroke Cerebrovasc Dis 2010;19(2):153–62.

57. Abbott AL, Adelman MA, Alexandrov AV, et al. Why calls for more routine carotid stenting are currently inappropriate: an international, multispecialty, expert review and position statement. Stroke 2013; 44(4):1186–90.

58. Landesberg G, Shatz V, Akopnik I, et al. Association of cardiac troponin, CK-MB, and postoperative myocardial ischemia with long-term survival after major vascular surgery. J Am Coll Cardiol 2003; 42(9):1547–54.

59. Stone GW, Mehran R, Dangas G, et al. Differential impact on survival of electrocardiographic Q-wave versus enzymatic myocardial infarction after percutaneous intervention: a device-specific analysis of 7147 patients. Circulation 2001;104(6):642–7.

60. Stilp E, Baird C, Gray WA, et al. An evidence-based review of the impact of periprocedural myocardial infarction in carotid revascularization. Catheter Cardiovasc Interv 2013. [Epub ahead of print].

61. Bonati LH, Lyrer P, Ederle J, et al. Percutaneous transluminal balloon angioplasty and stenting for carotid artery stenosis. Cochrane Database Syst Rev 2012;(9):CD000515.

62. Bonati LH, Ederle J, McCabe DJ, et al. Long-term risk of carotid restenosis in patients randomly assigned to endovascular treatment or endarterectomy in the Carotid and Vertebral Artery Transluminal Angioplasty Study (CAVATAS): long-term follow-up of a randomised trial. Lancet Neurol 2009;8(10):908–17.

63. Arquizan C, Trinquart L, Touboul PJ, et al. Restenosis is more frequent after carotid stenting than after endarterectomy: the EVA-3S study. Stroke 2011; 42(4):1015–20.

64. Attizzani GF, Jones MR, Given CA 2nd, et al. Frequency-domain optical coherence tomography assessment of very late vascular response after carotid stent implantation. J Vasc Surg 2013;58(1): 201–4.

65. Matsumura JS, Gray W, Chaturvedi S, et al. Results of carotid artery stenting with distal embolic protection with improved systems: Protected Carotid Artery Stenting in Patients at High Risk for Carotid

Endarterectomy (PROTECT) trial. J Vasc Surg 2012;55(4):968–76.e5.

66. Barr JD, Connors JJ 3rd, Sacks D, et al. Quality improvement guidelines for the performance of cervical carotid angioplasty and stent placement. AJNR Am J Neuroradiol 2003;24(10):2020–34.

67. Sidawy AN, Zwolak RM, White RA, et al. Risk-adjusted 30-day outcomes of carotid stenting and endarterectomy: results from the SVS Vascular Registry. J Vasc Surg 2009;49(1):71–9.

68. Jim J, Rubin BG, Ricotta JJ 2nd, et al. Society for Vascular Surgery (SVS) Vascular Registry evaluation of comparative effectiveness of carotid revascularization procedures stratified by Medicare age. J Vasc Surg 2012;55(5):1313–20 [discussion: 1321].

69. White CJ, Anderson HV, Brindis RG, et al. The Carotid Artery Revascularization and Endarterectomy (CARE) registry: objectives, design, and implications. Catheter Cardiovasc Interv 2008;71(6):721–5.

70. Longmore RB, Yeh RW, Kennedy KF, et al. Clinical referral patterns for carotid artery stenting versus carotid endarterectomy: results from the Carotid Artery Revascularization and Endarterectomy Registry. Circ Cardiovasc Interv 2011;4(1):88–94.

71. Anderson HV, Rosenfield KA, White CJ, et al. Clinical features and outcomes of carotid artery stenting by clinical expert consensus criteria: a report from the CARE registry. Catheter Cardiovasc Interv 2010;75(4):519–25.

72. Wimmer NJ, Yeh RW, Cutlip DE, et al. Risk prediction for adverse events after carotid artery stenting in higher surgical risk patients. Stroke 2012;43(12):3218–24.

Carotid Artery Stenting
Operator and Institutional Learning Curves

Siddharth A. Wayangankar, MD, MPH[a],
Herbert D. Aronow, MD, MPH[b],*

KEYWORDS

- Carotid artery stenting • Learning curve • Stroke

KEY POINTS

- Ideally, experience with carotid artery stenting (CAS) procedures should be sufficient to keep periprocedural death/stroke rates less than 3% for asymptomatic patients (<6% for symptomatic patients) in accordance with the American Heart Association's recommendations.
- Available data suggest that operators need to perform approximately 75 CAS cases before periprocedural complication rates decrease below this threshold, a level that would eliminate all but high-volume operators.
- Policies that would restrict the use of CAS to highly experienced operators might ensure the safety of CAS but would come at the expense of limited procedural access.
- Collaborative, cross-specialty dialogue around such policy decisions is urgently needed if CAS is to remain a viable treatment option for patients with carotid artery stenosis.
- Virtual reality simulated training initiatives might minimize the procedural volumes required to achieve proficiency, but that remains to be proven.

INTRODUCTION

Carotid artery stenting (CAS) is a unique interventional procedure. It requires an in-depth knowledge of vascular and intracranial anatomy, a robust experience with catheters and guidewires, and an understanding of disease pathology above and beyond that required for treating other vascular territories.[1,2] When compared with other end organs, the brain is distinctly sensitive to small errors in endovascular procedural technique that may culminate in distal microembolization. Unique hemodynamic consequences also occur commonly during the periprocedural period.[1,2] Standardizing CAS training has had its own inherent challenges in that the procedure is performed by operators from multiple specialties, including interventional cardiovascular medicine, interventional radiology, vascular surgery, neurosurgery, and interventional neurology,[1–3] specialists who possess varied clinical backgrounds and technical skill sets.

The utilization of CAS has increased significantly since the US Food and Drug Administration (FDA) approved the first carotid stent system in 2004.[4,5] Reasons for the rapid uptake of CAS into clinical practice are multifactorial. They include a growing evidence base of randomized trials supporting its equivalence/noninferiority for stroke prevention when compared with carotid endarterectomy (CEA) among high- and standard-surgical risk patients, patient preference for less invasive treatment options, and the presence of a diverse and

Relationship with Industry: H.D. Aronow is a nonpaid consultant for Silk Road Medical and chairman of the Clinical Events Committee for the Roadster trial; he is also a nonpaid consultant for the Medicines Company and a member of its ENDOMAX trial Executive Committee.
[a] University of Oklahoma Health Sciences Center, Oklahoma City, OK, USA; [b] St Joseph Mercy Hospital, Ann Arbor, MI, USA
* Corresponding author. 5325 Elliott Drive, Suite #202, Ypsilanti, MI 48197.
E-mail address: haronow@michiganheart.com

Intervent Cardiol Clin 3 (2014) 91–103
http://dx.doi.org/10.1016/j.iccl.2013.09.010
2211-7458/14/$ – see front matter © 2014 Elsevier Inc. All rights reserved.

interventional.theclinics.com

expanding group of physicians who are able to perform the procedure.[5,6] Despite its promise, concerns have been raised around the increasing use of CAS.[5] It is a technically demanding procedure for which there is a substantial learning curve, and this learning curve is an important determinant of both its technical success and periprocedural outcomes. In this article, the authors review existing data relating operator and institutional volumes to procedural outcomes and discuss the implications surrounding these relationships.

CAS LEARNING CURVE

Learning curves have been established for other catheter-based cardiovascular procedures, including atrial fibrillation ablation,[7] balloon valvuloplasty,[8] transcatheter aortic valve replacement,[9] transradial percutaneous coronary intervention,[10] complex endovascular interventions,[11] and intracranial angioplasty and stenting.[12] Accordingly, it should come as no surprise that a learning curve might exist for CAS.[13,14] Very poor clinical outcomes were observed in early studies of CAS, which included physicians and institutions with little or no relevant procedural experience (**Table 1**)[15,16]; and periprocedural complications were more common among inexperienced operators.[17] Other studies[18,19] have demonstrated a decrease in the incidence of periprocedural death and stroke over time (see **Table 1**). Both operator and institutional procedural experience likely influence this apparent learning curve.

OPERATOR LEARNING CURVE

Ahmadi and colleagues[20] found that greater experience seemed to overcome the initial learning curve associated with CAS. Among 4 groups of 80 consecutive symptomatic and asymptomatic patients undergoing CAS, they observed that the incidence of 30-day death and neurologic events for CAS procedures was 15% for the first 1 to 80 cases, 5% for cases 81 to 160, 6% for cases 161 to 240, and 5% for cases 241 to 320; the reduction in neurologic complications after the initial 80 interventions was statistically significant ($P = .03$). Similarly, Lin and colleagues[17] analyzed 200 consecutive CAS procedures in 182 patients followed over a 40-month period and observed increased technical success, reduced fluoroscopic time, less total procedure time, reduced contrast volume, and fewer procedure-related complications with the increasing number of CAS procedures performed by an operator (**Figs. 1** and **2**). The 30-day stroke and death rates after 0 to 50 cases and 51 to 100 CAS procedures were 8% and 2% ($P<.05$), respectively; after 101 to 150 and 151 to 200 CAS cases, the event rates were 0% ($P<.03$ compared with group 1) and 0% ($P<.01$ compared with group 1), respectively. Increasing procedural volume ($P = .03$) was identified as an independent predictor of reduced complication rates in Cox regression analysis.

In an observational study using administrative data from Medicare beneficiaries (n = 24,701) who underwent CAS between 2005 and 2007, Nallamothu and colleagues[5] found that only 11.6% of operators performed 12 or more CAS procedures per year (**Fig. 3**). Furthermore, these investigators identified annual operator volume and lifetime operator experience as important factors associated with 30-day mortality and with use of an embolic protection device (**Fig. 4**, **Table 2**).

In the Carotid ACCULINK/ACCUNET Post Approval Trial to Uncover Rare Events (CAPTURE-2), operator (n = 459)-related variables impacting CAS outcomes were evaluated at 180

Table 1
Observational studies suggesting the existence of procedure-related learning curve with CAS

Study Name	Study Period	Population	EPD	Sample Size	Event Rate
Naylor et al,[15]	1996	Sx	No	23	Periprocedural D/S CAS 45.5% vs CEA 0.0%, $P<.05$ Study halted prematurely
Alberts,[16,17]	Pre-2001	Sx	No	219	30-d D/S CAS 12.1% vs CEA 4.5% $P<.05$ Study stopped prematurely
Roubin et al,[18]	1994–1999	Asx + Sx	No	528	30-d D/S rates by year • 1994–1995, 9.3% • 1998–1999, 4.3%

Abbreviations: Asx, asymptomatic; D, death; EPD, embolic protection device; S, stroke; Sx, symptomatic.
  CAS-related complications clustered around physicians with little or no previous CAS experience.

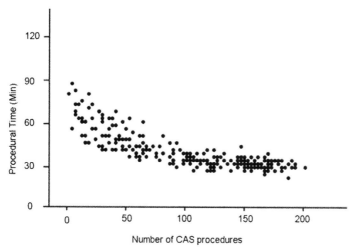

Fig. 1. Correlation of operator experience with procedural time. The procedural time in the first 30 CAS cases routinely exceeded 60 minutes, whereas it was performed within 30 to 40 minutes during the last 100 procedures. (*From* Lin PH, Bush RL, Peden EK, et al. Carotid artery stenting with neuroprotection: assessing the learning curve and treatment outcome. Am J Surg 2005;90(6):859; with permission.)

US hospitals between March 2006 and January 2009. In the asymptomatic, nonoctogenarian subgroup (n = 3388), 4 out of every 5 operators performed CAS without a periprocedural death or stroke. Among the remaining operators, more than 90% had periprocedural death or stroke rates greater than 3%.[21] Operator volume was inversely related to event rate in this cohort (**Fig. 5**), and results were consistent across all specialties (**Fig. 6**).

Institutional Learning Curve

Experienced centers can offer an ideal milieu for ensuring CAS safety even in the hands of new operators because of readily available technical mentoring and peer-to-peer feedback regarding the selection of patients, devices, and images and the prevention and management of complications. Despite the ability of experienced centers to mitigate a less-experienced operator's learning curve, institutional volume remains a major factor

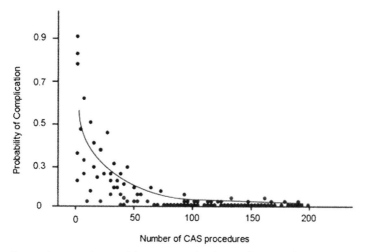

Fig. 2. Correlation of operator experience with postprocedural complications. (*From* Lin PH, Bush RL, Peden EK, et al. Carotid artery stenting with neuroprotection: assessing the learning curve and treatment outcome. Am J Surg 2005;90(6):859; with permission.)

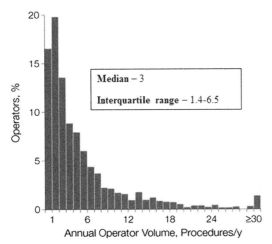

Fig. 3. Distribution of annual operator volume (N = 24,701 patients; operators, 2339); of these, 11,846 procedures were performed by 1792 operators who first performed carotid stenting after its national coverage decision. (*From* Nallamothu BK, Gurm HS, Ting HH, et al. Operator experience and carotid stenting outcomes in Medicare beneficiaries. JAMA 2011;306(12):1340; with permission.)

driving the periprocedural stroke/death risk associated with CAS.[22] In an international survey that included 12,392 CAS procedures performed at 53 centers from 1988 to 2002, the incidence of 30-day death and stroke declined in a stepwise fashion with increasing experience from 4% at centers that had performed only 20 to 50 cases to 1.6% at centers that had performed more than 500 procedures.[23] Verzini and colleagues[24] demonstrated that rates of major stroke and death as well as rates of any stroke and death decreased significantly between the 2001–2003

and 2004–2006 time periods (3.1% vs 0.9% [*P* = .047] and 8.2% vs 2.7% [*P* = .005], respectively) (**Fig. 7**).

In a study of[25] 5535 patients who underwent CAS between 1996 and 2009 in the German CAS Registry of the Arbeitsgemeinschaft Leitende Kardiologische Krankenhausärzte, centers that had performed 1 to 49, 50 to 99, 100 to 199, and more than 200 CAS procedures had respective in-hospital major stroke rates of 2.1%, 1.9%, 1.6%, and 0.9% (*P* = .014 for trend), ipsilateral stroke rates of 3.1%, 2.4%, 2.5%, and 1.6% (*P* = .019 for trend), and combined death or stroke rates of 4.0%, 3.2%, 3.4%, and 2.4% (*P* = .034 for trend) (**Fig. 8**). In a CAPTURE-2[21] subset analysis of asymptomatic nonoctogenarians, 66% of sites (118 of 180) had no death or stroke events. Among the remaining sites, 85% had death and stroke rates exceeding 3%, and an inverse relationship between site experience and event rates was apparent (**Fig. 9**).

In the Pro-CAS study, 5341 CAS procedures were entered into a prospective registry of 25 centers between 1999 and 2005.[26] In a multivariable logistic regression analysis, center experience (>151 superior to 51–150 superior to <50 cases) was found to be a significant and independent predictor of periprocedural stroke and death (**Fig. 10**). Finally, Parlani and colleagues[22] compared outcomes at their institution during 2 sequential time frames. In the first, leader-operators phase (n = 431, 2004–2006), only those operators who performed CAS with a risk for major stroke of less than 2% per year during an earlier (2001–2003) learning-curve period performed subsequent CAS procedures. During the second, expanded-team phase (n = 1026, 2006–2012), 5 new trainees began performing CAS; during this

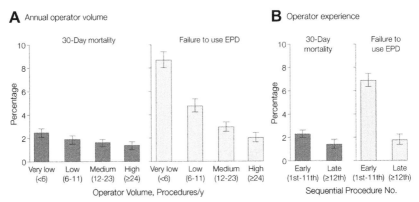

Fig. 4. Unadjusted patient outcomes by annual operator volume and operator experience at the time of the procedure. *P*<.001 for differences across categories for both outcomes. EPD, embolic protection device. Error bars indicate 95% confidence intervals. (*From* Nallamothu BK, Gurm HS, Ting HH, et al. Operator experience and carotid stenting outcomes in Medicare beneficiaries. JAMA 2011;306(12):1341; with permission.)

Table 2
Unadjusted and adjusted ORs of outcomes across categories of operator experience

Operator Experience	30-d Mortality					Failure to Receive Embolic Protection Device				
	No. of Deaths	Unadjusted OR (95% CI)	P Value	Adjusted OR (95% CI)[a]	P Value	No. of Events	Unadjusted OR (95% CI)	P Value	Adjusted OR (95% CI)[a]	P Value
Annual operator volume										
High (≥24) (n = 5127)	71	1 [Reference]	—	1 [Reference]	—	103	1 [Reference]	—	1 [Reference]	—
Medium (12–23) (n = 7059)	114	1.2 (0.8–1.6)	.40	1.2 (0.8–1.7)	.30	208	1.5 (0.8–2.9)	.24	1.6 (0.8–3.2)	.16
Low (6-11) (n = 5752)	109	1.4 (1.0–1.9)	.08	1.4 (1.0–2.0)	.06	274	2.6 (1.4–4.9)	.004	2.9 (1.5–5.6)	.001
Very low (<6) (n = 6763)	167	1.8 (1.3–2.5)	<.001	1.9 (1.4–2.7)	<.001	588	6.4 (3.5–11.7)	<.001	8.1 (4.4–14.9)	<.001
Operator experience at time of procedure										
Late (≥12th procedure) (n = 3732)	53	1 [Reference]	—	1 [Reference]	—	66	1 [Reference]	—	1 [Reference]	—
Early (1st-11th procedure) (n = 8114)	187	1 6 (1.1–2.2)	.005	1.7 (1.2–2.4)	.001	558	4.5 (3.2–6.2)	<.001	4.8 (3.4–6.8)	<.001

Abbreviations: CI, confidence interval; OR, odds rat o.

[a] Adjusted for age, sex, race, Elixhauser comorbidity score, acute stroke, or transient ischemic attack in the 180 days before carotid stenting, carotid endarterectomy in 1 year before carotid stenting, and date of operator's first procedure.

From Nallamothu BK, Gurm HS, Ting HH, et al. Operator experience and carotid stenting outcomes in Medicare beneficiaries. JAMA 2011;306(12):1341; with permission.

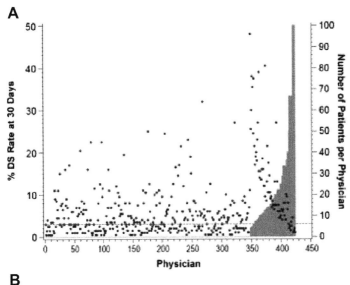

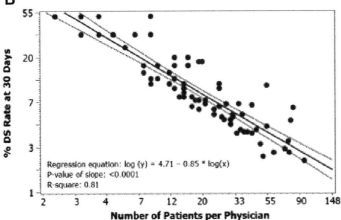

Fig. 5. (*A*) Death and stroke (DS) rate of nonoctogenarian asymptomatic patients and number of patients/physician (dotted horizontal line indicates American Heart Association guideline of 3% event rate for asymptomatic patients). (*B*) Linear regression of DS rate on number of patients/physician. (*From* Gray WA, Rosenfield KA, Jaff MR, et al, CAPTURE 2 Investigators and Executive Committee. Influence of site and operator characteristics on carotid artery stent outcomes: analysis of the CAPTURE 2 (Carotid ACCULINK/ACCUNET Post Approval Trial to Uncover Rare Events) clinical study. JACC Cardiovasc Interv 2011;4(2):243; with permission.)

phase, instruction was provided in a team-based setting on patient, device, and technique selection and all procedural steps and imaging were reviewed. These trainees were able to reproduce the results of leader operators such that periprocedural complication rates during the 2 time frames were statistically similar (stroke/death 3.0% vs 2.1%, $P = .35$). This study suggested that new operators could deliver similar outcomes to those of more experienced operators if they worked in an institutional environment that had already overcome its CAS learning curve for individual operators.[22]

IMPACT OF LEARNING CURVE ON RANDOMIZED CONTROL TRIALS

Although randomized controlled trials (RCTs) remain the gold standard for comparing the safety

and efficacy of revascularization modalities, such as CAS and CEA, the above-described operator- and institutional volume–outcome relationships or learning curves may have important implications for the interpretation of such studies. Although cross-trial comparisons are always difficult given the inherent differences in enrolled patient characteristics, substantially worse CAS outcomes have been apparent among RCTs that required less-experienced CAS operators. CAS operator requirements for comparative RCTs are highlighted in **Table 3** and demonstrate much lower 30-day major adverse event rates for trials with more rigorous CAS operator requirements, such as Stenting and Angioplasty with Protection in Patients at High risk for Endarterectomy (SAPPHIRE)[27,28] and Carotid Revascularization Endarterectomy vs Stenting Trial (CREST),[29] than for others with more liberal requirements, such as

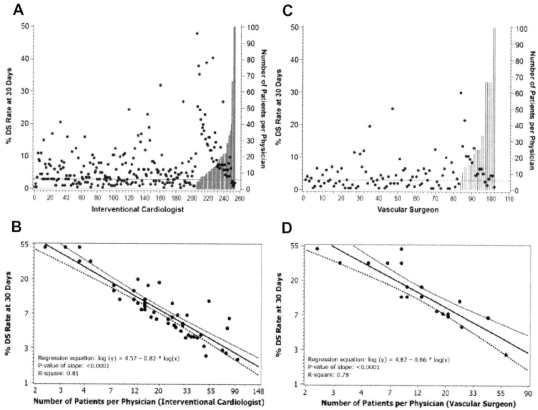

Fig. 6. (A) Death and stroke (DS) rate by number of patients/physician for interventional cardiologists (dotted horizontal line indicates American Heart Association guideline of 3% event rate for asymptomatic patients). (B) Linear regression of DS rate by number of patients for interventional cardiologists. (C) The DS rate by number of patients for vascular surgeons (dotted horizontal line indicates American Heart Association guideline of 3% event rate for asymptomatic patients). (D) Linear regression of DS rate by number of patients for vascular surgeons. (From Gray WA, Rosenfield KA, Jaff MR, et al, CAPTURE 2 Investigators and Executive Committee. Influence of site and operator characteristics on carotid artery stent outcomes: analysis of the CAPTURE 2 (Carotid ACCULINK/ACCUNET Post Approval Trial to Uncover Rare Events) clinical study. JACC Cardiovasc Interv 2011;4(2):244; with permission.)

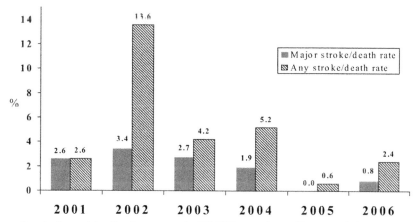

Fig. 7. Perioperative stroke and death rate per year in 627 CAS procedures. (From Verzini F, Cao P, De Rango P, et al. Appropriateness of learning curve for carotid artery stenting: an analysis of periprocedural complications. J Vasc Surg 2006;44(6):1208 [discussion: 1211–2]; with permission.)

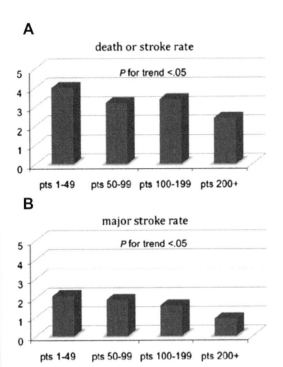

Fig. 8. In-hospital complications: death or stroke rate (*A*) and major stroke rate (*B*). (*From* Staubach S, Hein-Rothweiler R, Hochadel M, et al. The role of endovascular expertise in carotid artery stenting: results from the ALKK-CAS-Registry in 5535 patients. Clin Res Cardiol 2012;101(11):933; with permission.)

Endarterectomy versus Angioplasty in Patients with Symptomatic Severe Carotid Stenosis (EVA-3S),[30] Stent-Supported Percutaneous Angioplasty of the Carotid Artery versus Endarterectomy (SPACE),[31] and International Carotid Stenting Study (ICSS).[32] The importance of mandating adequate CAS operator training was evident from an analysis of CREST lead-in data in which catheter-based subspecialties (interventional radiology and cardiovascular medicine) had significantly lower rates of periprocedural complications when compared with vascular surgeons[33]; on completion of the required lead-in phase training and accrual of greater CAS experience, this cross-specialty quality gap evaporated.[1]

HOW MUCH VOLUME IS ADEQUATE?

Societal recommendations regarding volumes required to achieve and maintain CAS competency (including minimum numbers of proctored cases needed) are not uniform.[2,34] The Italian Consensus Carotid Stenting–SPREAD Joint Committee consensus document[34] recommends more than 75 CAS procedures (>50 as primary

operator). To maintain competence, this document recommends more than 50 CAS procedures annually. In contrast, the clinical competence statement of the Society for Cardiovascular Angiography and Interventions/Society for Vascular Medicine/Society for Vascular Surgery[2] recommends more than 25 CAS procedures in a supervised setting (half as primary operator). Studies relating minimum operator and institutional procedural volume requirements to favorable outcomes with CAS are summarized in **Tables 4** and **5**. These data, when reviewed in aggregate, suggest that operator minimum volume thresholds for achieving competency should be set at or around 75 CAS cases, with approximately 15 to 25 CAS cases required per year for maintenance. Institutional competency thresholds might be set anywhere from 30 to 200 CAS cases per year, depending on historical institutional outcomes.

SIMULATION IN CAS TRAINING

Virtual reality (VR) can help physicians master procedural skills without exposing patients to procedural risks.[37] The US FDA approved VR for CAS training in 2004,[38,39] and recent technological advances have made it feasible to incorporate patient-specific imaging data into VR simulation software, thereby allowing for procedural planning and rehearsal before the actual performance of CAS.[40,41] In a study of 33 operators (11 cardiologists, 19 radiologists, and 3 vascular surgeons), Willaert and colleagues[37] demonstrated that the use of a patient-specific simulator dry run favorably impacted the fluoroscopy time and equipment selection during complex CAS procedures. VR simulation most significantly impacted the fluoroscopy angle (46% of participants), choice of selective catheter (39%), and choice of sheath or guiding catheter (33%) (**Fig. 11**). Compared with experienced physicians (>15 CAS procedures), a numerically higher rate of equipment changes was observed among inexperienced physicians (5–20 CAS procedures). Although these and other differences were not statistically significant, they suggest that VR may allow preprocedural planning to identify the ideal fluoroscopy angles (potentially leading to less patient and operator radiation exposure and less contrast use) as well as selection of the most appropriate catheters before their actual use (potentially minimizing procedural time and catheter manipulation). If borne out in future studies, the institution of VR simulation training might go a long way to reduce the slope of the CAS learning curve.

A

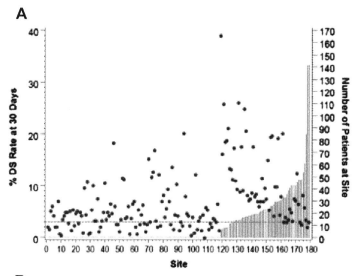

B

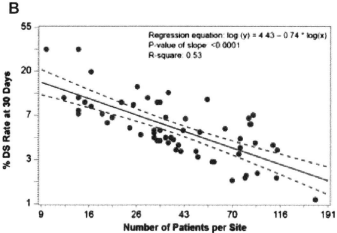

Fig. 9. (*A*) Death and stroke (DS) rate of nonoctogenarian asymptomatic patients by site and number of patients/site (dotted horizontal line indicates American Heart Association guideline of 3% event rate for asymptomatic patients). (*B*) Linear regression of DS on number of patients/site. (*From* Gray WA, Rosenfield KA, Jaff MR, et al, CAPTURE 2 Investigators and Executive Committee. Influence of site and operator characteristics on carotid artery stent outcomes: analysis of the CAPTURE 2 (Carotid ACCULINK/ACCUNET Post Approval Trial to Uncover Rare Events) clinical study. JACC Cardiovasc Interv 2011;4(2):241; with permission.)

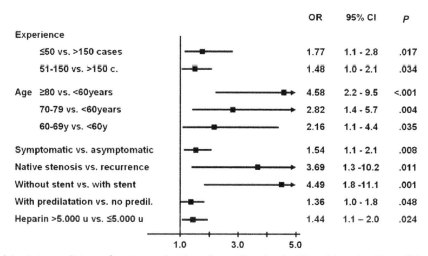

Fig. 10. Multivariate predictors of periprocedural stroke and/or death. OR, odds ratio; CI, confidence interval. (*From* Theiss W, Hermanek P, Mathias K, et al, for the German Society of Angiology/Vascular Medicine, the German Society of Radiology. Predictors of death and stroke after carotid angioplasty and stenting: a subgroup analysis of the Pro-CAS data. Stroke 2008;39(8):2327; with permission.)

Table 3
RCTs suggesting the existence of procedure-related learning curve with CAS

Study Name	Study Period	Population	EPD (%)	Sample Size	30-d Event Rate	Operator Experience
CREST[29]	2000–2008	Asx + Sx	96	2502	MACCE • CEA 4.5% • CAS 5.2% ($P = .38$)	CAS 20[a] CEA 50
SAPPHIRE[27,28]	2000–2002	Asx + Sx	Yes (96)	334	MACCE • CEA 9.8% • CAS 4.8% ($P = .09$)	CAS median 64 Cases per y (20–700) CEA median 30 cases per y (15–100)
EVA-3S[30]	2000–2005	Sx	78–98	527	D/S • CEA 3.9% • CAS 9.6% ($P<.01$)	CAS 12[b] or 5[b] if experience with 30 noncarotid supra-aortic stenting CEA 25
SPACE[31]	2001–2006	Sx	27	1200	D/S • CEA 6.3% • CAS 6.8% P value for noninferiority = .09	CAS 10[b] (perform or assist) CEA ≥25
ICSS[32]	2001–2008	Sx	72	1710	D/S • CEA 4.0% • CAS 7.4% ($P<.01$)	CAS 10[b] CEA 50

Abbreviations: Asx, asymptomatic; CREST, Carotid Revascularization Endarterectomy vs Stenting Trial; D, death; EPD, embolic protection device; EVA-3S, Endarterectomy versus Angioplasty in Patients with Symptomatic Severe Carotid Stenosis; ICSS, International Carotid Stenting Study; MACCE, Major Adverse Cardiac and Cerebrovascular Events; S, stroke; SAPPHIRE, Stenting and Angioplasty with Protection in Patients at High risk for Endarterectomy; SPACE, Stent-Supported Percutaneous Angioplasty of the Carotid Artery versus Endarterectomy; Sx, symptomatic.

[a] Those with more experience (≥30 cases) performed 5 to 10 procedures in the lead-in phase, and those with less experience (<30 cases) performed 10 to 20 procedures in the lead-in phase. Operators were selected by the Interventional Management Committee to participate in the randomized portion of the trial based on experience, training, and lead-in results.

[b] Tutoring for CAS was allowed.

Adapted from White CJ. Carotid artery stent placement. JACC Cardiovasc Interv 2010;3(5):467–74.

Table 4
Data on learning-curve thresholds for individual operators

Study	Period	Sample Size	Learning-Curve Thresholds
Ahmadi et al,[20]	1997–2000	320	30-d neurologic event and death rate 5% vs 15% ($P = .03$) comparing >80 vs <80 CAS procedures
Siena Score Study[35]	2000–2009	2124	OR for 30-d stroke 0.81 (95% CI 0.67–0.95) comparing >100 vs <100 CAS procedures
Lin et al,[17]	2002–2005	200	30-d stroke 2% vs 8% ($P<.05$) for >50 vs <50 CAS procedures
CAPTURE 2[21]	2006–2009	3388	To attain target 30-d D/S rate <3%: >72 CAS procedures
Vogel et al,[13]	2005–2006	18,599	Postprocedure stroke rates 1.5% vs 2.2%. ($P = .02$) comparing >30 CAS per 2 y vs <30 CAS per 2 y
Nallamothu et al,[5]	2005–2007	24,701	30-d mortality 1.4% vs 2.5% ($P<.001$) comparing >24 vs <6 CAS per y

Abbreviations: CI, confidence interval; D, death; OR, odds ratio; S, stroke.

Table 5
Data on learning-curve thresholds for institutions/centers

Study	Period	Sample Size	Learning-Curve Thresholds
Wholey & Al-Mubarek,[36]	1988–2002	53 centers 12,392 cases	30-d D/S 1.3% vs 4.0% comparing >100 CAS cases per center vs <100 cases per center
Pro-CAS Study[26]	1999–2005	25 centers 5341 cases	OR for periprocedural death and stroke 1.77 (CI 1.1–2.8, $P = .02$) comparing ≤50 CAS cases per center vs >150 CAS cases per center OR for periprocedural death and stroke 1.48 (CI 1.0–2.1, $P = .03$) comparing 50–150 CAS cases per center vs >150 CAS cases per center
Vogel et al,[13]	2005–2006	18,599 patients from NIS	Postprocedure stroke rates 1.8% vs 2.4%. ($P = .02$) comparing >60 CAS per center per 2 y vs <60 CAS per center per 2 y
Verzini et al,[24]	2001–2006	627 patients	To attain D/S rates <2% - >195 CAS cases

Abbreviations: CI, confidence interval; D, death; NIS, nationwide inpatient sample; OR, odds ratio; S, stroke. Updated review of the Global CAS Registry.

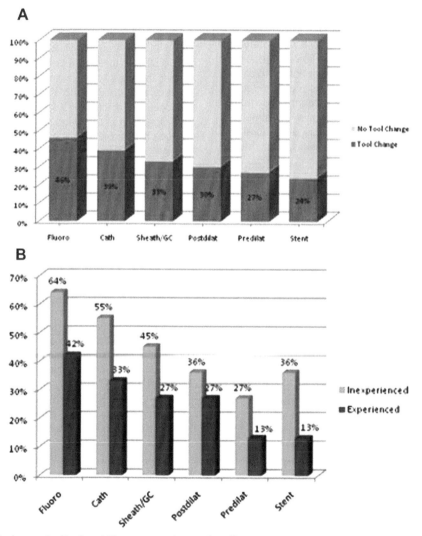

Fig. 11. (*A*) Endovascular Tool and Fluoroscopy change for all participants combined. (*B*) Endovascular Tool and Fluoroscopy change for the inexperienced CAS interventionalists vs the highly experienced interventionalists. Fluoro, fluoroscopy angle; Cath, selective catheter; GC, guiding catheter; Postdilat, balloon postdilation; Predilat, balloon predilation. (*From* Willaert WI, Aggarwal R, Van Herzeele I, et al, European Virtual Reality Endovascular Research Team EVEResT. Patient-specific endovascular simulation influences interventionalists performing carotid artery stenting procedures. Eur J Vasc Endovasc Surg 2011;41(4):497; with permission.)

SUMMARY

There is a clear learning curve, or volume-outcome relationship, for both operators and institutions that perform CAS procedures. This observation has important implications for physician training, operator and site credentialing, and for the interpretation of RCTs comparing CAS with CEA or medical therapy. Ideally, CAS procedural experience should be sufficient to keep periprocedural death/stroke rates less than 3% for asymptomatic patients (<6% for symptomatic patients) in accordance with the American Heart Association's recommendations.[42] Available data suggest that operators need to perform approximately 75 CAS cases before periprocedural complication rates decreased below this threshold, a level that would eliminate all but high-volume operators. Policies that would restrict the use of CAS to highly experienced operators might ensure CAS safety but would come at the expense of limited procedural access. Collaborative, cross-specialty dialogue around such policy decisions is urgently needed if CAS is to remain a viable treatment option for patients with carotid artery stenosis. VR-simulated training initiatives might minimize procedural volume required to achieve proficiency, but that remains to be proven.

REFERENCES

1. White CJ. Carotid artery stent placement. JACC Cardiovasc Interv 2010;3(5):467–74.
2. Rosenfield K, Babb JD, Cates CU, et al. Clinical competence statement on carotid stenting: training and credentialing for carotid stenting–multispecialty consensus recommendations: a report of the SCAI/SVMB/SVS Writing Committee to develop a clinical competence statement on carotid interventions. J Am Coll Cardiol 2005;45(1):165–74.
3. Nallamothu BK, Lu M, Rogers MA, et al. Physician specialty and carotid stenting among elderly Medicare beneficiaries in the United States. Arch Intern Med 2011;171(20):1804–10.
4. Goodney PP, Travis LL, Malenka D, et al. Regional variation in carotid artery stenting and endarterectomy in the Medicare population. Circ Cardiovasc Qual Outcomes 2010;3(1):15–24.
5. Nallamothu BK, Gurm HS, Ting HH, et al. Operator experience and carotid stenting outcomes in Medicare beneficiaries. JAMA 2011;306(12):1338–43.
6. Halm EA. The good, the bad, and the about-to-get ugly: national trends in carotid revascularization: comment on "geographic variation in carotid revascularization among Medicare beneficiaries, 2003-2006". Arch Intern Med 2010;170(14):1225–7.
7. Calvo N, Nadal M, Berruezo A, et al. Improved outcomes and complications of atrial fibrillation catheter ablation over time: learning curve, techniques, and methodology. Rev Esp Cardiol (Engl Ed) 2012; 65(2):131–8.
8. Rihal CS, Nishimura RA, Holmes DR Jr. Percutaneous balloon mitral valvuloplasty: the learning curve. Am Heart J 1991;122(6):1750–6.
9. Feldman T. Learning curve for transcatheter aortic valve replacement. Catheter Cardiovasc Interv 2011;78(7):985–6.
10. Goldberg SL, Renslo R, Sinow R, et al. Learning curve in the use of the radial artery as vascular access in the performance of percutaneous transluminal coronary angioplasty. Cathet Cardiovasc Diagn 1998;44(2):147–52.
11. Riga CV, Bicknell CD, Sidhu R, et al. Advanced catheter technology: is this the answer to overcoming the long learning curve in complex endovascular procedures. Eur J Vasc Endovasc Surg 2011;42(4):531–8.
12. Cai Q, Li Y, Xu G, et al. Learning curve for intracranial angioplasty and stenting in single center. Catheter Cardiovasc Interv 2013. [Epub ahead of print].
13. Vogel TR, Dombrovskiy VY, Graham AM. Carotid artery stenting in the nation: the influence of hospital and physician volume on outcomes. Vasc Endovascular Surg 2010;44(2):89–94.
14. Fiehler J, Jansen O, Berger J, et al. Differences in complication rates among the centres in the SPACE study. Neuroradiology 2008;50(12):1049–53.
15. Naylor AR, Bolia A, Abbott RJ, et al. Randomized study of carotid angioplasty and stenting versus carotid endarterectomy: a stopped trial. J Vasc Surg 1998;28(2):326–34.
16. Bangalore S, Kumar S, Wetterslev J, et al. Carotid artery stenting vs carotid endarterectomy: meta-analysis and diversity-adjusted trial sequential analysis of randomized trials. Arch Neurol 2011;68(2): 172–84.
17. Lin PH, Bush RL, Peden EK, et al. Carotid artery stenting with neuroprotection: assessing the learning curve and treatment outcome. Am J Surg 2005;190(6):850–7.
18. Roubin GS, New G, Iyer SS, et al. Immediate and late clinical outcomes of carotid artery stenting in patients with symptomatic and asymptomatic carotid artery stenosis: a 5-year prospective analysis. Circulation 2001;103(4):532–7.
19. Diethrich EB, Ndiaye M, Reid DB. Stenting in the carotid artery: initial experience in 110 patients. J Endovasc Surg 1996;3(1):42–62.
20. Ahmadi R, Willfort A, Lang W, et al. Carotid artery stenting: effect of learning curve and intermediate-term morphological outcome. J Endovasc Ther 2001;8(6):539–46.
21. Gray WA, Rosenfield KA, Jaff MR, et al, CAPTURE 2 Investigators and Executive Committee. Influence of

site and operator characteristics on carotid artery stent outcomes: analysis of the CAPTURE 2 (Carotid ACCULINK/ACCUNET Post Approval Trial to Uncover Rare Events) clinical study. JACC Cardiovasc Interv 2011;4(2):235–46.

22. Parlani G, De Rango P, Verzini F, et al. Safety of carotid stenting (CAS) is based on institutional training more than individual experience in large-volume centres. Eur J Vasc Endovasc Surg 2013;45(5): 424–30.

23. D'Ayala M, Toursarkissian B, Ferral H, et al. Endovascular treatment of innominate artery stenosis in a bovine aortic arch–a case report. Vasc Endovascular Surg 2003;37(4):279–82.

24. Verzini F, Cao P, De Rango P, et al. Appropriateness of learning curve for carotid artery stenting: an analysis of periprocedural complications. J Vasc Surg 2006;44(6):1205–11 [discussion: 1211–2].

25. Staubach S, Hein-Rothweiler R, Hochadel M, et al. The role of endovascular expertise in carotid artery stenting: results from the ALKK-CAS-Registry in 5,535 patients. Clin Res Cardiol 2012;101(11):929–37.

26. Theiss W, Hermanek P, Mathias K, et al, for the German Society of Angiology/Vascular Medicine, the German Society of Radiology. Predictors of death and stroke after carotid angioplasty and stenting: a subgroup analysis of the Pro-CAS data. Stroke 2008;39(8):2325–30.

27. Yadav JS, Wholey MH, Kuntz RE, et al. Protected carotid-artery stenting versus endarterectomy in high-risk patients. N Engl J Med 2004;351(15): 1493–501.

28. Gurm HS, Yadav JS, Fayad P, et al. Long-term results of carotid stenting versus endarterectomy in high-risk patients. N Engl J Med 2008;358(15): 1572–9.

29. Brott TG, Hobson RW 2nd, Howard G, et al. Stenting versus endarterectomy for treatment of carotid-artery stenosis. N Engl J Med 2010;363(1):11–23.

30. Mas JL, Chatellier G, Beyssen B, et al. Endarterectomy versus stenting in patients with symptomatic severe carotid stenosis. N Engl J Med 2006; 355(16):1660–71.

31. Ringleb PA, Allenberg J, Bruckmann H, et al. 30 day results from the SPACE trial of stent-protected angioplasty versus carotid endarterectomy in symptomatic patients: a randomised non-inferiority trial. Lancet 2006;368(9543):1239–47.

32. Ederle J, Dobson J, Featherstone RL, et al. Carotid artery stenting compared with endarterectomy in patients with symptomatic carotid stenosis (International Carotid Stenting Study): an interim analysis of a randomised controlled trial. Lancet 2010; 375(9719):985–97.

33. Hopkins LN, Roubin GS, Chakhtoura EY, et al. The Carotid Revascularization Endarterectomy versus Stenting Trial: credentialing of interventionalists and final results of lead-in phase. J Stroke Cerebrovasc Dis 2010;19(2):153–62.

34. Cremonesi A, Setacci C, Bignamini A, et al. Carotid artery stenting: first consensus document of the ICCS-SPREAD Joint Committee. Stroke 2006;37(9): 2400–9.

35. Setacci C, Chisci E, Setacci F, et al. Siena carotid artery stenting score: a risk modelling study for individual patients. Stroke 2010;41(6):1259–65.

36. Wholey MH, Al-Mubarek N. Updated review of the global carotid artery stent registry. Catheter Cardiovasc Interv 2003;60(2):259–66.

37. Willaert WI, Aggarwal R, Van Herzeele I, et al, European Virtual Reality Endovascular Research Team EVEResT. Patient-specific endovascular simulation influences interventionalists performing carotid artery stenting procedures. Eur J Vasc Endovasc Surg 2011;41(4):492–500.

38. US FDA, Center for Devices and Radiological Health, Medical Devices Advisory Committee. Circulatory System Devices Panel meeting. Available at: http://www.fda.gov/ohrms/dockets/ac/04/transcripts/4033t1.htm. Accessed September 10, 2013.

39. Gallagher AG, Cates CU. Approval of virtual reality training for carotid stenting: what this means for procedural-based medicine. JAMA 2004;292(24): 3024–6.

40. Cates CU, Patel AD, Nicholson WJ. Use of virtual reality simulation for mission rehearsal for carotid stenting. JAMA 2007;297(3):265–6.

41. Hislop SJ, Hedrick JH, Singh MJ, et al. Simulation case rehearsals for carotid artery stenting. Eur J Vasc Endovasc Surg 2009;38(6):750–4.

42. Brott TG, Halperin JL, Abbara S, et al. 2011 ASA/ACCF/AHA/AANN/AANS/ACR/ASNR/CNS/SAIP/SCAI/SIR/SNIS/SVM/SVS guideline on the management of patients with extracranial carotid and vertebral artery disease. executive summary. A report of the American College of Cardiology Foundation/American Heart Association Task Force on Practice Guidelines, and the American Stroke Association, American Association of Neuroscience Nurses, American Association of Neurological Surgeons, American College of Radiology, American Society of Neuroradiology, Congress of Neurological Surgeons, Society of Atherosclerosis Imaging and Prevention, Society for Cardiovascular Angiography and Interventions, Society of Interventional Radiology, Society of NeuroInterventional Surgery, Society for Vascular Medicine, and Society for Vascular Surgery. Circulation 2011;124(4):489–532.

Complications and Solutions with Carotid Stenting

Robert D. Safian, MD

KEYWORDS

- Carotid artery stenting • Complications • Embolic protection devices

KEY POINTS

- Complications of carotid stenting can be classified as neurologic, cardiovascular, death, carotid, access site, device malfunctions, and general and late complications.
- The risk of most complications is related to readily identifiable patient and anatomic factors.
- Management and outcome of complications require immediate recognition and a team-based approach to patient care.

INTRODUCTION

Patient selection for percutaneous and surgical revascularization for carotid artery stenosis is highly dependent on assessment of the risk/benefit ratio. Carotid artery stenting (CAS) may be associated with a variety of complications (**Box 1**); some are similar to complications arising after carotid endarterectomy (CEA), and some are unique to CAS. Since the introduction of CAS more than 20 years ago, there has been a decline in the risk of most complications due to improvements in operator experience, patient selection, technique, and equipment. Accordingly, this article focuses on the most mature CAS experience when possible, highlighting robust data from large randomized trials and registry studies that included more than 1000 patients, mandatory use of embolic protection devices (EPDs), independent neurologic assessment before and after CAS, and adjudication of all major events by an independent clinical events committee.

NEUROLOGIC COMPLICATIONS

Because the primary purpose of carotid revascularization is stroke prevention, it is compelling that the most important and dreaded complication is stroke. Most published studies of CAS enrolled specific patient populations designated as standard risk (patients considered reasonable candidates for CEA) or high risk (patients considered high risk for CEA on the basis of established clinical and anatomic criteria). The reported risk of stroke for standard and high-risk patients is 1.0% to 4.8%, including ipsilateral major stroke in 0.5% to 2%, ipsilateral minor stroke in 0.5% to 2.9%, and other types of stroke (contralateral or bilateral) in 0.3% to 0.4% (**Table 1**). In the Carotid Revascularization Endarterectomy versus Stenting Trial (CREST), 2502 standard-risk patients were randomized to CAS with distal EPD (n = 1262 patients) or CEA (n = 1240 patients). The risk of procedure-related stroke after CAS (defined as stroke within 30 days) was 4.1%, which included major ipsilateral stroke in 0.9%, minor ipsilateral stroke in 2.9%, and other types of stroke in 0.3%.[1] In another study of 1300 unselected standard-risk and high-risk patients, the risk of procedure-related stroke after CAS with proximal EPD was 0.9%, equally divided between major and minor stroke.[2] Among 4 large registries of high-risk patients, the risk of stroke was 2.8% to 4.8%, including major ipsilateral stroke in 0.8% to 2.0%, minor ipsilateral stroke in 1.4% to 2.9%, and other strokes in 0.4%.[3–5]

Disclosure Statement: No relationships to disclose.
Center for Innovation and Research in Cardiovascular Diseases (CIRC), Beaumont Health System, Oakland University William Beaumont School of Medicine, Royal Oak, MI 48073, USA
E-mail address: rsafian@beaumont.edu

Intervent Cardiol Clin 3 (2014) 105–113
http://dx.doi.org/10.1016/j.iccl.2013.09.004

interventional.theclinics.com

Box 1
Complications of carotid artery stenting

Neurologic complications

  Transient ischemic attack

  Ischemic stroke

  HPS

  ICH

Cardiovascular complications

  VVRs

  VDRs

  AMI

Death

Carotid artery complications

  Dissection

  Perforation

  Thrombosis

  Vasospasm

  Injury to ECA

Device malfunction

  Stent migration

  Stent deformation

General complications

  Access site injury

  Contrast nephropathy

Late complications

  Restenosis

  TVR

  Stent fracture

  Death

  Stroke

  Cognitive dysfunction

Most neurologic complications associated with CAS and CEA can be broadly classified as ischemic injury, hyperperfusion syndrome (HPS), and intracranial hemorrhage (ICH), depending on the primary cause (**Table 2**).[6] This classification is somewhat arbitrary, however, because these conditions often coexist in the same patient. CREST investigators performed a detailed analysis of clinical and imaging characteristics of patients who developed procedure-related stroke (**Table 3**).[7] Clinical characteristics included major and minor strokes in 20.8% and 79.2% of patients, respectively, and 91.7% were identified as ischemic strokes and 8.3% as ICH. Although more than 90% of neurologic deficits were located in the ipsilateral cerebral hemisphere, 9.2% of patients had bilateral or contralateral deficits, suggesting that atheroembolism may originate from the aortic arch and brachiocephalic circulation. Furthermore, catheter or guide wire manipulation, placement and retrieval of EPDs, balloon inflation, and stent deployment may cause cerebral embolization. Imaging findings indicate that 83% of abnormalities involve the anterior circulation, 3% involve the posterior circulation, and 14% involve both circulations. Patterns of ischemic injury include scattered emboli in 38%, isolated cortical infarction in 31%, subcortical infarction in 17%, and bilateral infarction in 14%. These data indicate that most strokes after CAS are minor ischemic ipsilateral injuries, but there is a potentially broad spectrum of clinical and imaging abnormalities.

Approximately two-thirds of strokes after CAS occur during the day of the procedure[7]; most of these are minor and are due to atheroembolism. Complete or partial occlusion of a filter EPD is an important cause of acute neurologic injury that occurs during the CAS procedure and results from accumulation of atherosclerotic debris in the EPD. Clinically, filter occlusion may be indistinguishable from atheroembolic stroke, but this distinction is important because patients with filter occlusion usually respond immediately to filter aspiration and removal. Filter occlusion can usually be distinguished from other causes of cerebral ischemia by angiographic demonstration of impaired blood flow at the level of the filter itself.[8] In contrast, acute intracranial embolization during CAS is usually established by clinical examination of the patient and by anteroposterior and lateral projections of the intracranial circulation with digital subtraction angiography. Angiographic findings may include abrupt cutoff of one or more branches of the anterior or middle cerebral artery or more subtle wedge-shaped defects in the brain blush, visualized best in a lateral projection.

When acute neurologic injuries are recognized after CAS, activation of an institution's comprehensive stroke team is recommended, and individuals with expertise in the management of acute stroke should be consulted immediately. CT imaging of the brain is required to exclude ICH; further treatment recommendations depend on the imaging findings and on the extent of neurologic impairment.

Most strokes that occur on the day of CAS are minor and do not require acute stroke intervention. In contrast, major strokes, including ICH, tend to occur several days after CAS.[7] HPS and ICH are

Table 1
Procedure-related stroke reported in major CAS publications

Study,[Ref] Year	N	Risk	Stroke	Major	Minor	Other
CREST,[1] 2010	2502	SR	4.1	0.9	2.9	0.3
Stabile,[2] 2010	1300	SR, HR	1.0	0.5[a]	0.5[a]	—
CAPTURE-2,[3] 2009	4175	HR	2.8	0.8	1.6	0.4
XACT,[3] 2009	2145	HR	3.6	1.0	2.2	0.4
CASES-PMS,[4] 2007	1493	HR	3.0	1.1	1.4	0.4
CAPTURE,[5] 2007	3500	HR	4.8	2.0	2.9	—

Abbreviations: CAPTURE, Carotid Acculink/Accunet Post-Approval Trial to Uncover Unanticipated or Rare Events; CASES-PMS, CAS with Emboli Protection Surveillance-Post-Marketing Study; HR, high-risk patients; Major, major ipsilateral stroke; Minor, minor ipsilateral stroke; N, number of patients; Other, contralateral or bilateral strokes; Ref, reference number; SR, standard-risk patients; Stroke, all strokes; XACT, Xact Post-Approval Carotid Stent Trial.
   [a] Major and minor strokes not characterized as ipsilateral, contralateral, or bilateral.

inter-related neurologic syndromes with early mortality of nearly 60%. Typical HPS occurs in fewer than 1% of CAS patients and is characterized by a spectrum of neurologic manifestations, ranging from headache, seizures, altered consciousness, focal neurologic deficits, and to cerebral edema, with or without ICH.[9–12] Carotid revascularization may disturb normal autoregulation of intracranial blood flow leading to HPS, particularly in patients with critical bilateral carotid artery stenosis/occlusion and severe hypertension. There seems to be bimodal timing of HPS and ICH after CAS—one occurs within 24 hours of intervention and another occurs several days to weeks after revascularization. A relationship between procedure-related anticoagulation, dual antiplatelet therapy, and HPS/ICH has been postulated but not established. The diagnosis of HPS is based on the presence of clinical features and identification of cerebral edema or ICH by imaging studies. Management includes optimal regulation of blood pressure, treatment of cerebral edema, and anticonvulsant therapy in a neurologic intensive care unit.

Compared with patients without stroke, those with stroke have worse long-term outcome, including a 3-fold greater risk of mortality and a greater likelihood of physical disability; most of the impact on late mortality was due to prior major stroke rather than minor stroke.[7] Accordingly, several studies have evaluated demographic, clinical, anatomic, and procedural variables that seem associated with procedural success, procedure-related complications, and late mortality. Symptomatic carotid stenosis, age greater than 80 years, anatomic complexity of the aortic arch and brachiocephalic circulation, and baseline

Table 2
Neurologic complications after CAS

Complication	Incidence (%)	Risk Factors	Diagnosis	Treatment
Ischemic Stroke	Major 0.5–2.0 Minor 0.5–2.9	Symptomatic stenosis, age >80, complex arch and carotid anatomy, calcified stenosis, baseline cognitive dysfunction	Clinical findings, HCT, MRI	See article by Panagiotis et al elsewhere in this issue
HPS/ICH	<1	Severe HTN, critical bilateral carotid stenosis	Clinical findings, HCT	BP control; treat cerebral edema, anticonvulsant treatment

Abbreviations: BP, blood pressure; HCT, CT of the brain; HTN, hypertension; MRI, MRI of the brain.
   Data from Goldberg JB, Goodney PP, Kumbhani SR, et al. Brain injury after carotid revascularization: outcomes, mechanisms, and opportunities for improvement. Ann Vasc Surg 2011;25:270–86.

Table 3
Clinical and imaging characteristics of stroke patients in CREST

Characteristic	Incidence (%)
Timing of stroke	
Day of CAS	60.5
1–7 d after CAS	20.8
8–30 d after CAS	18.7
Extent of injury	
Major	20.8
Minor	79.2
Etiology	
Ischemic	91.7
ICH	8.3
Neurologic deficits	
Ipsilateral	90.8
Contralateral	4.6
Bilateral	4.6
Location of imaging abnormalities	
Anterior circulation	83
Posterior circulation	3
Anterior and posterior	14
Ischemic pattern by imaging	
Scattered emboli	38
Cortical infarction	31
Subcortical infarction	17
Bilateral infarction	14

Data from Hill MD, Brooks W, Mackey A, et al. Stroke after carotid stenting and endarterectomy in the carotid revascularization endarterectomy versus stenting trial (CREST). Circulation 2012;126:3054–61.

cognitive dysfunction are consistent determinants of neurologic injury after CAS.[13–19] Furthermore, there may be a strong interaction between age greater than 80, anatomic complexity, and baseline cognitive dysfunction, creating less cerebral reserve in the elderly.[13] Although it seems intuitive that EPDs with larger pore diameters and stents

with open cell designs may predispose patients to more cerebral embolization, a clear impact on CAS outcome has not yet been demonstrated.[20,21] Recently, 3 small randomized trials suggested that compared with distal EPDs, proximal EPDs provide better cerebral protection when evaluated by diffusion-weighted magnetic resonance imaging or transcranial Doppler, although both studies were not powered to evaluate the risk of stroke. Nevertheless, these data suggest that more widespread use of proximal EPDs may reduce the risk of stroke, especially in high-risk patients such as the elderly and those with symptomatic carotid stenosis.[22–24] Several clinical tools have been developed and validated, one using anatomic variables to predict procedural success and aid in case selection,[17] one relying on readily available baseline clinical characteristics to predict in-hospital death and stroke,[18] and another relying on clinical characteristics to predict late mortality after CAS.[19]

CARDIOVASCULAR COMPLICATIONS

Most cardiovascular complications associated with carotid stenting are due to dynamic changes in heart rate and blood pressure and can be classified as vasovagal reactions (VVRs) and vasodepressor reactions (VDRs) (**Table 4**). VVRs are characterized by acute bradycardia and hypotension, whereas VDRs are characterized by acute hypotension without bradycardia. VVRs and VDRs are related to stimulation of the carotid baroreceptors, activation of the baroreceptor reflex, enhancement of parasympathetic nerve activity mediated by the glossopharyngeal nerve, and inhibition of sympathetic nerve activity, leading to hypotension. Dynamic changes in heart rate and blood pressure may occur in up to 65% of patients after CAS and CEA, but only 10% to 20% of patients require atropine or transient pressor therapy[25–27]; temporary pacemaker implantation and mechanical hemodynamic support are not required in most patients. Some patients experience sustained hypotension for 12 to 36 hours

Table 4
Cardiovascular complications after CAS

Complication	Incidence (%)	Etiology	Treatment
VVR/VDR	10–20	Stimulation of baroreceptor reflex	Fluid, atropine, and pressors if needed
AMI	0.9–2.4	Type 2 injury; ST elevation is rare	Usually conservative

Data from Refs.[27–29]

and should be maintained on low-dose pressor agents to avoid hypoperfusion by achieving systolic blood pressure 100 to 130 mm Hg. Patients with preexisting hypertension who develop sustained hypotension after carotid stenting should be observed closely to prevent rebound hypertension.

Acute myocardial infarction (AMI) has been reported in 0.9% to 2.4% of patients after CAS (see **Table 4**),[27–29] but more contemporary studies suggest that the risk is less than or equal to 1.1% (**Table 5**).[1–5] Admittedly, the incidence of AMI after CAS is dependent on the patient population (standard risk vs high risk), whether cardiac biomarkers and ECG are obtained after intervention, and the definition of AMI. In CREST, AMI required evidence of myocardial ischemia by symptoms or ECG changes plus elevated cardiac biomarkers; the choice of biomarkers was left to institutional protocols.[30] The risk of AMI after CAS was 1.1% (including 1 patient with ST elevation), and an additional 0.6% had isolated biomarker elevation without symptoms or ECG changes. Biomarker elevation alone, or with associated ECG changes or symptoms of myocardial ischemia, was associated with 3 to 4 times higher risk of late mortality compared with those without biomarker elevation. Furthermore, compared with patients with minor stroke, there was a 5.2-fold greater risk of late mortality in patients with procedure-related AMI. The cause of AMI has not been clearly defined but is most likely a type 2 (demand-induced) myocardial injury.

Table 5
Procedure-related death and AMI reported in major CAS publications

Study,[Ref] Year	N	Risk	Death	AMI
CREST,[1] 2010	2502	SR	0.7	1.1
Stabile,[2] 2010	1300	SR, HR	0.6	0.1
CAPTURE-2,[3] 2009	4175	HR	0.9	0.4
XACT,[3] 2009	2145	HR	0.9	0.2
CASES-PMS,[4] 2007	1493	HR	0.3	0.7
CAPTURE,[5] 2007	3500	HR	1.8	0.9

Abbreviations: CAPTURE, Carotid Acculink/Accunet Post-Approval Trial to Uncover Unanticipated or Rare Events; CASES-PMS, Carotid Artery Stenting with Emboli Protection Surveillance-Post-Marketing Study; HR, high-risk patients; N, number of patients; Ref, reference number; SR, standard-risk patients; XACT, Xact Post-Approval Carotid Stent Trial.

DEATH

Procedure-related mortality is reported in 0.3% to 1.8% of patients (see **Table 5**)[1–5] and may be due to fatal stroke, AMI, bleeding complications, pneumonia, and multiorgan system failure.

CAROTID ARTERY COMPLICATIONS

Local injury to the carotid artery may result in dissection, perforation, and thrombosis; all are rare in contemporary CAS (**Table 6**).[5,27–29,31–36] Dissection of the common carotid artery (CCA) is usually due to the guiding catheter or interventional sheath, particularly if the CCA is tortuous or angulated, and is readily managed in most patients by implantation of a self-expanding stent. Dissection (and rarely perforation) of the internal carotid artery (ICA) may occur in heavily calcified or angulated lesions by an oversized angioplasty balloon (balloon:artery ratio >1). Acute and subacute stent thromboses are probably related to inadequate antiplatelet therapy, problems with stent expansion due to heavily calcified lesions and extrinsic stent compression, and edge dissection. Edge dissections should be corrected with additional stents if possible. Vasospasm in the ICA occurs in 10% to 15% of CAS procedures, is a benign angiographic observation in most cases, and is usually related to the distal EPD. Severe vasospasm generally responds readily to intra-arterial nitroglycerin. Injury or compromise in flow to the external carotid artery (ECA) is probably under-reported and well tolerated. In exceptional circumstances, occlusion of the ECA may result in jaw claudication.

DEVICE MALFUNCTION

Stent malfunction, including stent migration and malformation, is rare in contemporary CAS practice, and occurs in less than 1% of patients.

GENERAL COMPLICATIONS

As is true with other endovascular procedures relying on a retrograde femoral arterial approach, access site complications occur in fewer than 5% of patients.[13,37–39] The most common access sites complications are inguinal hematoma, femoral artery pseudoaneurysm, and retroperitoneal hemorrhage; blood transfusion or vascular repair is required in 2% to 3% of patients.

LATE COMPLICATIONS

Late complications after CAS include (1) anatomic carotid artery problems, such as restenosis, target vessel revascularization (TVR), and stent fracture,

Table 6
Carotid artery complications after CAS

Complication	Incidence (%)	Etiology	Treatment
Dissection (CCA)	<1	Injury from guiding catheter or interventional sheath	Stent
Dissection/perforation (ICA)	<1	Overdistension of calcified stenosis by oversized balloon	Stent for dissection; covered stent for perforation; surgery consultation
Thrombosis	<1	Interruption of DAPT, edge dissection, extrinsic stent compression	Surgery consultation, stent edge dissection if acute
Vasospasm	10–15	Usually from movement of the distal EPD	Intra-arterial NTG if needed
Injury to ECA	10–15	Sidebranch injury; rarely may result in jaw claudication	None

Abbreviations: DAPT, dual antiplatelet therapy; NTG, nitroglycerin.
   Data from Refs.[5,27–29,31–36]

and (2) late adverse outcomes, such as stroke, death, and cognitive dysfunction (**Table 7**). Restenosis after CAS, like restenosis after other endovascular procedures and CEA, is typically due to neointimal proliferation. The risk of restenosis is low: 4% to 6.8% at 1 to 2 years and 6% to 8% at 10 years.[40–43] In CREST, restenosis was defined as peak systolic velocity greater than 300 cm/s by duplex ultrasound, as measured by an independent core laboratory,[43] and was identified in 5.3% of CAS patients at 2 years. Risk factors for restenosis include hyperlipidemia, diabetes, and female gender. Most patients with restenosis are asymptomatic; the best management is unclear,

Table 7
Late complications of CAS

Complication	Incidence (%)	Comment
Restenosis	4–6.8 (1–2 y) 6–8 (10 y)	Most patients are asymptomatic; need for treatment is controversial unless patient is symptomatic.
TVR	0.6–1.8 (1–2 y) 2.4 (3 y)	Symptomatic restenosis is treated by repeat CAS.
Stent fracture	20–30 (18 mo)	Significance is uncertain; diagnosis is overestimated by plain radiograph; fluoroscopy is more specific.
Stroke	10.2[a]	Approximately 50% of late strokes are due to ipsilateral stroke.
Death	10%–30% (5 y)	The risk of later death is dependent on the patient risk profile; high-risk patients have more heart failure and ischemic heart disease and have worse later outcomes.
Cognitive dysfunction	Unknown	Further study is needed. There is evidence that silent atheroembolization can lead to late cognitive impairment, especially in patients with limited cerebral reserve.

[a] Includes all strokes from time of CAS to late follow-up.
   Data from Brott TG, Hobson RW, Howard G, et al. Stenting versus endarterectomy for treatment of carotid-artery stenosis. N Engl J Med 2010;363:11–23; and Gurm HS, Yadav JS, Fayad P, et al. Long-term results of carotid stenting versus endarterectomy in high-risk patients. N Engl J Med 2008;358:1572–9.

but many physicians recommend conservative therapy and close follow-up. Symptomatic restenosis is unusual but, if present, is usually treated with repeat CAS. The risk of TVR after CAS is 0.6% to 1.8% at 1 to 2 years and 2.4% at 3 years.[42,44,45] Stent fractures have been observed in up to 29% of patients at 18 months when specifically sought by plain radiographs,[46] and some occur at sites associated with heavy calcification. Plain radiographs may overestimate the presence of stent fracture; fluoroscopy is reasonable if more accurate diagnosis is required. The relationship between stent fracture, restenosis, and late stroke is poorly defined. There are individual case reports of symptoms associated with severe stent fracture; further study is needed to better define this association.

The most important late complications after CAS are death and stroke (see **Table 7** and **Table 8**).[1,45] A vast majority of late deaths are unrelated to stroke and are due to cardiac causes, pulmonary disease, and cancer; cardiovascular mortality is particularly prevalent among high-risk patients. Approximately 50% to 70% of late strokes after CAS are due to ischemic events in the distribution of the ipsilateral carotid artery, and most are minor strokes. Although not yet reported in clinical trials of CAS or CEA, there is growing interest in the problem of asymptomatic incidental cerebral embolization that occurs during a large variety of invasive procedures and its relationship to cognitive dysfunction, memory loss, and dementia.[47]

Table 8
Late outcomes after CAS in CREST and SAPPHIRE[a]

	CREST	SAPPHIRE
N	2502	334
Risk profile	Standard risk	High risk
Follow-up duration	4 y	3 y
Death	11.3	18.6[b]
Stroke	10.2	9.0
Major ipsilateral	1.4	1.2
Minor ipsilateral	4.5	5.4
Other	4.9	3.0
Death/stroke	6.4	—
Symptomatic patients	8.0	—
Asymptomatic patients	4.5	—
Primary endpoint[c]	7.2	24.6
Annual risk of ipsilateral stroke	1.4	2.2

Abbreviations: N, number of patients enrolled in trial; SAPPHIRE, Stenting and Angioplasty with Protection in Patients at High Risk for Endarterectomy.

[a] Late outcomes include periprocedural adverse events within 30 days after CAS.

[b] Cardiac death in 9%, fatal stroke in 1.8%, and other deaths in 7.8%.

[c] Defined as 30-day risk of death, any stroke, AMI plus death, and ipsilateral stroke at last follow-up.

Data from Brott TG, Hobson RW, Howard G, et al. Stenting versus endarterectomy for treatment of carotid-artery stenosis. N Engl J Med 2010;363:11–23; and Gurm HS, Yadav JS, Fayad P, et al. Long-term results of carotid stenting versus endarterectomy in high-risk patients. N Engl J Med 2008;358:1572–9.

REFERENCES

1. Brott TG, Hobson RW, Howard G, et al. Stenting versus endarterectomy for treatment of carotid-artery stenosis. N Engl J Med 2010;363:11–23.
2. Stabile E, Salemme L, Sorropago G, et al. Proximal endovascular occlusion for carotid artery stenting. J Am Coll Cardiol 2010;55:1661–7.
3. Gray WA, Chaturvedi S, Verta P, et al. Thirty-day outcomes for carotid artery stenting in 6320 patients from 2 prospective, multicenter, high-surgical-risk registries. Circ Cardiovasc Interv 2009;2:159–66.
4. Katzen BT, Criado FJ, Ramee SR, et al. Carotid artery stenting with emboli protection surveillance study: thirty-day results of the CASES-PMS study. Catheter Cardiovasc Interv 2007;70:316–23.
5. Gray WA, Yadav JS, Verta P, et al. The CAPTURE registry: results of carotid stenting with embolic protection in the post approval setting. Catheter Cardiovasc Interv 2007;69:341–8.
6. Goldberg JB, Goodney PP, Kumbhani SR, et al. Brain injury after carotid revascularization: outcomes, mechanisms, and opportunities for improvement. Ann Vasc Surg 2011;25:270–86.
7. Hill MD, Brooks W, Mackey A, et al. Stroke after carotid stenting and endarterectomy in the carotid revascularization endarterectomy versus stenting trial (CREST). Circulation 2012;126:3054–61.
8. Casserly IP, Abou-Chebl A, Fathi RB, et al. Slow-flow phenomenon during carotid artery intervention with embolic protection devices. J Am Coll Cardiol 2005;46:1466–72.
9. Moulakakis KG, Myloras SN, Syfroeras GS, et al. Hyperperfusion syndrome after carotid revascularization. J Vasc Surg 2009;49:1060–8.
10. Abou-Chebl A, Yadav JS, Reginelli JP, et al. Intracranial hemorrhage and hyperperfusion syndrome following carotid artery stenting. J Am Coll Cardiol 2004;43:1596–601.
11. Henry M, Gopalakrishnan L, Rajagopal S, et al. Bilateral carotid angioplasty and stenting. Catheter Cardiovasc Interv 2005;64:275–82.

12. Brantley HP, Kiessling JL, Milteer HB Jr, et al. Hyperperfusion syndrome following carotid artery stenting: the largest single-operator series to date. J Invasive Cardiol 2009;21:27–30.

13. Werner M, Bausback Y, Sven Braunlich S, et al. Anatomic variables contributing to a higher periprocedural incidence of stroke and TIA in carotid artery stenting: Single center experience of 833 consecutive cases. Catheter Cardiovasc Interv 2012;80: 321–8.

14. Khatri R, Chaudhry SA, Vazquez G, et al. Age differential between outcomes of carotid angioplasty and stent placement and carotid endarterectomy in general practice. J Vasc Surg 2012;55:72–8.

15. Naggara O, Touzé E, Beyssen B, et al. Anatomical and technical factors associated with stroke or death during carotid angioplasty and stenting. Stroke 2011;42:380–8.

16. Zhou W, Hitchner E, Gillis K, et al. Prospective neurocognitive evaluation of patients undergoing carotid interventions. J Vasc Surg 2012;56:1571–8.

17. Macdonald S, Lee R, Williams R, et al. Towards safer carotid artery stenting a scoring system for anatomic suitability. Stroke 2009;40:1698–703.

18. Hawkins BM, Kennedy KF, Giri J, et al. Pre-procedural risk quantification for carotid stenting using the CAS score. J Am Coll Cardiol 2012;60:1617–22.

19. Hoke M, Ljubuncic E, Steinwender C, et al. A validated risk score to predict outcomes after carotid stenting. Circ Cardiovasc Interv 2012;5:841–9.

20. Longhmanpour NA, Siewiorek GM, Wanamaker KM, et al. Assessing the impact of distal protection filter design characteristics on 30-day outcomes of carotid artery stenting procedures. J Vasc Surg 2013; 57:309–17.

21. Tadros RO, Spyris CT, Vouyouka AG, et al. Comparing the embolic potential of open and closed cell stents during carotid angioplasty and stenting. J Vasc Surg 2012;56:89–95.

22. Bijuklic K, Wandler A, Hazizi F, et al. The PROFI Study (Prevention of Cerebral Embolization by Proximal Balloon Occlusion Compared to Filter Protection During Carotid Artery Stenting): a prospective randomized trial. J Am Coll Cardiol 2012;59: 1383–91.

23. Montorsi P, Caputi L, Galli S, et al. Microembolization during carotid artery stenting in patients with high-risk, lipid-rich plaque: a randomized trial of proximal versus distal embolic protection. J Am Coll Cardiol 2011;58:1656–63.

24. Leal I, Orgaz A, Flores A, et al. A diffusion-weighted magnetic resonance imaging-based study of transcervical carotid stenting with flow reversal versus transfemoral filter protection. J Vasc Surg 2012;56: 1585–90.

25. Cayne NS, Faries PL, Trocciola SM, et al. Carotid angioplasty and stent-induced bradycardia and hypotension: impact of prophylactic atropine administration and prior carotid endarterectomy. J Vasc Surg 2005;41:956–61.

26. Leisch F, Kerschner K, Hofmann R, et al. Carotid sinus reactions during carotid artery stenting: predictors, incidence, and influence on clinical outcome. Catheter Cardiovasc Interv 2003;58: 516–23.

27. Coward LJ, Featherstone RL, Brown MM. Percutaneous transluminal angioplasty and stenting for carotid artery stenosis. Cochrane Database Syst Rev 2004;(2):CD000515.

28. Gray WA, Hopkins LN, Yadav S, et al. Protected carotid stenting in high-surgical-risk patients: the ARCHeR results. J Vasc Surg 2006;44:258–68.

29. Coward LJ, Featherstone RL, Brown MM. Safety and efficacy of endovascular treatment of carotid artery stenosis compared with carotid endarterectomy: a Cochrane systematic review of the randomized evidence. Stroke 2005;36:905–11.

30. Blackshear JL, Cutlip DE, Roubin GS, et al. Myocardial infarction after carotid artery stenting and carotid endarterectomy: results from the Carotid Revascularization Endarterectomy Stenting Trial. Circulation 2011;123:2571–8.

31. Roubin GS, Yadav S, Iyer SS, et al. Carotid stent-supported angioplasty: a neurovascular intervention to prevent stroke. Am J Cardiol 1996;78:8–12.

32. Dietrich EB, Ndiaye M, Reid DB. Stenting in the carotid artery: initial experience in 100 patients. J Endovasc Surg 1996;3:42–62.

33. Tong FC, Cloft HJ, Joseph GJ, et al. Abciximab rescue in acute carotid stent thrombosis. AJNR Am J Neuroradiol 2000;21:1750–2.

34. Chaturvedi S, Sohrab S, Tselis A. Carotid stent thrombosis: report of 2 fatal cases. Stroke 2001;32: 2700–2.

35. Buhk JH, Wellmer A, Knauth M. Late in-stent thrombosis following carotid angioplasty and stenting. Neurology 2006;66:1594–6.

36. Kwon BJ, Han MH, Kang HS, et al. Protection filter-related events in extracranial carotid artery stenting: a single-center experience. J Endovasc Ther 2006; 13:711–22.

37. Cil BE, Turkbey B, Canyigit M, et al. An unusual complication of carotid stenting: spontaneous rectus sheath hematoma and its endovascular management. Diagn Interv Radiol 2007;13:46–8.

38. Zorger N, Finkenzeller T, Lenhart M, et al. Safety and efficacy of the Perclose suture-mediated closure device following carotid artery stenting under clopidogrel platelet blockade. Eur Radiol 2004; 14:719–22.

39. Gupta A, Bhatia A, Ahuja A, et al. Carotid stenting in patients older than 65 years with inoperable carotid artery disease: a single-center experience. Catheter Cardiovasc Interv 2000;50:1–8.

40. Gröschel K, Riecker A, Schulz JB, et al. Systematic review of early recurrent stenosis after carotid angioplasty and stenting. Stroke 2005;36:367–73.

41. Bergeron P, Roux M, Khanoyan P, et al. Long-term results of carotid stenting are competitive with surgery. J Vasc Surg 2005;41:213–21.

42. CaRESS Steering Committee. Carotid Revascularization Using Endarterectomy or Stenting Systems (CaRESS) phase I clinical trial: 1-year results. J Vasc Surg 2005;42:213–9.

43. Lal BK, Beach KW, Roubin GS, et al. Restenosis after carotid artery stenting and endarterectomy: a secondary analysis of CREST, a randomized controlled trial. Lancet Neurol 2012;11:755–63.

44. Yadav JS, Wholey MH, Kunt RE, et al. Protected carotid-artery stenting versus endarterectomy in high-risk patients. N Engl J Med 2004;351:1493–501.

45. Gurm HS, Yadav JS, Fayad P, et al. Long-term results of carotid stenting versus endarterectomy in high-risk patients. N Engl J Med 2008;358:1572–9.

46. Ling AJ, Mwipatayi P, Gandhi T, et al. Stenting for carotid artery stenosis: fractures, proposed etiology and the need for surveillance. J Vasc Surg 2008;47:1220.

47. Gress D. The problem with asymptomatic cerebral embolic complications in vascular procedures. J Am Coll Cardiol 2012;60:1614–6.

Percutaneous Treatment of Vertebral Artery Stenosis

J. Stephen Jenkins, MD, FSCAI, FSVM

KEYWORDS

- Vertebrobasilar insufficiency • Vertebral artery stenosis • Vertebrobasilar system
- Endovascular intervention • Vertebral artery angioplasty • Vertebral artery stent
- Peripheral vascular disease

KEY POINTS

- Endovascular treatment of the ostial and proximal portion of the vertebral artery is a safe and effective technique for alleviating symptoms and improving cerebral blood flow to the posterior circulation.
- Vertebral artery angioplasty can be performed with high technical and clinical success rates, low complication rates and durable long-term results.
- Although restenosis rates vary widely, the durability of vertebral artery angioplasty is evidenced by low restenosis rates in several large series reported in the literature using multiple treatment options, including balloon angioplasty alone, bare metal stents, and drug-coated stents.
- Endovascular stenting of vertebral artery atherosclerotic disease in patients who fail medical therapy should be considered first-line therapy despite the absence of randomized trials demonstrating superiority of endovascular therapy.

 Videos of stent deployment accompany this article at http://www.interventional.theclinics.com/

INTRODUCTION

Eighty percent of strokes are ischemic in origin, the vertebrobasilar system (VBS) responsible for approximately 25% of cases, and they manifest symptoms or posterior circulation ischemia.[1,2] Atherosclerotic occlusion or thrombosis of the VBS carries a poor prognosis, with mortality rates approximating 80%.[3,4] Vertebral artery insufficiency and stenosis with posterior circulation symptoms refractory to medical therapy carry a 5% to 11% incidence of stroke or death at 1 year.[5] Reversible neurologic deficits caused by extracranial vertebral artery disease carry a 5-year stroke rate of 30%.[6–8]

Patients with documented peripheral vascular disease or positive markers for atherosclerosis have a 40% incidence of vertebral artery stenosis (VAS).[9] Clinical presentation of symptomatic posterior circulation ischemia correlates with a 25% to 40% incidence of VAS. In a large series of 3800 patients who were referred for angiography because of symptomatic cerebrovascular disease, there was a 40% incidence of unilateral VAS and a 10% incidence of total occlusion of 1 vertebral artery.[10] Another large series of 4748 patients with ischemic stroke demonstrated extracranial VAS present in 18% of cases on the right and 22.5% on the left. VAS was the second most common location for extracranial arterial stenosis behind carotid bifurcation disease.[11]

Despite this increased incidence of VAS in patients with documented peripheral artery disease

Disclosures: None.
Interventional Cardiology, John Ochsner Heart and Vascular Institute, 1514 Jefferson Highway, New Orleans, LA 70121, USA
E-mail address: sjenkins@ochsner.org

Intervent Cardiol Clin 3 (2014) 115–122
http://dx.doi.org/10.1016/j.iccl.2013.09.005

(PAD), posterior circulation symptoms are frequently unrecognized and underdiagnosed. Noninvasive ultrasound imaging of the proximal portion of the vertebral artery is often difficult and incomplete, requiring invasive testing to demonstrate stenosis in the most common location for disease to occur in this vessel.[12] Computed tomographic angiography and magnetic resonance angiography has been used more recently to evaluate the proximal vertebral artery, but their ability to reliably detect vertebral disease is not available.[13]

INDICATIONS AND PATIENT SELECTION

Patients should be considered for vertebral artery revascularization if symptoms do not resolve despite maximal medical therapy.

Symptoms consistent with posterior circulation ischemia include dizziness, drop attacks, diplopia, gait disturbance, dysphasia, and bilateral hemianopia.[14]

Less common symptoms of posterior circulation ischemia include confusion, global amnesia, syncope, occipital headaches, nausea, vomiting, nystagmus, bilateral facial numbness, cortical blindness, and altered mental status.[15]

Revascularization therapy for symptomatic vertebrobasilar insufficiency (VBI) is reasonable in patients with bilateral vertebral stenosis greater than 70; unilateral vertebral stenosis greater than 70 in the presence of an occluded or hypoplastic contralateral vertebral artery; or artery-to-artery embolism even in the presence of unilateral stenosis.[16,17] It should also be considered if vertebral angioplasty would increase total cerebral blood flow to patients with diffuse atherosclerotic disease involving occlusions of both carotid arteries.[18]

Revascularization of the vertebral artery should not be attempted if the vessel is totally occluded.

Even though technical success could be accomplished in some percentage of total occlusions, the distal embolic debris would be clinically devastating due to territory supplied by V4 and the basilar artery. Revascularization of vertebral artery total occlusions should be avoided to prevent cerebellar, midbrain, pons, medullary, or brainstem infarctions. Therefore, total occlusion of the vertebral artery is a contraindication to endovascular treatment.[19]

RELEVANT ANATOMY

Anatomy of the anterior and posterior circulation and the circle of Willis should be defined prior to any decision regarding percutaneous revascularization of the vertebral artery (**Fig. 1**). Diagnostic angiography of the aortic arch with selective carotid and vertebral artery angiography is then correlated with the posterior circulation symptom complex to determine which artery requires revascularization.

The vertebral artery originates at a 90° angle as the first branch of the subclavian artery and is divided into 4 segments defined by bony landmarks illustrated in **Fig. 2**. These 4 segments are designated V1 to V4, and the ostium is designated as VO. The ostium and V1 segment are the most frequent locations of disease in this vessel treated with percutaneous intervention.

The V1 segment courses between the longus colli and scalenus anterior muscles until it enters the transverse foramina of either the fifth or sixth cervical vertebrae and becomes the V2 segment. The V1 segment can be treated percutaneously with ease provided it is not tortuous or redundant.[20]

The V2 segment begins as it enters the transverse foramina of C5 or C6, courses through the

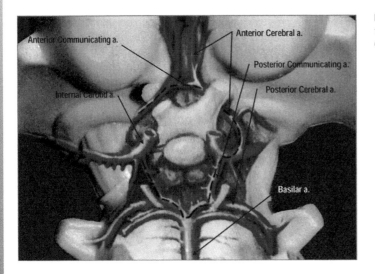

Fig. 1. Circle of Willis anatomy. (*Courtesy of* J. Stephen Jenkins, MD, New Orleans, LA.)

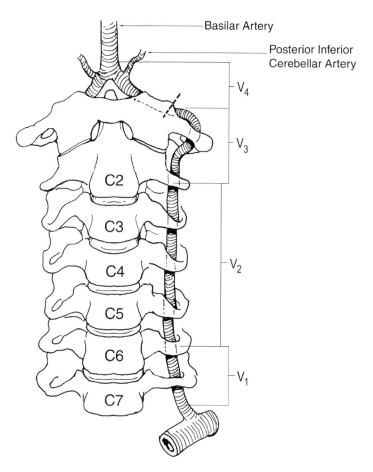

Basilar Artery

Posterior Inferior
Cerebellar Artery

V_4

V_3

C2

C3

C4 — V_2

C5

C6 — V_1

C7

Fig. 2. Vertebral artery anatomy. (*From* Jenkins JS, Collins TJ. Vertebrobasilar insufficiency. In: Jaff MR, White CJ, editors. Textbook of vascular disease, diagnostic and therapeutic approaches. Minneapolis (MN): Cardiotext Publishing, LLC; 2011. p. 99; with permission.)

bony canal of the transverse foramina C6 to C2, and ends when it exits the transverse foramina of C2. The V2 segment is also easily treated with percutaneous intervention due to favorable anatomic features such as its short distance from the subclavian artery and a straight course through the transverse foramina of the cervical vertebra.

The V3 segment begins as it exits the transverse foramina of C2 and ends as the vessel penetrates the dura mater through the foramen magnum and becomes an intracranial vessel. Percutaneous intervention in the V3 segment is more difficult, as this segment is extremely tortuous to allow mobility of the alanto-axial and the alanto-occipital joint. Balloon expandable stents should be avoided in this flexible joint region. Avoiding extreme tortuosity and use of short self-expanding stents increases success in this segment.

The V4 segment extends along the inferior portion of the pons and joins the contra lateral vertebral artery to form the basilar artery. Anterior spinal communicator arteries originate from the V4 segments bilaterally, join in the midline, and perfuse the anterior two-thirds of the spinal cord.

Therefore, percutaneous intervention in the V4 segment is extremely risky and is rarely attempted except for acute stroke intervention or severe symptoms unresponsive to medical therapy. Occlusion of the anterior spinal communicators can cause major deficits and brain stem infarcts.

There are several anatomic variants to consider when performing selective vertebral artery angiography. The left vertebral artery origin is anomalous in 5% to 10% of the population arising from the aortic arch just proximal to the left subclavian artery or from the proximal left subclavian artery.[21,22] The right vertebral artery arises from the aorta distal to the left subclavian artery or from the right carotid artery in 0.18% of the population.[23] Hypoplasia of 1 vertebral artery with congenital absence of the V4 segment and termination in the posterior inferior cerebellar artery occurs is 6% or the population.[24]

PREPROCEDURE PLANNING

Digital subtraction contrast angiography is the gold standard to identify vertebral basilar atherosclerotic disease. A complete angiographic evaluation includes an aortic arch and 4-vessel study with selective angiography of bilateral carotid and vertebral arteries including intracranial imaging. The intracranial anatomy of the anterior and posterior circulation and the circle of Willis should also be defined in several views making certain to identify any collateral blood supply. Vertebral artery anatomy and collateral flow is then correlated with the posterior circulation symptom complex to determine which artery requires revascularization. A team approach is advantageous, utilizing a neurologist, a neuro-interventional radiologist, and a cardiologist to make revascularization decisions. Unilateral VAS or occlusion is well tolerated in the absence of proximal atherosclerotic occlusive disease.

DESCRIPTION OF PROCEDURE
Access Site

Femoral is used 80% of the time. Ipsilateral brachial or radial artery access is used 20% of the time if the proximal vertebral artery is acutely angulated when imaged from the femoral access. A combination of femoral and upper extremity access is used in complex cases involving subclavian artery atherosclerotic disease.

Sheath Sizes

4F diagnostic catheters do not provide adequate visualization when performing selective vertebral or carotid artery angiography; therefore, a 5F diagnostic sheath is used. A 6F to 8F sheath is used for vertebral artery interventions.

Angiographic Catheter

A 5F or 6F pigtail catheter is used to perform an aortic arch angiogram in the left anterior oblique view to rule out anomalous vertebral artery origin. A 5F Berenstein is the diagnostic catheter of choice. Note: 5F or 6F Judkins right, internal mammary, or Vitek curve catheters are acceptable; multipurpose curves are used for the brachial of radial access. A 6F to 8F Judkins right or multipurpose guiding catheter can be used to perform most vertebral interventions. A curve similar to the diagnostic imaging catheter should be chosen.

Diagnostic Guidewire

0.035″ glide wire or J-wire is used to advance the diagnostic catheter distal to the vertebral artery ostium. Continuous pressure is monitored while engaging the vertebral artery ostium.

Interventional Guidewire

A 0.014″ soft guide wire is recommended with a rapid exchange (RX), or monorail balloon. An embolic protection device should be used in all vertebral arteries with an adequate landing zone distal to the index lesion. There are no embolic protection devices with US Food and Drug Administration (FDA) approval for use in the vertebral artery.

Percutaneous Transluminal Angioplasty Balloons

Balloon length is determined by the lesion length and should cover the lesion completely. Balloon diameter should be 0.5 mm less that the reference vessel diameter.

Stent

Balloon expandable coronary or peripheral stents on a 0.014 platform work well in the vertebral artery ostium (Videos 1–8). Proximal vertebral artery stents are commonly extended into the subclavian artery by 1 to 2 mm to assure complete coverage of the ostium. Both balloon expandable and self-expanding stents are acceptable in the V1 and V2 segment if the vertebral artery ostium is not involved.

Interventional Tips

Embolic protection devices are not FDA approved for use in the vertebral artery; however, it is reasonable to use these devices with a comfortable landing zone distal to the index lesion. The guide wire should be kept within view at all times during the procedure to prevent perforation and causing fatal intracranial hemorrhage. Particular care should be exercised when using a hydrophilic guide wire.

Imaging

Digital subtraction techniques are essential when imaging intracranial anatomy. A minimum image intensifier size of 12 in is necessary to adequately image the intracranial vessels. The technique of digital subtraction rotational angiography limits contrast and provides up to 180° of angles with which to view vessels. Nonionic, iso-osmolar contrast should be used for intracranial angiography.

IMMEDIATE POSTPROCEDURAL CARE

Low-dose weight-adjusted heparin to maintain an activated clotting time greater than 200 seconds is the procedural anticoagulant of choice for vertebral artery intervention. Bivalirudin is an acceptable alternative in patients with heparin-induced thrombocytopenia. All patients should be loaded with aspirin (325 mg) and plavix (300 mg) at least 1 day prior to the procedure. Plavix (75 mg daily) should be continued for 1 month after the procedure if bare metal stents are used, and aspirin (81 mg daily) should be continued indefinitely. If drug-eluting stents are used, dual antiplatelet therapy should be continued at least 1 year. Dual antiplatelet therapy is frequently continued indefinitely with the use of drug eluting stents to prevent the occurrence of late stent thrombosis.

Duplex ultrasound should be performed at 3, 6, and 12 months and yearly thereafter, if VBI symptoms resolve. Patients with recurrent VBI symptoms should undergo repeat angiography to identify restenosis or progression of atherosclerotic disease. Intracranial intervention above the V3 segment is followed with mandatory 1-year selective angiography.

CLINICAL RESULTS IN LITERATURE

Since the first successful treatment of a VAS with balloon angioplasty by Sundt and colleagues[25] in 1980, multiple case reports and case series have been reported describing the successful use of endovascular techniques to treat posterior circulation atherosclerotic disease. Endovascular treatment of VAS still remains a major challenge today due to a lack of randomized controlled trials and a nonpayment decision by Medicare in 1984.

Table 1
Review of results of endovascular stent for VAS

Author,[Ref] Year	n	Technical Success Rate (%)	Procedural Complications	Improvement in Symptoms	Mean Follow-up (mo)	Late Stroke	Restenosis
Jenkins et al,[15] 2001	32	100	TIA (1)	31/32	10.6	0/32	1/32
Albuquerque et al,[29] 2003	33	97	CVA (1)	27/33	16.2	1/33	43%
Chastain et al,[30] 1999	50	98	None	48/50	25	1/50	10%
Lin et al,[31] 2004	58	100	CVA (3)	56/58	31.3	0/58	25%
Weber et al,[32] 2005	38	95	TIA (1)	23/26	11	0/26	36%
Cloud et al,[33] 2003	14	100	TIA (1)	13/14	33.6	1/14	36%
SSYLVIA Study Investigators,[34] 2004	18	100	None	—	6	2/18	43%
Jenkins et al,[78] 2010	112	100	TIA (1)	95/105	29	5/105	13%
Hatano et al,[35] 2011	117	99	TIA (2)	113/116	6	2/117	10%
Lin et al,[36] 2006	80	100	CVA (3)	78/80	12	0/80	28%
Karameshev et al,[37] 2010	10	100	TIA (1)	10/10	10	0/10	10%
Lin et al,[38] 2008	11	100	None	11/11	8	0/11	0%
Zhou et al,[39] 2011	61	100	None	—	12	—	27%
Gupta et al,[40] 2006	31	100	None	31/31	4	0/31	7%
Vajda et al,[41] 2009	48	100	None	48/48	7	0/48	12%

Abbreviations: CVA, cerebral vascular accident; TIA, transient ischemic attack.

Despite these challenges, review of previous studies demonstrates that endovascular treatment of the vertebral artery is safe, feasible, and durable, with high technical success rates and low clinical complication rates (**Table 1**).

Only one, small, prospective randomized trial comparing VAS with medical therapy (Carotid and Vertebral Artery Transluminal Angioplasty Study [CAVATAS] n = 16 patients) has been published. In this trial, 8 patients were randomized to medical therapy, and 8 patients underwent successful endovascular stenting with no strokes or deaths occurring within 30 days in either group. There were no vertebral strokes in either group at mean follow-up of 4.7 years. Because no patient in either arm had recurrent stroke, there was no difference in outcomes among either group in this small, randomized trial.[26]

In the Cochrane Review, 173 cases of VAS stenting were identified out of 313 cases of vertebral artery intervention. Meta-analysis of these 20 studies found a 30-day major stroke and death rate of 3.2% and a 30-day transient ischemic attack (TIA) and nondisabling stroke rate of 3.2%. These data would suggest that vertebral artery stenting is safe and effective, although an obvious selection bias exists.[3]

In another meta-analysis of 300 proximal vertebral artery interventions at a mean follow-up of 14.2 months, the risk of death was 0.3%; the risk of peri-procedural neurologic complications was 5.5%, and the risk of posterior stroke was 0.7%. After a mean of 12 months (range 3–25 months), restenosis occurred in 26% of cases (range 0%–43%); however, this did not correlate with recurrent symptoms.[27]

A review of long-term results of previous series with at least 10 patients on endovascular stent treatment for extracranial vertebral artery stenosis is shown in **Table 1**.

POTENTIAL COMPLICATIONS/MANAGEMENT

Peri-procedural complications of vertebral artery stenting include both adverse events associated with vertebral angioplasty as well all other complications that accompany percutaneous procedures, including death, access site bleeding, vessel rupture, and renal failure. Major/minor stroke and TIA prior to hospital discharge are considered direct complications of the endovascular procedure, and management of these complications requires repeat imaging to treat mechanical complications of the angioplasty procedure or catheter-directed thrombolysis for thromboembolic events. The frequencies of these major adverse events are shown in **Table 2**.[27,28]

Table 2 Major adverse events associated with vertebral angioplasty	
Event	Frequency (%)
TIA	1–2
Major stroke	1–2
Myocardial infarction	0
Death	<1

Data from Eberhardt O, Naegele T, Raygrotzki S, et al. Stenting of vertebrobasilar arteries in symptomatic atherosclerotic disease and acute occlusion: case series and review of the literature. J Vasc Surg 2006;43: 1145–54; and Jenkins JS, Patel SN, White CJ, et al. Endovascular stenting for vertebral artery stenosis. J Am Coll Cardiol 2010;55:538–42.

SUMMARY

In summary, defining the anatomy of the vertebral artery, including proximal inflow and collateral pathways, is necessary to determine the appropriate vessel to treat that will provide the best revascularization to the posterior circulation. The use of coronary angioplasty equipment and proper guide selection will allow safe and effective treatment of complex vertebral lesions. If vertebral artery anatomy is suitable, embolic protection devices should be used to prevent distal embolic complications. Endovascular treatment of the proximal vertebral artery is safe, can be performed with high technical success rates, and is effective for alleviating symptoms and improving cerebral blood flow to the posterior circulation. Although restenosis rates vary widely, the durability of endovascular treatment is evidenced by low restenosis rates in multiple large series reported in the literature with both balloon angioplasty alone, bare metal stent placement, and drug eluting stent placement. Vertebral stenting is a less morbid alternative than open surgery and should become the preferred therapy for symptomatic vertebral artery atherosclerotic obstructive disease.

VIDEOS

Videos related to this article can be found online at http://dx.doi.org/10.1016/j.iccl.2013.09.005.

REFERENCES

1. Bamford J, Sandercock P, Dennis M, et al. Classification and natural history of clinically identifiable subtypes of cerebral infarction. Lancet 1991;337: 1521–6.

2. Bogousslavsky J, Van Melle G, Regli F. The Lausanne Stroke Registry: analysis of 1,000 consecutive patients with first stroke. Stroke 1988;19: 1083–92.

3. Coward LJ, Featherstone RL, Brown MM. Percutaneous transluminal angioplasty and stenting for vertebral artery stenosis. Cochrane Database Syst Rev 2005;(2):CD000516.

4. Higashida RT, Hieshima GB, Tsai FY, et al. Transluminal angioplasty of the vertebral and basilar artery. AJNR Am J Neuroradiol 1987;8:745–9.

5. Qureshi AI, Ziai WC, Yahia AM, et al. Stroke-free survival and its determinants in patients with symptomatic vertebrobasilar stenosis: a multicenter study. Neurosurgery 2003;52:1033–9 [discussion: 1039–40].

6. Crawley F, Brown MM. Percutaneous transluminal angioplasty and stenting for vertebral artery stenosis. Cochrane Database Syst Rev 2000;(2):CD000516.

7. Imparato AM. Vertebral arterial reconstruction: a nineteen-year experience. J Vasc Surg 1985;2: 626–34.

8. Spetzler RF, Hadley MN, Martin NA, et al. Vertebrobasilar insufficiency. Part 1: microsurgical treatment of extracranial vertebrobasilar disease. J Neurosurg 1987;66:648–61.

9. Phatouros CC, Higashida RT, Malek AM, et al. Endovascular treatment of noncarotid extracranial cerebrovascular disease. Neurosurg Clin N Am 2000; 11:331–50.

10. Fields WS, North RR, Hass WK, et al. Joint study of extracranial arterial occlusion as a cause of stroke. I. Organization of study and survey of patient population. JAMA 1968;203:955–60.

11. Hass WK, Fields WS, North RR, et al. Joint study of extracranial arterial occlusion. II. Arteriography, techniques, sites, and complications. JAMA 1968; 203:961–8.

12. Long A, Lepoutre A, Corbillon E, et al. Critical review of non- or minimally invasive methods (duplex ultrasonography, MR and CT-angiography) for evaluating stenosis of the proximal internal carotid artery. Eur J Vasc Endovasc Surg 2002;24:43–52.

13. Rocha-Singh K. Vertebral artery stenting: ready for prime time? Catheter Cardiovasc Interv 2001; 54:6–7.

14. Whisnant JP, Cartlidge NE, Elveback LR. Carotid and vertebral-basilar transient ischemic attacks: effect of anticoagulants, hypertension, and cardiac disorders on survival and stroke occurrence–a population study. Ann Neurol 1978;3:107–15.

15. Jenkins JS, White CJ, Ramee SR, et al. Vertebral artery stenting. Catheter Cardiovasc Interv 2001; 54:1–5.

16. Henry M, Polydorou A, Henry I, et al. Angioplasty and stenting of extracranial vertebral artery stenosis. Int Angiol 2005;24:311–24.

17. Jenkins JS, White CJ, Ramee SR, et al. Vertebral insufficiency: when to intervene and how? Curr Interv Cardiol Rep 2000;2:91–4.

18. Wehman JC, Hanel RA, Guidot CA, et al. Atherosclerotic occlusive extracranial vertebral artery disease: indications for intervention, endovascular techniques, short-term and long-term results. J Interv Cardiol 2004;17:219–32.

19. Chimowitz MI, Lynn MJ, Howlett-Smith H, et al. Prognosis of patients with symptomatic vertebral or basilar artery stenosis. The Warfarin-Aspirin Symptomatic Intracranial Disease (WASID) Study Group. Stroke 1998;29:1389–92.

20. Nomura M, Hashimoto N, Nishi S, et al. Percutaneous transluminal angioplasty for intracranial vertebral and/or basilar artery stenosis. Clin Radiol 1999; 54:521–7.

21. Lemke AJ, Benndorf G, Liebig T, et al. Anomalous origin of the right vertebral artery: review of the literature and case report of right vertebral artery origin distal to the left subclavian artery. AJNR Am J Neuroradiol 1999;20:1318–21.

22. Gluncic V, Ivkic G, Marin D, et al. Anomalous origin of both vertebral arteries. Clin Anat 1999;12:281–4.

23. Palmer FJ. Origin of the right vertebral artery from the right common carotid artery: angiographic demonstration of three cases. Br J Radiol 1977;50: 185–7.

24. Wholey MH, Wholey MH. The supraaortic and vertebral endovascular interventions. Tech Vasc Interv Radiol 2004;7:215–25.

25. Sundt TM Jr, Smith HC, Campbell JK, et al. Transluminal angioplasty for basilar artery stenosis. Mayo Clin Proc 1980;55:673–80.

26. Coward LJ, McCabe DJ, Ederle J, et al. Long-term outcome after angioplasty and stenting for symptomatic vertebral artery stenosis compared with medical treatment in the Carotid And Vertebral Artery Transluminal Angioplasty Study (CAVATAS): a randomized trial. Stroke 2007;38:1526–30.

27. Eberhardt O, Naegele T, Raygrotzki S, et al. Stenting of vertebrobasilar arteries in symptomatic atherosclerotic disease and acute occlusion: case series and review of the literature. J Vasc Surg 2006;43: 1145–54.

28. Jenkins JS, Patel SN, White CJ, et al. Endovascular stenting for vertebral artery stenosis. J Am Coll Cardiol 2010;55:538–42.

29. Albuquerque FC, Fiorella D, Han P, et al. A reappraisal of angioplasty and stenting for the treatment of vertebral origin stenosis. Neurosurgery 2003;53:607–14 [discussion: 614–6].

30. Chastain HD 2nd, Campbell MS, Iyer S, et al. Extracranial vertebral artery stent placement: in-hospital and follow-up results. J Neurosurg 1999;91:547–52.

31. Lin YH, Juang JM, Jeng JS, et al. Symptomatic ostial vertebral artery stenosis treated with tubular

coronary stents: clinical results and restenosis analysis. J Endovasc Ther 2004;11:719–26.

32. Weber W, Mayer TE, Henkes H, et al. Efficacy of stent angioplasty for symptomatic stenoses of the proximal vertebral artery. Eur J Radiol 2005;56: 240–7.

33. Cloud GC, Crawley F, Clifton A, et al. Vertebral artery origin angioplasty and primary stenting: safety and restenosis rates in a prospective series. J Neurol Neurosurg Psychiatry 2003;74:586–90.

34. SSYLVIA Study Investigators. Stenting of Symptomatic Atherosclerotic Lesions in the Vertebral or Intracranial Arteries (SSYLVIA): study results. Stroke 2004;35:1388–92.

35. Hatano T, Tsukahara T, Miyakoshi A, et al. Stent placement for atherosclerotic stenosis of the vertebral artery ostium: angiographic and clinical outcomes in 117 consecutive patients. Neurosurgery 2011;68:108–16 [discussion: 116].

36. Lin YH, Liu YC, Tseng WY, et al. The impact of lesion length on angiographic restenosis after vertebral artery origin stenting. Eur J Vasc Endovasc Surg 2006;32:379–85.

37. Karameshev A, Schroth G, Mordasini P, et al. Long-term outcome of symptomatic severe ostial vertebral artery stenosis (OVAS). Neuroradiology 2010;52:371–9.

38. Lin YH, Hung CS, Tseng WY, et al. Safety and feasibility of drug-eluting stent implantation at vertebral artery origin: the first case series in Asians. J Formos Med Assoc 2008;107:253–8.

39. Zhou Z, Yin Q, Xu G, et al. Influence of vessel size and tortuosity on in-stent restenosis after stent implantation in the vertebral artery ostium. Cardiovasc Intervent Radiol 2011;34:481–7.

40. Gupta R, Al-Ali F, Thomas AJ, et al. Safety, feasibility, and short-term follow-up of drug-eluting stent placement in the intracranial and extracranial circulation. Stroke 2006;37:2562–6.

41. Vajda Z, Miloslavski E, Guthe T, et al. Treatment of stenoses of vertebral artery origin using short drug-eluting coronary stents: improved follow-up results. AJNR Am J Neuroradiol 2009;30:1653–6.

Common Cervical and Cerebral Vascular Variants

Peter C. Thurlow, MD[a], Jason M. Andrus, MD[a],
Mark H. Wholey, MD[a,b,c],*

KEYWORDS

- Vascular variants • Carotid stenting • Aortic arch • Internal carotid artery
- Persistent carotid-vertebrobasilar anastomoses • Circle of Willis

KEY POINTS

- Successful open and endovascular carotid artery intervention depends on a thorough foundational knowledge of cervical and intracranial vascular anatomy.
- Variant vascular anatomy is frequently observed during preprocedural evaluation and endovascular intervention.
- Alterations in the normal patterns of blood supply to the cerebral vascular territories often occur as a consequence of variant vascular anatomy.
- Recognition of cervical and intracranial vascular variants, and the corresponding changes in blood supply, is essential to successful and complication-free endovascular carotid interventions.

INTRODUCTION

Successful open and endovascular carotid artery intervention depends on a thorough foundational knowledge of cervical and intracranial vascular anatomy. It is essential for the carotid interventionalist to be familiar with the common and rare vascular variants in the head and neck, and to understand the implications of these variants for the performance of carotid intervention with protection of the distal circulation. The purpose of this article is to provide interventionalists with a basic description of the normal and relevant variant vascular anatomy from the aortic arch to the circle of Willis, and outline the potential difficulties that specific variants may present for endovascular therapy.

ANOMALIES OF THE AORTIC ARCH
Normal Anatomy

In approximately 70% of individuals, the innominate artery, left common carotid artery (CCA), and left subclavian arteries arise in sequence from a left-sided arch of the aorta. The innominate artery then branches into the right subclavian artery and the right CCA. The bilateral vertebral arteries arise as proximal branches of their respective subclavian artery.[1] A frequently used classification system for the normal aortic arch is based on the relationships of the origins of the great vessels to a tangent across the top of the aortic arch. The aortic arch is defined as type I if the origin of the innominate artery is less than 1 diameter of the left CCA from the top of the aortic arch in the vertical plane, type II if between 1 and 2 left CCA diameters, and type III if greater than 2 left CCA diameters. This classification system is designed to predict the difficulty of arch vessel intubation, and may help to guide catheter selection.[2] True variation of the normal aortic arch anatomy occurs frequently, and can present a challenge for catheterization. These variants are best classified according to the direction of the aortic arch (**Box 1**).

The authors have nothing to disclose.
[a] Department of Radiology, Allegheny General Hospital, 320 East North Avenue, Pittsburgh, PA 15212, USA;
[b] Center for Vascular and Neurovascular Interventions, Cardiovascular Institute, Allegheny General Hospital, 320 East North Avenue, Pittsburgh, PA 15212, USA; [c] Department of Biomedical Engineering, Carnegie Mellon University, Pittsburgh, PA 15213, USA
* Corresponding author. Center for Vascular and Neurovascular Interventions, Cardiovascular Institute, Allegheny General Hospital, 320 East North Avenue, Pittsburgh, PA 15212.
E-mail address: mwholey@wpahs.org

Intervent Cardiol Clin 3 (2014) 123–134
http://dx.doi.org/10.1016/j.iccl.2013.09.002
2211-7458/14/$ – see front matter © 2014 Elsevier Inc. All rights reserved.

Box 1
Branching patterns of aortic arches

Arch Type

  Left-sided aortic arch

    Normal branching

    Common origin of the right brachioce-phalic trunk and left common carotid artery

    Vertebral artery as a direct branch of the aorta

    Aberrant right subclavian artery

    Bilateral brachiocephalic trunks

    Arteria thyroidea ima

  Right-sided aortic arch

    Mirror-image branching (type I)

    Aberrant left subclavian artery (type II)

    Isolation of the left subclavian artery (type III)

  Double aortic arch

  Cervical aortic arch

Left-Sided Aortic Arch

Common origin of the right brachiocephalic trunk and left common carotid artery

The second most common pattern of aortic arch branching consists of a common origin of the right brachiocephalic trunk and the left CCA, and is identified in 13% of the population.[1] Consequently, only 2 vessels arise directly from the aortic arch. A similar variant, in which the left CCA originates as a branch of the right brachiocephalic trunk, occurs in 9% of the population.[1] These variants have at times been erroneously referred to as a "bovine arch" or "bovine anatomy."[3] However, the branching pattern of the aortic arch found in cattle consists of a single brachiocephalic trunk that subsequently gives rise to the bilateral subclavian arteries and a bicarotid trunk. This true bovine arch does not occur in humans.

Vertebral artery as a direct branch of the aortic arch

Although the aforementioned 3 branching patterns represent the vast majority of aortic arch variants, numerous less common but clinically significant anomalies have been reported. In approximately 4% of the population, the left vertebral artery arises as a direct branch of the aorta, most often as the third branch arising between the left CCA and the left subclavian artery.[1] Therefore, 4 vessels arise from the aortic arch.

Aberrant right subclavian artery

Although well known, the aberrant right subclavian artery (ARSA) arising as the last branch of the aortic arch distal to the left subclavian artery is observed in only 1% of the population.[4] An association has been made with Down syndrome.[5] Also termed arteria lusoria, this variant may result in dysphagia or dyspnea when the ARSA courses anterior to the trachea as it crosses the midline. This variant can also present unique technical challenges to reaching the coronary sinus or great vessels when encountered during the right trans-radial approach.[6]

Other anomalies

Although more than 20 anomalies associated with left-sided aortic arch branching have been reported in cadaveric or imaging studies, most anomalies are exceedingly rare. Right and left brachiocephalic trunks that give rise to right and left subclavian arteries and CCAs may occur with a frequency as high as 1% of the population. The lowest thyroid artery, or arteria thyroidea ima, may arise as a second branch from the aortic arch in approximately 1% of the population. Although this artery is only present in 6% of individuals, recognition of its presence is important before surgical dissection caudal to the thyroid isthmus is attempted.[1]

Right-Sided Aortic Arch

Right-sided aortic arch (RAA) is a rare anomaly (0.04%–0.1% on necropsy series) and has an association with congenital heart defects, esophageal atresia, and tracheoesophageal fistula.[4,7] The most common classification system divides right-sided aortic arch branching into 3 types. Type I represents RAA with mirror-image branching, whereby a left brachiocephalic trunk arises as the first branch of the aorta and gives rise to the left subclavian artery and left CCA, followed by right CCA and right subclavian arteries branching from the aortic arch. RAA with an aberrant left subclavian artery (ALSA) (type II), in which the ALSA arises as the last branch of the RAA, is the most common type of RAA. RAA with isolation of the left subclavian artery (type III) occurs when the left subclavian artery does not connect directly to the aortic arch. The left subclavian artery instead fills through collateral circulation, potentially resulting in arm ischemia or a steal phenomenon.[8]

Double Aortic Arch

The double aortic arch is a rare anomaly (<0.1%) that occurs when the bilateral fourth branchial aortic arches and dorsal aortas persist, forming a vascular ring where the left and right aortic arches connect the ascending and descending aorta.[4] The right aortic arch is dominant in 75% of patients, with either hypoplasia or atresia of the left aortic arch.[9] Each arch will usually give rise to a CCA and subclavian artery. Although the anatomy varies greatly, important angiographic factors include the position of the ductus arteriosus, the side and degree of hypoplasia or atresia, and the side of descent of the aorta.[5]

Cervical Aortic Arch

When the aortic arch is shifted cranially from its mediastinal position and extends above the clavicles, the aortic arch is termed a cervical arch. Although the cervical aortic arch is usually an incidental finding, it may also present as a pulsatile neck mass or with symptoms from tracheal or esophageal compression.[4] This anomaly is thought to be caused by a lack of caudal migration following fusion of the third and fourth branchial aortic arches.[10]

ANOMALIES OF THE COMMON CAROTID ARTERY

The normal and common variant branching patterns of the paired CCA origins are described in an earlier section. The CCA does not typically have any major branches, except in the presence of common carotid bifurcation variants. In 62% of individuals, the bifurcation of the CCA is near the upper margin of the thyroid cartilage at C3-C4.[11] The typical anatomic landmark used during carotid catheterization is the angle of the mandible. However, variation exists, and the bifurcation can be found as low as T2 or as high as C2.[1,5] Low carotid bifurcations may be at high risk of unintentional catheterization above the bifurcation during angiography. Both high and low bifurcations present a challenge for endarterectomy, and should be considered for angioplasty and stenting.[12]

In the setting of a bifurcation at levels above C4-C5, the ascending pharyngeal or superior thyroid arteries may rarely arise directly from the CCA, below the carotid bifurcation.[13] The vertebral, inferior thyroid, and occipital arteries have also been reported as anomalous CCA branches.[14] In congenital absence of either the external carotid artery (ECA) or internal carotid artery (ICA), the so-called nonbifurcating carotid trunk will be seen. A third pattern of anomalous branching may occur when the ECA and ICA arise separately and directly from the aortic arch or brachiocephalic artery, an exceedingly rare anomaly.

ANOMALIES OF THE EXTERNAL CAROTID ARTERY
Normal Anatomy

The proximal ECA arises from either the third aortic arch or aortic pouch, with contributions of the distal branches from the first aortic arch. Eight to 9 major branches from the ECA are typically described, and these are named according to their respective territories, without consideration of the site of origin from the ECA.[5] Extensive anastomoses for collateral flow exist between ECA branch territories. For this reason, an understanding of the naming system according to vascular territory (not the simple origin of the ECA), and the potential for dangerous collateral pathways between branch vessels and with the ICA or ophthalmic artery, are essential before ECA branch embolization. Failure to do so can have disastrous consequences. A complete discussion of the ECA anatomy is beyond the scope of this review.

Absence of the External Carotid Artery

Absence of the external carotid artery is an extremely rare anomaly, with fewer than 10 cases published in the literature.[15] Overall, this anomaly is thought to be of little clinical importance, as collateral circulation, including anomalous ECA branches arising from the ICA, prevents arterial insufficiency.[11]

Lateral Position of the External Carotid Artery

The ECA initially lies anteromedial to the ICA. As the ICA ascends, it courses medial to the main ECA trunk. An anomalous initial lateral position of the external carotid artery (LPECA) is thought to arise from either an excessive embryologic rotation of the external carotid artery or from an acquired rotation of the CCA resulting from aging and atherosclerotic disease.[11,16] The incidence of this anomaly is between 5% and 16%, and is more common on the right.[16,17] Clinically it is important that this anomaly is identified before performing carotid endarterectomy so as to preserve the hypoglossal, vagus, and internal laryngeal nerves during ICA exposure.[18]

ANOMALIES OF THE INTERNAL CAROTID ARTERY
Normal Anatomy

The ICA provides the majority of the blood supply to the cerebral hemispheres. The Bouthillier classification is the system most widely used to describe the anatomy of the ICA. This system divides the ICA into 7 segments according to the direction of blood flow and various anatomic boundaries (**Fig. 1**).[19]

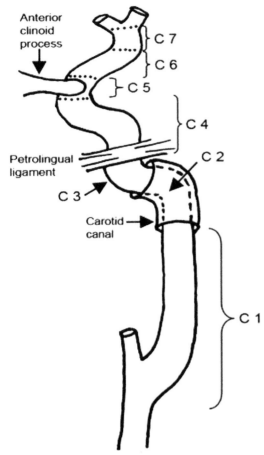

Fig. 1. Anatomic segments of the internal carotid artery (ICA). C1, cervical segment; C2, petrous segment; C3, lacerum segment; C4, cavernous segment; C5, clinoidal segment; C6, ophthalmic segment; C7, communicating segment. (*From* Buerke B, Puesken M, Wittkamp G, et al. Bone subtraction CTA for transcranial arteries: intra-individual comparison with standard CTA without bone subtraction and TOF-MRA. Clin Radiol 2010;65(6):442; with permission.)

The cervical segment is formed from the fetal third aortic arch, and the remaining segments are from the cranial extensions of the embryonic dorsal aortas.[20]

The cervical segment (C1) has 2 parts, the carotid bulb and the ascending cervical segment, both of which are contained within the carotid sheath. This segment begins at the level of the CCA bifurcation and ends at the entrance of the osseous petrous carotid canal. There are normally no branches off of the cervical ICA. The petrous segment (C2) begins at the inferior osseous petrous carotid canal and ends inferomedial to the Meckel cave at the posterior edge of the foramen lacerum. The caroticotympanic artery and, occasionally, the vidian artery arise from this

segment. The lacerum segment (C3) begins at the superior edge of the carotid canal at the level of the foramen lacerum and extends to the superior margin of the petrolingual ligament. The cavernous segment (C4) begins at the superior margin of the petrolingual ligament and ends at the proximal dural ring at the level of the clinoid process. It is surrounded by the cavernous sinus. The meningohypophyseal artery and the inferolateral trunk arise from this segment. The clinoid segment (C5) begins at the proximal dural ring and ends at the distal dural ring. It is at this point that the ICA becomes intradural. There are no branches arising from this segment. The ophthalmic segment (C6) begins at the distal dural ring and ends proximal to the origin of the posterior communication artery (PComm). The ophthalmic and superior hypophyseal arteries arise from this segment. The communicating segment (C7), the last segment of the ICA, begins just proximal to the PComm and ends at the ICA bifurcation. The PComm and anterior choroidal arteries are its primary branches.

Absence of the Internal Carotid Artery

Congenital absence of the ICA, including aplasia, hypoplasia, and agenesis, is a rare congenital anomaly, occurring in less than 0.01% of the population.[21] Collateral flow is through the circle of Willis or, less commonly, through persistent embryonic vessels or from transcranial collaterals originating from the ECA system. Slightly more than 100 cases of congenital absence of the ICA have been reported in the literature.[21] True congenital absence of the ICA will be reflected by an absence or hypoplasia of the bony carotid canal, thus differentiating it from an acquired occlusion. Though primarily asymptomatic, there have been reports of increased prevalence of associated abnormalities such as aneurysm.[20]

Anomalous Branches of the Internal Carotid Artery

Anomalous ICA branches are rare. Reports of anomalous branches include those normally arising from the ECA, such as the occipital and ascending pharyngeal arteries. Occasionally, anomalous branches may arise off of the cervical segment (C1) from other segments, and rarely from the vertebrobasilar circulation (such as the cerebellar or posterior marginal arteries).[20] In the setting of congenital absence of the ECA, all of the normal ECA branches will arise from the cervical ICA.

Aberrant Internal Carotid Arteries

There are multiple types of aberrant internal carotid arteries, determined by cervical segment and persistence of their corresponding fetal precursors.[22] The most common and clinically relevant are the intratympanic and lateral pharyngeal types.

Intratympanic aberrant ICA

This type arises when the cervical segment of the carotid artery fails to develop. The petrous portion is reconstituted via the inferior tympanic artery, which arises from the ascending pharyngeal artery of the ECA and connects to the caroticotympanic (embryonic hyoid artery) of the ICA (**Fig. 2**). On imaging, this can be recognized as an abnormal soft-tissue mass in the middle ear and absent tympanic portion of the ICA. This variant can be associated with a persistent stapedial artery. Its clinic importance lies in the fact that if not recognized, it can lead to potential catastrophic consequences during myringotomy and middle ear surgery.[23]

Aberrant lateral pharyngeal ICA

The lateral pharyngeal type is a common variant that results in an anomalous vessel, which runs midline to the course of the normal pharyngeal ICA. This variant places the patient at risk during

surgeries such as tonsillectomy and resection of oropharyngeal tumor.[22]

Persistent dorsal ophthalmic artery

Two primitive ophthalmic arteries exist during the early embryologic stage. In normal development the dorsal artery regresses, and the ventral artery persists and enters the orbit through the optic canal. By contrast, a persistent dorsal artery arises off of the supraclinoid ICA and enters into the orbit through the superior orbital fissure.[24]

PERSISTENT CAROTID-VERTEBROBASILAR ANASTOMOSES

Persistent carotid-basilar and carotid-vertebral anastomoses are relatively rare but potentially clinically relevant anomalies of the cervical and intracranial vasculature (**Fig. 3**).[25] When performing a carotid angiogram, the presence of carotid-vertebrobasilar anastomoses may be suggested by simultaneous filling of the basilar artery, alone or together with the vertebral artery. In a series of 4400 cerebral angiograms studied by Yilmaz and colleagues,[26] the incidence of persistent primitive carotid-basilar and carotid-vertebral anastomoses was 0.14% and 0.023%, respectively. Their persistence has been associated with neuralgias and paralysis caused by local compressive effects. Their association with other vascular pathologic conditions, such as aneurysms, remains unclear.[26]

Carotid-Basilar Anastomoses

Carotid-basilar anastomoses develop in the 4-mm embryo between the ICAs extending from the dorsal aortic arches and the parallel primitive vertebrobasilar system. These anastomoses usually regress after the formation of the posterior communicating artery.[11] The persistence of these arteries correlates with variations of absent or hypoplastic posterior communicating arteries.

Persistent trigeminal artery

The persistent trigeminal artery is the most common persistent carotid-vertebrobasilar anastomosis, with an incidence of 0.1% to 0.6%.[27] It is also the most cephalad and last of the carotid-basilar anastomoses to regress. Persistent trigeminal artery arises from the cavernous segment of the ICA and anastomoses with the proximal basilar artery (**Fig. 4**). It is classified according to the location (medial or lateral) and the absence or presence of the posterior communicating artery (Salzman type 1 and Salzman type 2, respectively). It is clinically important to identify this anomaly in patients undergoing transsphenoidal surgery for pituitary adenoma so as to avoid accidental transection.[23]

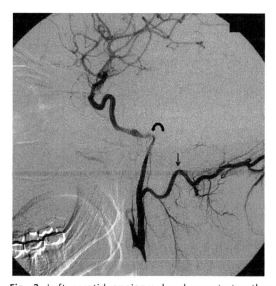

Fig. 2. Left carotid angiography demonstrates the characteristic lateral posterior temporal bone course of the intratympanic aberrant ICA (*curved arrow*). The occipital artery (*arrow*) can be seen arising from the aberrant segment, which represents enlargement of the inferior tympanic artery. (*Adapted from* Knox WJ, Milburn JM, Dawson R. Bilateral aberrant internal carotid arteries: treatment of a hemorrhagic complication. Am J Otolaryngol 2007;28(3):215; with permission.)

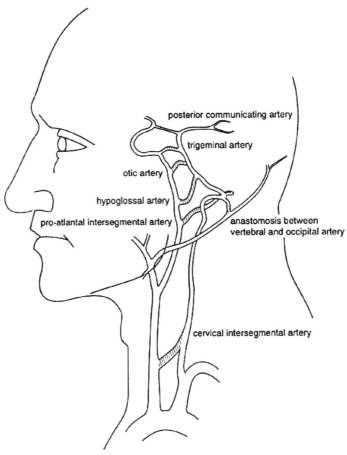

Fig. 3. Carotid-basilar and carotid-vertebral anastomoses. (*From* Fantini GA, Reilly LM, Stoney RJ. Persistent hypoglossal artery: diagnostic and therapeutic considerations concerning carotid thromboendarterectomy. J Vasc Surg 1994;20(6):995–9; with permission.)

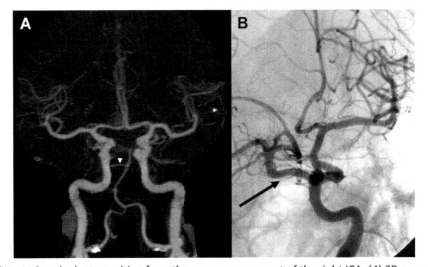

Fig. 4. Persistent trigeminal artery arising from the cavernous segment of the right ICA. (*A*) 3D reconstruction of an intracranial CT angiogram in the frontal view demonstrates an anomalous vessel (*arrowhead*) extending from the cavernous right ICA to the proximal basilar artery, consistent with a persistent right trigeminal artery. (*B*) Left internal carotid angiogram in a separate patient shows filling of the distal basilar artery by a persistent trigeminal artery (*arrow*). ([*B*] *Adapted from* Heran MKS, Abruzzo TA. Diagnostic Cerebral Angiography and the Wada Test in Pediatric Patients. Tech Vasc Interv Radiol 2011;14(1):48; with permission.)

Persistent hypoglossal artery

The persistent hypoglossal artery is the second most common persistent carotid-vertebrobasilar anastomosis, with an incidence of 0.02% to 0.10%.[23] It is the most caudal of the 3 carotid-basilar anastomoses and is the first to regress. It arises from the cervical carotid at C1-C3 and courses through the hypoglossal canal to the level of the midbasilar artery (**Fig. 5**). There is a significant association with hypoplasia of both the vertebral artery and the posterior communicating artery. In most cases (78%) the basilar artery will originate from this artery. Clinically these patients have been reported as having associated glossopharyngeal and hypoglossal nerve paralysis.[23,26]

Persistent otic artery

The persistent otic artery is such a rare anomaly that its very existence has been debated.[28] Theoretically this artery arises from the petrous ICA to the midbasilar artery. Its clinical significance is negligible, and it is only mentioned because it is almost always included in discussion of the 3 so-called presegmental arteries.[11]

Carotid-Vertebral Anastomoses

The carotid-vertebral anastomoses develop from persistence of intersegmental arteries arising from dorsal extensions of the primitive ICA. The distal segments later coalesce into the vertebral arteries. The most common of the persistent carotid-vertebral anastomoses is the proatlantal intersegmental artery.

Proatlantal intersegmental artery

The proatlantal artery is the first and embryonically most prominent of the intersegmental arteries. Although it represents the most common of this type of anastomosis, it is still extremely rare, with fewer than 40 cases presented in the literature.[23] It originates at the level of C2-C4; type 1 arises from the dorsal portion of the proximal internal carotid (38%), and type 2 arises from the ECA (50%) (**Fig. 6**).[23] Occasionally it can arise from the carotid bifurcation and can give rise to the occipital artery. It then joins the suboccipital horizontal portion of the vertebral artery. The anomaly is associated with proximal vertebral artery hypoplasia or aplasia in 50% of cases, and has been reported to have an association with intracranial vascular abnormalities such as aneurysm.[29,30]

Congenital Anastomoses Between the External and Internal Carotid Arteries

Persistent stapedial artery

The persistent stapedial artery is a failed regression of the embryologic anastomosis between the distal internal artery and the ECA. It originates from the embryologic hyoid artery off the petrous

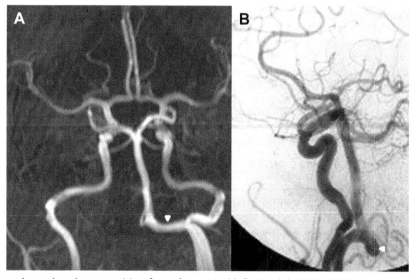

Fig. 5. Persistent hypoglossal artery arising from the cervical left ICA. (*A*) 3D-TOF-MRA reconstruction displayed in the frontal projection demonstrates a large vessel (*arrowhead*) arising from the C1 segment of the left ICA and supplying the basilar artery. The bilateral vertebral arteries are hypoplastic, a frequent finding in the setting of persistent hypoglossal artery. (*B*) Lateral carotid DSA in a separate patient demonstrating the persistent hypoglossal artery (*arrowhead*) arising from the cervical internal carotid artery and supplying the basilar artery. ([*B*] *Adapted from* Perez-Carrillo GJ, Hogg JP. Intracranial vascular lesions and anatomical variants all residents should know. Curr Probl Diagn Radiol 2010;39(3):95; with permission.)

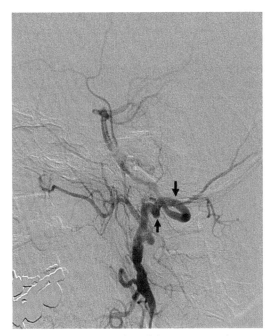

Fig. 6. Persistent proatlantal intersegmental artery, type II. Left external carotid angiogram in the lateral view demonstrates an anastomotic vessel (*arrows*) arising from the external carotid and passing posteriorly to become the vertebral artery. (*Adapted from* Nakashima K, Itokawa H, Oishi A, et al. Persistent primitive first cervical intersegmental artery (proatlantal artery II) associated with subarachnoid hemorrhage of unknown origin. Clin Neurol Neurosurg 2012;141(1):91; with permission.)

ICA, where it passes through the foramen of the stapes and terminates as the middle meningeal artery.[11] Clinically these anomalies may manifest as pulsatile tinnitus, and should be recognized preoperatively because they can complicate middle ear surgery or cochlear implantation. In addition, they should not be mistaken for a glomus tumor.[23,31]

ANOMALIES OF THE VERTEBRAL ARTERIES
Normal Anatomy

The normal vertebral artery (VA) can be divided into 4 segments. The V1, or extraosseous, segment arises as the first branch of the subclavian artery and enters into the C6 transverse foramen. The V2, or foraminal, segment ascends through the C6 to C3 transverse foramina, then turns sharply superolaterally through the C2 transverse foramen and ascends through the more laterally positioned C1 transverse foramen. The V3, or extraspinal, segment extends from the top of the C1 transverse foramen to the foramen magnum, where the VA pierces the dura and

enters the subarachnoid space. The point of dural penetration is seen as a circumferential cincture. The V4, or intradural, segment courses from the foramen magnum superomedially behind the clivus, uniting with the contralateral VA at the pontomedullary junction to form the basilar artery.

Extradural Vertebral Artery Anomalies

Anomalous origins of the VA are relatively rare, with most types having been published in only a limited number of case reports. The only anomaly occurring with notable frequency is the origin of the left VA from the aortic arch, usually between left CCA and left superior cerebellar artery (SCA), found in 2.4% to 5.8% of individuals.[32] In this variant, the left V1 segment enters the transverse foramen at C4 instead of C6, and results from the persistence of segmental arteries more cranial than the sixth cervical artery. The other notable anomaly of vertebral artery origin occurs in the setting of the ARSA, where a right VA arises from the right CCA.[32] Additional anomalies of vertebral origin have been documented in case reports, but all are exceedingly rare.

Intradural Vertebral Artery Anomalies

In 5% to 10% of individuals, the distal intradural VA is hypoplastic or absent, ending in a posterior inferior cerebellar artery (PICA) terminal branch. The angiographer, therefore, should be aware of this anomaly before injection because of the potential disastrous consequences of a full-volume vertebral injection into the PICA.[5]

Anterior Spinal Artery and the Artery of Cervical Enlargement

The anterior spinal artery (ASA) is classically thought of as originating from the fusion of paired bilateral spinal arteries arising from the V4 segments. In fact, these diminutive feeding vessels to the ASA supply only the first 2 or 3 cervical segments, with anterior radicular arteries arising from the VA, costocervical trunk, and thyrocervical trunk, reinforcing the ASA in its cervical segments.[28,33] The largest of the radicular arteries is often referred to as the artery of cervical enlargement, and may arise from branches from the bilateral VAs between C4 and C6.[28] Similar to concerns with the artery of Adamkiewicz during repair of abdominal aortic aneurysm, it is essential to identify and preserve these feeding vessels to the ASA, given the potential for disastrous complications.

ANOMALIES OF THE INTRACRANIAL VASCULATURE
Normal Anatomy

As described earlier, the ICA ascends through the skull base and is classically divided into 7 segments (see **Fig. 1**). The C7 communicating segment then divides at the ICA terminus into the M1 segment of the middle cerebral artery (MCA) and A1 segment of the anterior cerebral artery (ACA). The bilateral A1 segments course toward the midline, where the anterior communicating artery (AComm) connects the ACAs and marks the division between the A1 and A2 segments of the ACA.

The intradural V4 segment of the vertebral arteries normally gives rise to the ASA and PICA, which then join at the pontomedullary junction to form the basilar artery. The anterior inferior cerebellar artery (AICA) and SCA arise from the basilar artery as it courses in the midline to the circle of Willis, where the basilar artery divides to give rise to bilateral P1 segments of the posterior cerebral arteries. If the circle of Willis is complete, the PComm then merges with the P1 segment, defining the beginning of the P2 segment.

Normal Variants of the Circle of Willis

When approaching endovascular interventions in the carotid and vertebral arteries, knowledge of the patient's intracranial vascular anatomy is essential in avoiding cerebrovascular insufficiency and potentially catastrophic neurologic complications. In their totality, anatomic variants at and above the circle of Willis are relatively frequent. Consequently, significant differences in the source vessels for the cerebral vascular territories may exist between patients. A discussion of the most common and critical vascular variants with proximity to the circle of Willis follows (**Box 2**).

Box 2
Common variants of the circle of Willis^a

ACA

  Azygous ACA

  Bihemispheric ACA

  ACA trifurcation

  A1 segment absence or hypoplasia

AComm

  AComm absence

  ACA segmental lateral anastomosis

MCA

  Accessory MCA

  MCA originating from the contralateral A1 segment or basilar artery

PCA/PComm

  Fetal origin of the PCA

  PComm infundibulum

Abbreviations: ACA, anterior cerebral artery; AComm, anterior communicating artery; MCA, middle cerebral artery; PCA, posterior cerebral artery; PComm, posterior communicating artery.

  ^a Arterial fenestration and duplication at the circle of Willis is common but is excluded from the table.

Fenestrations and duplications

Fenestrations and duplications are the most commonly observed anomalies of the intracranial vasculature, and are often detected incidentally during computed tomographic angiography or autopsy (**Fig. 7**). Fenestration is the division of a single artery into 2 separate lumens, which share an adventitia but with each branch retaining its own intima and media, and having distal arterial convergence.[34] Duplication is defined as 2 distinct

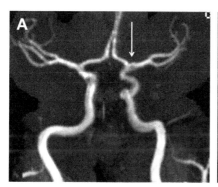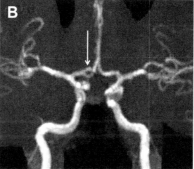

Fig. 7. Fenestrations of the intracranial vasculature. (*A*) 3D-TOF-MRA reconstruction demonstrates a fenestration of the left M1 segment of the left MCA. (*B*) 3D-TOF-MRA reconstruction demonstrates a fenestration of the right A1 segment of the right ACA.

arteries with separate origins and no distal arterial convergence.[35] An association between aneurysm formation and fenestration, but not duplication, has been observed, and has been attributed to focal defects in the media at the proximal and distal ends of the fenestration.[36]

Intracranial arterial duplication and fenestration is most prevalent in the anterior communicating artery, occurring in 18% and 12% to 21% of the population, respectively.[1,37] MCA duplication has a reported prevalence of 0.2% to 2.9%, with the duplicate vessel often supplying the anterior temporal lobe.[38,39] Fenestration of the MCA has a reported prevalence as high as 1%, and most commonly presents in the proximal M1 segment. Although vertebrobasilar duplication is exceedingly rare, fenestration of the intracranial vertebral and basilar arteries has a reported prevalence as high as 2% and 5%, respectively. Fenestration of the ACA, posterior cerebral artery (PCA), PComm, and distal ICA is extremely rare, with only a few case reports in the published literature.[23]

Normal Variants of the Anterior Circulation

Azygous and bihemispheric ACA
Azygous ACA (0.2%–4.0%) occurs when the bilateral A1 segments join to form a single midline A2 trunk that supplies the bilateral ACA territories. A similar anomaly, the bihemispheric ACA (2%–7%), occurs when there is hypoplasia of 1 A2 segment, resulting in arterial supply to the bilateral ACA territory solely from the contralateral A2 trunk. Injury or occlusion in the setting of either anomaly will result in bilateral ACA-territory ischemia.

ACA trifurcation
ACA trifurcation arises when a persistent median callosal artery arises from the AComm, resulting in 3 A2 segments. The prevalence of ACA trifurcation is approximately 10%.[1,20,23]

A1 segment absence or hypoplasia
Unilateral absence or hypoplasia of an A1 segment of the ACA has a prevalence of approximately 10%.[1,23,37] The anterior communicating artery is often enlarged in this setting.

AComm anomalies
Definitive absence of the AComm is relatively rare (1%), but carries important clinical consequences because of the absence of a collateral arterial supply in the event of A1 occlusion. More frequently, the AComm is replaced by a lateral anastomosis between the 2 anterior cerebral arteries. This condition manifests as either a short-segment lateral anastomosis (3%) or longer-segment common

trunk that later divides again to form bilateral ACAs (5%).[1]

Normal variants of the middle cerebral artery
Early branching of the MCA, whereby the M1 segment bifurcates or trifurcates at the insula, is a common variant and of little clinical significance. Accessory MCA (1%–2.7%) occurs when a small MCA branch arises from the A1 segment of the ACA and courses parallel to the M1 segment of the MCA. When present, this branch supplies the anterior inferior frontal lobe. An aneurysm may arise from the origin of the accessory MCA. In the setting of unilateral congenital absence of the ICA, the MCA may originate from the basilar artery or from the contralateral ICA as a branch of an enlarged A1 segment.[1]

Hyperplastic anterior choroidal artery
The anterior choroidal artery arises from the supraclinoid ICA distal to the PComm to provide arterial supply to the cerebral peduncle and optic tract. In 1.1% to 2.3% of individuals, the anterior choroidal artery gives rise to the temporo-occipital branches of the PCA and becomes hyperplastic.[40]

Normal Variants of the Posterior Circulation

Fetal origin of the PCA
A hyperplastic PComm supplying the PCA, with absent or negligible flow through the ipsilateral P1 segment of the PCA, is termed fetal origin of the PCA. This anomaly occurs unilaterally in approximately 10% and bilaterally in 5% to 8% of individuals.[1,23,41] Ten percent of individuals will also demonstrate unilateral fetal origin of the PCA with contralateral absence of the PComm.[1]

PComm infundibulum
A funnel-shaped origin of the PComm from the ICA is termed an infundibulum. It is important that infundibular widening of the PComm is not confused with aneurysmal dilatation of the PComm origin. Criteria for infundibular widening of the PComm include round or conical shape, size less than 3 mm in diameter, and the PComm arising from the apex of the segment of dilatation.[5,42] Infundibular widening of the PComm is observed in approximately 7% of individuals.[43] Although defined as a normal variant, care must be taken in an individual with a prominent PComm infundibulum and otherwise unexplained subarachnoid hemorrhage.[5]

SUMMARY

Variant vascular anatomy can have profound implications for cervical and intracranial endovascular intervention. The potential exists for significant morbidity and mortality if there is a failure to recognize these vascular variants. This article provides a foundational knowledge of the common and critical variants that may be encountered, and briefly outlines the implications of these variants for approaches to endovascular therapy.

REFERENCES

1. Lippert H, Pabst R. Arterial variations in man: classification and frequency. Munich (Germany): J F Bergmann; 1985.
2. Bhatt DL. Peripheral and cerebrovascular intervention. New York: Springer; 2011.
3. Layton KF, Kallmes DF, Cloft HJ, et al. Bovine aortic arch variant in humans: clarification of a common misnomer. AJNR Am J Neuroradiol 2006;27(7): 1541–2.
4. Stojanovska J, Cascade PN, Chong S, et al. Embryology and imaging review of aortic arch anomalies. J Thorac Imaging 2012;27(2):73–84.
5. Morris PP. Practical neuroangiography. 2nd edition. Philadelphia: Lippincott Williams & Wilkins; 2007.
6. Yiu KH, Chan WS, Jim MH, et al. Arteria lusoria diagnosed by transradial coronary catheterization. JACC Cardiovasc Interv 2010;3(8):880–1.
7. Hastreiter AR, D'Cruz IA, Cantez T, et al. Right-sided aorta. I. Occurrence of right aortic arch in various types of congenital heart disease. II. Right aortic arch, right descending aorta, and associated anomalies. Br Heart J 1966;28(6):722–39.
8. Hara M, Kitase M, Satake M, et al. A case of right-sided aortic arch with isolation of the left subclavian artery: CT findings. Radiat Med 2001;19(1):33–6.
9. McElhinney DB, Hoydu AK, Gaynor JW, et al. Patterns of right aortic arch and mirror-image branching of the brachiocephalic vessels without associated anomalies. Pediatr Cardiol 2001;22(4):285–91.
10. Haughton VM, Fellows KE, Rosenbaum AE. The cervical aortic arches. Radiology 1975;114(3):675–81.
11. Lie TA. Congenital anomalies of the carotid arteries. Including the carotid-basilar and carotid-vertebral anastomoses. An angiographic study and a review of the literature. Amsterdam: Excerpta Medica; 1968.
12. Gailloud P, Murphy KJ, Rigamonti D. Bilateral thoracic bifurcation of the common carotid artery associated with Klippel-Feil anomaly. AJNR Am J Neuroradiol 2000;21(5):941–4.
13. Cho L, Mukherjee D. Basic cerebral anatomy for the carotid interventionalist: the intracranial and extracranial vessels. Catheter Cardiovasc Interv 2006; 68(1):104–11.
14. Jinkins JR. Atlas of neuroradiologic embryology, anatomy, and variants. Philadelphia: Lippincott Williams & Wilkins; 2000.
15. Rodriguez HE, Ziauddin MF, Podbielski FJ, et al. Congenital absence of the external carotid artery:
atherosclerosis without a bifurcation. J Vasc Surg 2002;35(3):573–5.
16. Teal JS, Rumbaugh CL, Bergeron RT, et al. Lateral position of the external carotid artery: a rare anomaly? Radiology 1973;108(1):77–81.
17. Trigaux JP, Delchambre F, Van Beers B. Anatomical variations of the carotid bifurcation: implications for digital subtraction angiography and ultrasonography. Br J Radiol 1990;63(747):181–5.
18. Bailey MA, Scott DJ, Tunstall RG, et al. Lateral external carotid artery: implications for the vascular surgeon. Eur J Vasc Endovasc Surg 2007;34(4):492.
19. Buerke B, Puesken M, Wittkamp G, et al. Bone subtraction CTA for transcranial arteries: intra-individual comparison with standard CTA without bone subtraction and TOF-MRA. Clin Radiol 2010;65(6): 440–6.
20. Osborn AG, Jacobs JM, Osborn AG. Diagnostic cerebral angiography. 2nd edition. Philadelphia: Lippincott-Raven; 1999.
21. Given CA 2nd, Huang-Hellinger F, Baker MD, et al. Congenital absence of the internal carotid artery: case reports and review of the collateral circulation. AJNR Am J Neuroradiol 2001;22(10):1953–9.
22. Okahara M, Kiyosue H, Mori H, et al. Anatomic variations of the cerebral arteries and their embryology: a pictorial review. Eur Radiol 2002;12(10): 2548–61.
23. Dimmick SJ, Faulder KC. Normal variants of the cerebral circulation at multidetector CT angiography. Radiographics 2009;29(4):1027–43.
24. Uchino A, Nomiyama K, Takase Y, et al. Anterior cerebral artery variations detected by MR angiography. Neuroradiology 2006;48(9):647–52.
25. Fantini GA, Reilly LM, Stoney RJ. Persistent hypoglossal artery: diagnostic and therapeutic considerations concerning carotid thromboendarterectomy. J Vasc Surg 1994;20(6):995–9.
26. Yilmaz E, Ilgit E, Taner D. Primitive persistent carotid-basilar and carotid-vertebral anastomoses: a report of seven cases and a review of the literature. Clin Anat 1995;8(1):36–43.
27. Hahnel S, Hartmann M, Jansen O, et al. Persistent hypoglossal artery: MRI, MRA and digital subtraction angiography. Neuroradiology 2001;43(9):767–9.
28. Harrigan MR, Deveikis JP. Handbook of cerebrovascular disease and neurointerventional technique. 2nd edition. Dordrecht (The Netherlands): Humana Press; 2013.
29. Luh GY, Dean BL, Tomsick TA, et al. The persistent fetal carotid-vertebrobasilar anastomoses. AJR Am J Roentgenol 1999;172(5):1427–32.
30. Kolbinger R, Heindel W, Pawlik G, et al. Right proatlantal artery type I, right internal carotid occlusion, and left internal carotid stenosis: case report and review of the literature. J Neurol Sci 1993;117(1–2): 232–9.

31. Silbergleit R, Quint DJ, Mehta BA, et al. The persistent stapedial artery. AJNR Am J Neuroradiol 2000; 21(3):572–7.

32. Lemke AJ, Benndorf G, Liebig T, et al. Anomalous origin of the right vertebral artery: review of the literature and case report of right vertebral artery origin distal to the left subclavian artery. AJNR Am J Neuroradiol 1999;20(7):1318–21.

33. Sherman PM, Gailloud P. Artery of the cervical enlargement originating from the inferior thyroid artery: an angiographic observation. J Vasc Interv Radiol 2004;15(6):648–50.

34. Parmar H, Sitoh YY, Hui F. Normal variants of the intracranial circulation demonstrated by MR angiography at 3T. Eur J Radiol 2005;56(2):220–8.

35. Lesley WS, Dalsania HJ. Double origin of the posterior inferior cerebellar artery. AJNR Am J Neuroradiol 2004;25(3):425–7.

36. Sanders WP, Sorek PA, Mehta BA. Fenestration of intracranial arteries with special attention to associated aneurysms and other anomalies. AJNR Am J Neuroradiol 1993;14(3):675–80.

37. Perlmutter D, Rhoton AL Jr. Microsurgical anatomy of the anterior cerebral-anterior communicating-recurrent artery complex. J Neurosurg 1976;45(3):259–72.

38. Uchino A, Kato A, Takase Y, et al. Middle cerebral artery variations detected by magnetic resonance angiography. Eur Radiol 2000;10(4):560–3.

39. Komiyama M, Nishikawa M, Yasui T. The accessory middle cerebral artery as a collateral blood supply. AJNR Am J Neuroradiol 1997;18(3):587–90.

40. Takahashi S, Suga T, Kawata Y, et al. Anterior choroidal artery: angiographic analysis of variations and anomalies. AJNR Am J Neuroradiol 1990;11(4):719–29.

41. Caldemeyer KS, Carrico JB, Mathews VP. The radiology and embryology of anomalous arteries of the head and neck. AJNR Am J Neuroradiol 1998; 170(1):197–203.

42. Taveras JM, Wood EH. Diagnostic neuroradiology. 2nd edition. Baltimore (MD): Williams & Wilkins Co; 1976.

43. Saltzman GF. Infundibular widening of the posterior communicating artery studied by carotid angiography. Acta Radiol 1959;51(6):415–21.

Percutaneous Treatment of Severe Intracranial Carotid and Middle Cerebral Artery Stenosis

Alex Abou-Chebl, MD

KEYWORDS

- Intracranial stenting • MCA stenosis • Intracranial atherosclerosis

KEY POINTS

- Symptomatic intracranial MCA stenosis carries a high risk of stroke despite medical therapy and is generally not amenable to surgical bypass.
- Due to the lack of efficacy and durability data from prospective, randomized, multicenter trials, intracranial stenting remains investigational and should be used only in carefully selected patients after thorough evaluation of their clinical and anatomic factors.
- Stenting should not be performed in chronic total occlusions and asymptomatic lesions and generally should be avoided in very old patients, especially those with underlying dementia and severe calcification of their vessels.
- Symptomatic patients with angiographically documented greater than 70% stenosis and who have failed medical therapy are appropriate candidates for intracranial angioplasty and stenting and should be enrolled in clinical trials when possible.

INTRODUCTION

Intracranial atherosclerosis disease (ICAD) accounts for 8% to 10% of ischemic stroke in the United States but is more prevalent in Asia.[1–4] The exact prevalence is unknown because many patients with the condition are asymptomatic and the intracranial location has limited noninvasive imaging as well as pathologic analysis. In addition, other causes of intracranial stenosis, such as vasculitis, dissection, embolism undergoing recanalization, moyamoya arteriopathy, postradiation arteriopathy, and infectious vasculitides, may all mimic ICAD and need to be carefully excluded in all symptomatic patients.[5]

Cerebral ischemia is caused primarily by limitation of flow as well as by vessel thrombosis and occlusion with or without distal embolization. The Warfarin-Aspirin for Symptomatic Intracranial Disease (WASID) trial demonstrated that a significant proportion (up to 22% annually) of symptomatic patients with significant intracranial disease (defined as angiographic stenosis between 70% and 99%) who were treated medically experienced recurrent ischemia.[2,6] Surgical bypass has proved ineffective in a randomized trial and endarterectomy is exceedingly difficult to perform.[7]

With advancements in stent technology, endovascular therapy has emerged as a feasible and potentially highly effective means of treating patients with ICAD. The primary goal of endovascular therapy is to improve flow through the stenosis and the increase in lumen diameter need not be significant for clinical benefit. Although desirable, an angiographic endpoint of a smooth, normal caliber lumen is not necessary; because the cerebral vessels are so fragile, the pursuit of such a goal may lead to dissection, arterial rupture, or intracerebral hemorrhage (ICH), which is often catastrophic and not amenable to treatment. This concept is of paramount importance, especially compared with the goals of epicardial coronary

The author has nothing to disclose.
Department of Neurology, University of Louisville School of Medicine, Room 114, 500 South Preston Street, Louisville, KY 40202, USA
E-mail address: a0abou03@Louisville.edu

Intervent Cardiol Clin 3 (2014) 135–143
http://dx.doi.org/10.1016/j.iccl.2013.09.003

intervention, for which there are data supporting a more "aggressive" endpoint.

INDICATIONS AND PATIENT SELECTION

The indication for intracranial stenting is the presence of an intracranial atherosclerotic stenosis that is producing symptoms despite optimal medical therapy (OMT) (**Box 1**). The stipulation that patients fail OMT first is based on anecdotal experience that many patients become asymptomatic on initiation of antithrombotic therapy. Treatment of asymptomatic stenoses is not recommended and is generally not performed because the risk of transient ischemic attack (TIA) or stroke is thought to be low. In patients with symptomatic, angiographically proved greater than 50% intracranial stenoses measured via the WASID method, the risk of recurrent stroke is approximately 12% annually regardless of treatment with aspirin or warfarin.[6] In those who have a greater than 70% stenosis, however, the risk of stroke is approximately 22% annually.[8] Therefore, an ideal candidate for intracranial intervention is a patient with a symptomatic, greater than 70% stenosis who has failed OMT.

Additionally a patient's symptoms should be attributable to the territory distal to the stenotic segment rather than to the territory of a perforator arising from the stenosis.[9] In cases of perforator stroke as the sole manifestation of ischemia, angioplasty and stenting have (anecdotally) a high likelihood of causing complete occlusion of and subsequent infarction in the territory of the perforator. In addition, those patients are effectively asymptomatic in the territory distal to the stenosis if their only manifestation is perforator ischemia and, therefore, they are less likely to benefit from revascularization. Recently symptomatic patients, especially those with a large or disabling infarct, may have an increased risk of ICH.[10,11] Unless

the need is pressing, some investigators have advocated delaying treatment for 6 weeks or more in these patients.[12] Functional imaging to assess cerebrovascular reserve (ie, collateral competence) may also be used to select patients at highest risk of stroke with medical therapy and, therefore, those patients most likely to benefit from percutaneous transluminal angioplasty and/or stenting (PTAS).[9,13] Such tests can consist of the widely available acetazolamide single-photon emission CT, breath-holding transcranial Doppler ultrasound studies, or the less widely available acetazolamide perfusion CT and positron emission tomography scanning.

Lesion characteristics play an important role in the likelihood of success and complications. Although the data on this subject are limited in comparison to those in the cardiac literature, it is the author's belief, based on personal experience and supported by some small case series, that the same risk factors for complications with percutaneous transluminal coronary angioplasty (PTCA) are also applicable to intracranial interventions.[9,14] Lesion length, eccentricity, calcification, and angulation as well as small vessel size, proximity to a bifurcation, and large adjacent branches are all risk factors for complications. Given the fragility of the cerebral vessels, these factors are even more relevant than in the thicker, more muscular coronary arteries.

Another important selection criterion is the feasibility of gaining access to the site to perform the intervention. This was of somewhat greater importance when a majority of patients were treated with coronary stents that were difficult to deliver intracranially. With the availability of the self-expanding cerebral stent systems, deliverability has been less of an issue but remains important.[15] Vessel tortuosity, especially of the internal carotid artery (ICA) or vertebral artery (VA), can be so severe that a guide catheter can not be placed in the parent artery or even prevent intracranial delivery of a balloon. Under such circumstances, the risk of complications (eg, guide catheter–induced dissections and intracranial artery perforation or dissection) increases significantly. Hence, a rule of thumb is if a stent cannot be delivered safely, then an intervention probably should not be performed, in case there is vessel dissection or abrupt closure after PTA, necessitating provisional stenting.

CEREBROVASCULAR ANATOMY

The intracranial vessels most often associated with ICAD and are the most amenable to endovascular therapy are the paired ICA, middle cerebral

---

Box 1
Patient selection criteria for intracranial stenting

Presence of an intracranial atherosclerotic stenosis that produces symptoms despite OMT

Patient symptoms attributable to the territory distal to the stenotic segment rather than to the territory of a perforator arising from the stenosis

Lesion characteristics amenable to PTAS

Feasibility of gaining access to the site to perform the intervention arteries (MCAs), anterior cerebral arteries, VA, and the singular basilar artery (BA). The intracranial arteries present several challenges. First, they course in the subarachnoid space (with the exception of the petrous and cavernous segments of the ICA). Second, they are thin with no external elastic lamina and have a thin tunica muscularis and a very thin adventitia. Third, there is significant tortuosity in their proximal segments. These factors greatly increase the risk of vessel injury and perforation during endovascular therapy. Such complications are often catastrophic (fatal in up to 80%) because ICH or subarachnoid hemorrhage (SAH) can result in a rapid increase in intracranial pressure leading to herniation or cessation of cerebral blood flow and death. The brain is also very sensitive to embolic debris, even if nearly microscopic in size, and emboli that in other vascular beds would be of no clinical significance could in the brain cause devastating deficits (eg, lenticulostriate artery occlusion causing internal capsular stroke and complete hemiplegia).

Other important anatomic considerations include the competence of the circle of Willis, a potential source of collateral flow for the major vessels of the brain. Flow can be directed either anterior-posterior (or the reverse) via the posterior communicating (PCOM) or right to left (or the reverse) via the anterior communicating (ACOM) arteries. A complete circle is present in only approximately 25% of individuals, with most individuals harboring a normal variant, such as a fetal posterior cerebral artery (PCA) (approximately 20%) or an absent or atretic PCOM or ACOM artery (approximately 50%). These collaterals are important as sources of flow in cases of occlusion of the proximal BA or the ICA. Vessels over the surface of the brain (ie, pial collaterals) may also supply collaterals that may be robust but usually are only adequate to perfuse a portion of a territory. These pial collaterals are important to note in cases of MCA intervention in particular because the PCOM or ACOM artery is proximal and cannot typically supply collateral flow directly to the MCA.

Lastly, there are essential perforating arteries that emanate from the MCA, BA, and PCA trunks. These vessels supply critical structures and, although small (50–200 μm), their occlusion can cause major and disabling neurologic deficits. These vessels are at risk of occlusion with PTAS especially if they were the cause of the presenting symptoms. Furthermore, they are particularly vulnerable to wire perforation and its disastrous consequences. They arise from the dorsal (superiorly in anterior-posterior view) aspect of the MCA and (posteriorly in anterior-posterior view) BA.

PREPROCEDURE PLANNING

First, the appropriateness of the treatment should be determined without doubt. Patients must be adequately pretreated with a dual antiplatelet regimen consisting of aspirin and clopidogrel. As a rule, any patient who cannot receive both for the necessary duration should not undergo stenting. Use of other agents is unproved and is discouraged. Balloon angioplasty alone may be performed using treatment with a single agent if necessary. Although of unproved benefit, anecdotal experience suggests that confirmation of adequate platelet inhibition preprocedure decreases ischemic complications. A full understanding of each patient's cerebrovascular anatomy is essential and can be gleaned by noninvasive imaging, such as CT angiography or magnetic resonance angiography. The purpose is to determine not only the best approach (ie, femoral vs radial) but also the possibility of being able to deliver a stent through the tortuous segments and to understand the potential sources of collateral flow (discussed previously). Thorough, multiplanar digital subtraction angiography is also essential for understanding the anatomy, lesion configuration, sources of collateral flow, and presence of other pathologies or anatomic variants. For example, the presence of a persistent trigeminal artery in the setting of a "stenotic" proximal BA or V4 segment of a VA indicates that those segments are congenitally hypoplastic, and dilation is contraindicated.

ENDOVASCULAR APPROACH

A femoral approach is preferred, especially for MCA and ICA procedures, but brachial or radial access should be considered for vertebrobasilar interventions if there is severe and unfavorable innominate, subclavian, or VA angulation. Heparin is given to achieve an activated clotting between 250 and 300 seconds. Routine use of glycoprotein IIb/IIIa receptor antagonists is discouraged unless patients are inadequately premedicated with antiplatelet agents and the intervention is urgent. A 6 French (F) guide catheter should be placed distally in the cervical ICA or distal V2 segment of the VA if safe and feasible. If there is severe tortuosity, then a 6F to 8F sheath may be placed in the common carotid or subclavian arteries to provide additional support for the guide catheter. The newer generation of highly flexible guide catheters (eg, Neuron [Penumbra Inc, Alameda, CA]), or so-called intermediate catheters, may sometimes overcome severe tortuosity and facilitate balloon or stent delivery. The lesion should then be crossed with a soft, neuro-microwire with an atraumatic tip, such as a Synchro (Stryker) or Transcend (Stryker). The guide wire should be advanced with great care to avoid cannulating small branches or perforators and this is best performed with road-mapping technology. For terminal ICA and MCA treatment, the wire should be passed into the second or proximal third-order MCA branches.

No randomized data show superiority of stenting over angioplasty; yet, similar to coronary disease, stenting is generally preferred.[16,17] The author's approach is to predilate the lesion with an undersized over-the-wire balloon; oversizing or too-aggressive performance of inflation can lead to vessel rupture or dissection.[12] This approach permits adequate sizing of the vessel and observation of lesion response to angioplasty as well as patient pain response. A headache with submaximal balloon inflation suggests that a patient's vessel may not tolerate a stent much larger than the predilation balloon or that inflation rates need to be slower.[18] Nitroglycerin (200–400 µg) should then be given through the guide catheter, followed by angiography. If there is an excellent result after PTA, with less than 30% residual stenosis, stenting need not be performed depending on the circumstances. Otherwise, stenting should be strongly considered, selecting a stent sized no larger than the smallest normal segment into which the stent will be placed. Stent length should be kept to the minimum needed to cover the lesion or angioplasty segment.

Stent delivery, particularly to the terminal ICA or MCA, is the most challenging aspect of these procedures.[19] The latest generation of cobalt-chromium coronary stents has proved highly deliverable, but in 8% to 10% of patients even these stents cannot be delivered safely, especially through the severe angulation of the cavernous carotid artery.[20] Better guide catheter support, exchanging for medium support wires, buddy wires, and other tricks, may sometimes facilitate stent delivery.[21] Very stiff wires should never be used in the intracranial vessels due to increased propensity to cause vessel dissection and perforation. Throughout, close observation of the patient and monitoring for headache should be carried out.[18]

Two stents that have been developed specifically for the cerebral vasculature have been tested in humans. The balloon-expandable Neurolink (Guidant Corp.) balloon-expandable stent (BES) was evaluated in a 43-patient trial (Stenting of Symptomatic Atherosclerotic Lesions in the Vertebral or Intracranial Arteries).[22] It was highly deliverable with a low complication rate (6.6% stroke at 30 days), but it demonstrated a high restenosis rate of 32.4% and is not approved in the United States. The more recent device, the Wingspan (Stryker) self-expanding, nitinol, highly flexible

and deliverable stent, was tested in a 45-patient study and approved by the Food and Drug Administration (FDA) under a humanitarian device exemption.[23] Although highly deliverable, the clinical results with Wingspan have not been as good as expected (discussed later). Therefore, the ideal device for the treatment of intracranial stenosis has yet to be developed; clinicians must decide on a case-by-case basis which device to use.

Poststenting dilation is rarely needed unless a self-expanding stent (SES) is used; this is controversial because the instructions for use of the Wingspan stent warn against postdilation. Based on the author's (anecdotal) experience, postdilation of the Wingspan is almost always needed to avoid leaving behind a very small residual lumen. Postdilation is always performed, however, with a compliant balloon no larger than the smallest segment into which it is placed. After treatment, thorough angiographic assessment is performed, looking for any evidence of distal embolization, branch occlusion, dissection, or perforation. A brief neurologic examination is also performed. The author prefers to keep the wire across the lesion and repeat angiography 10 to 15 minutes later to monitor for evidence of in-stent thrombus formation. If all is clear and the patient is neurologically normal, then the procedure is terminated.

PERIOPERATIVE MANAGEMENT

The author recommends that these procedures be performed under local rather than general anesthesia to permit frequent intraoperative neurologic assessments.[18,19] Headache can be an important marker for impending vessel injury and should prompt a reassessment of wire position, balloon inflation rate and pressure, amount of force used to deliver a stent, and so forth. Such maneuvers may avert disaster.[18] Close observation of neurologic status and monitoring of blood pressure are critical. Generally speaking, blood pressure should be kept in the low normal range for at least 14 days (complications discussed later). Dual antiplatelet therapy should be continued for at least 30 days, but the author's approach is to continue them for 6 to 12 months (1–2 years for a drug-eluting stent [DES]) or until a follow-up angiogram confirms there is no restenosis.[20] This is controversial because of a lack of long-term safety data and the presence of evidence that dual therapy increases the risk of ICH in some stroke patients.[24,25]

CLINICAL RESULTS

A majority of published series of intracranial angioplasty and stenting have been retrospective series of patients treated with BESs. The reported outcomes with these stents have been highly variable because of differences in patient selection, technique, operator experience, and a lack of adequate angiographic and clinical follow-up.[5] Therefore, no firm conclusions regarding long-term safety, efficacy, and durability can be drawn from these data. Most studies have reported 30-day stroke, ICH, and death rates of 8% to 20% but some have had rates as high as 50%, with an average rate of 10% to 12%.[11,12,18,26-38] The author and other investigators have reported on the limited use of DESs for intracranial stenoses, with excellent success. The ultimate safety of this approach remains, however, unclear.[28,39]

Two registries of real world experience with the Wingspan stent system have been published. In the first of those studies, which included 78 patients, the major periprocedural complication rate was 6.1%. In-stent restenosis ($\geq$50% narrowing) was seen in 34.5% of patients and stent thrombosis rate was 4.1%.[40] The largest prospective registry studied 129 patients with symptomatic 70% to 99% stenoses; the technical success rate was 96.7%, but the 30-day stroke/death rate was 9.6%.[41] Restenosis was seen in 24.5% of those who underwent follow-up imaging. When compared with the event rates in patients on medical therapy in the WASID trial beyond 3 months, the recurrent event rate was lower for those stented.[6] Restenosis rates seem high with the Wingspan stent and its management is generally repeat angioplasty.[42]

The only randomized trial data regarding intracranial stenting come from the Stenting versus Aggressive Medical Management for Preventing Recurrent Stroke in Intracranial Arterial Stenosis (SAMMPRIS) trial.[10] SAMMPRIS randomized 451 patients with a recently symptomatic 70% to 99% stenosis to OMT or OMT plus PTAS with the Wingspan stent system. OMT consisted of aspirin (325 mg/d) plus clopidogrel (75 mg/d) for 90 days, rosuvastatin (target low-density lipoprotein <70 mg/dL), systolic blood pressure [SBP] lowering to less than 140 mm Hg (<130 mm Hg for diabetics), and lifestyle modification. Enrollment was stopped early because the 30-day stroke/death rate was 14.7% with PTAS but only 5.8% with AMT ($P = .002$).[10] The 30-day risk of PTAS was approximately twice as high as previously assumed and the 30-day risk under OMT alone was approximately half of that predicted from WASID.[6,40,41] These results have severely curtailed the practice of intracranial stenting. Although SAMMPRIS was the best and largest trial to date, it had many limitations.[9,43] A full discussion of the limitations is beyond the scope of this article, but

the major criticisms consist of the following: (1) inclusion of patients who had not failed OMT and who were many days or weeks from the primary event, thus creating selection bias for patients who would do well with OMT; (2) the operators not having had experience with the Wingspan stent or with treatment of ICAD; (3) patients not selected based on the presence of decreased flow reserve; (4) patients enrolled with perforator ischemia, thus increasing the risk of complications (a majority of ischemic complications were due to perforator occlusion) with minimal potential for benefit; and (5) the procedures performed under general anesthesia, thus preventing assessment of neurologic status or pain and possibly contributing to a high number of wire perforations and ICH.[9,43]

There has been one randomized trial (VISSIT) of a BES (Pharos Vitesse stent [Codman]) for ICAD but that trial was stopped early due to futility and the results have not been published or presented.[44] Other than the issue of deliverability, there are many reasons that BESs may be preferred for ICAD, much like for coronary PTCA. Given the SAMMPRIS data, however, the current medical-legal environment, and the fact that Wingspan is FDA approved for this (limited) indication but BESs are not, the use of BESs is problematic. There is a pressing need for prospective clinical trials of intracranial PTAS with standardized patient and lesion selection criteria, experienced operators, standardized perioperative medical management, balloons and stents designed for the cerebral vasculature, and comprehensive postoperative management criteria and follow-up.[9]

Direct comparisons of BESs versus SESs have been lacking until recently. In the largest registry of PTAS published, Jiang and colleagues[15] from 5 centers retrospectively reviewed the outcomes of 670 treated lesions in 637 patients. Of the total, 454 (68%) lesions were treated with BESs and 216 (32%) lesions with SESs. The 30-day periprocedural complication rate was 6.1% and was similar between the two groups. A major predictor of complications was treatment within 24 hours of the index event (odds ratio [OR] 4.0; 95% CI, 1.7–6.7; $P<.007$). Focal lesions, however, were associated with lower perioperative events (OR 0.31; 95% CI, 0.13–0.72; $P<.001$). Importantly, the midterm restenosis rate was lower in patients with a lower post-treatment residual stenosis (OR 0.97; 95% CI, 0.95–0.99; $P<.006$) and in patients treated with BES (20%) compared with SES (28%). These data are reassuring that, in the real world, PTAS may be performed safely but must be reconciled with the results of the randomized trials. In addition, the consequences and management of restenosis are not well understood.

Long-term follow-up after intracranial stenting has generally been lacking. Only one series has reported long-term follow-up; this cohort included 53 patients with 69 arterial lesions treated with a mix of angioplasty, bare-metal stents, and DES.[20] They were followed for up to 7 years with a median follow-up duration of 24 months. The procedural success rate was 98.6%; 30-day death/stroke rate was 10.1%, with only 1 death. The 2-year stroke/death/TIA rate was 15.9%, significantly lower than the 22% to 23% annual rate of stroke expected with medical therapy. Restenosis at 1 year was reported in 15.9% of patients and was symptomatic in 18.2% of these. Factors associated with restenosis were vessel size less than 2.5 mm (hazard ratio = 4.78; 95% CI, 1.35–16.93) and interventions performed in the setting of an acute stroke (hazard ratio = 6.36; 95% CI, 1.78–22.56).

POTENTIAL COMPLICATIONS AND THEIR MANAGEMENT

Chief among the risk factors for complications are the tortuosity and fragility of the cerebral vessels and the maneuvers needed to overcome them (**Box 2**). The cerebral vessels may have extensive calcification like the coronary arteries; therefore, lesion characteristics considered high risk for coronary PTCA should likewise be considered high risk if present in the cerebral vessels.[14] Advancing age is also a marker for decreasing cerebral neuronal reserve and, along with preexisting neurologic dysfunction, is a marker for increased risk of ischemic injury and reduced potential for recovery. In patients with recent ischemic stroke or those with severely stenotic lesions, hypertension is a major risk factor for ICH

Box 2
Factors Associated with Complications

Tortuosity and fragility of the cerebral vessels

Lesion characteristics associated with high risk with coronary PTCA (ie, small vessels, lesion length, eccentricity, calcification, angulation, and presence of side branches or a bifurcation)

Advanced age

Significant hypertension

Recent (<4 weeks) brain infarction affecting more than one-third of the territory supplied by the vessel or associated with a disabling deficit

Presence of ICH on a CT scan

History of ICH

---

due to the hyperperfusion syndrome.[45,46] Recent (<4 weeks) brain infarction affecting more than one-third of the territory supplied by the vessel or associated with a disabling deficit should be a relative contraindication to treatment, which should be delayed 4 to 6 weeks if possible.[10,11] The presence of ICH on a CT scan or a history of ICH should be considered a contraindication to PTAS.

ISCHEMIC COMPLICATIONS

Embolism and thrombosis are the most likely causes of ischemia during PTAS, but dissection and vasospasm may also occur and cause symptoms. If a new neurologic deficit is found during the intervention, an immediate cerebral angiogram of the likely culprit vessel should be performed in multiple orthogonal planes and reviewed closely. If an arterial occlusion is noted, the likely cause should be determined and addressed (eg, if inadequate anticoagulation is the culprit, then more heparin may be considered as long as the occlusion is small and the operator is able to perform rescue therapy). Physicians performing intracranial intervention should generally be trained and equipped to perform rescue therapy. If the patient has more than a trivial deficit and the operator is unable to perform rescue therapy (and no other interventionist is available who might do so), then intravenous (IV) tissue plasminogen activator (tPA) or a small quantity of tPA infused through the guide catheter should be considered. If a large vessel occlusion is seen (eg, ICA, MCA trunk, or first-order branch occlusion) or if a patient has a severe neurologic deficit, then rescue therapy must be rapidly performed. Ideally, catheterization of the occluded segment with a 2F to 2.3F microcatheter should be performed if a small thrombus burden is noted and the patient can safely receive fibrinolytics. If the occluded segment is very small (<2 mm), it may be worthwhile to attempt clot disruption with the microwire or microcatheter. If this is not effective or feasible, then through the microcatheter, small aliquots of a fibrinolytic (1–5 mg tPA, 1 U reteplase, and so forth) should be given directly into the clot. If a platelet-rich thrombus is suspected, intra-arterial (or IV) abciximab or eptifibatide can be given in low doses (ie, no more than one-quarter to one-half of the usual IV bolus).[47,48] The dosage should be adjusted based on the risk factors for ICH (noted previously), especially the presence of other anticoagulants or fibrinolytics.

Alternatively, particularly if there is a large thrombus burden, mechanical embolectomy may be performed. The commercially available embolectomy devices (Merci Retriever [Stryker Inc,

Kalamazoo, Michigan], Penumbra aspiration catheter [Penumbra Inc, Alameda, CA], Solitaire FR [Covidien Inc, Mansfield, MA], and Trevo [Stryker Inc, Kalamazoo, Michigan]) have between 50% and 90% recanalization efficacy.[49–52] The choice of device is dependent on the status of the parent vessel and location of the occlusion relative to the stenotic segment being treated. Most of the embolectomy devices result in loss of wire access to the lesion, a factor that needs to be considered if the stenosis is difficult to cannulate or a dissection flap is suspected. In addition, the stent-retriever systems should be avoided if a stent is already deployed, because they can become ensnared. If embolectomy is not successful or if the occlusion is suspected to be in a severely stenotic segment, then angioplasty and/or stenting may be successful.

If there is a severe or rapidly expanding dissection, treatment should be initiated. Once the lesion is crossed with an appropriate wire, stenting should be performed using an SES, if possible. An exception to the SES recommendation is dissection localized to the VA ostium, where a BES is preferred because of ease of placement and preservation of access to the subclavian artery distal to the VA. In the remainder of the VA, which is highly mobile, SESs are preferred. If a dissection extends intracranially or primarily involves the intracranial vessels, then the situation becomes more dire. In the author's experience, these complications are rarely benign and are often associated with ischemia or SAH.[53] The most common cause of iatrogenic dissection is the attempted delivery of stiff devices, which almost by definition suggests that there is severe tortuosity or severe atherosclerosis, and stenting of the dissected segment may be difficult. Accordingly, treatment must be individualized in such situations. Often in these cases, the SESs designed for the brain are ideal, because they do not require balloon inflation and thus reduce the chance for vessel rupture. If the dissection is noted post-stenting, then it can typically be watched as long as there is no perforation of the vessel.

Cerebral vasospasm is common and is commonly transient and asymptomatic and generally does not require treatment. Severe vasospasm can cause ischemia, however, and may lead to dissection or vessel perforation and should be treated with nitroglycerin, verapamil, or cardene.

INTRACEREBRAL HEMORRHAGE

If there is any clinical deterioration and angiography does not show an occlusion, an expanding ICH should be suspected and intraoperative CT should be performed immediately. If there is frank extravasation of contrast on angiography, immediate blood pressure reduction, heparin reversal, and transfusion of coagulation factors and platelets should be implemented. Temporary balloon occlusion should be considered. Rarely, embolization and vessel sacrifice may be needed to save a patient's life. For the most part, there is no treatment of ICH and SAH and what treatment exists is either ineffective or associated with a high-risk of ischemia. The author has seen a minority of patients survive an ICH despite all of these measures.[54] The single greatest obstacle in the treatment of cerebrovascular disease is that all treatment of cerebral ischemia carries a risk of ICH and all treatment of ICH carries a risk of cerebral ischemia. Neurosurgical ICH evacuation may be appropriate in selected cases but is generally of no benefit or even harmful especially in the presence of potent antithrombotic therapy. Nevertheless, in cases of marked elevation of intracranial pressure and hydrocephalus, external ventricular drain placement may be life saving.

Cerebral hyperperfusion syndrome can occur with any cerebral revascularization procedure and most commonly causes delayed headache, seizures, cerebral edema, or ICH 3 to 5 days postoperatively.[45,46,55] The mainstay of treatment and prevention of the hyperperfusion syndrome is aggressive blood pressure control postoperatively; in the author's experience SBP less than 120 mm Hg or even lower is often needed.[56] A detailed discussion of the neurologic critical care of such patients is beyond the scope of this article but neurologic consultants expert in stroke and neurologic critical care, which has been shown to improve survival and neurologic outcomes, should follow these patients.

SUMMARY

Due to the lack of efficacy and durability data from prospective, randomized, multicenter trials, intracranial stenting remains investigational and should be used only in carefully selected patients after thorough evaluation of their clinical and anatomic factors. Stenting should not be performed in chronic total occlusions and asymptomatic lesions and generally should be avoided in very old patients, especially those with underlying dementia and severe calcification of their vessels. Symptomatic patients with angiographically documented greater than 70% stenosis and who have failed medical therapy are, however, appropriate candidates for intracranial angioplasty and stenting and should be enrolled in clinical trials when possible.

REFERENCES

1. Sacco RL, Kargman DE, Gu Q, et al. Race-ethnicity and determinants of intracranial atherosclerotic cerebral infarction. The northern manhattan stroke study. Stroke 1995;26:14–20.

2. Thijs VN, Albers GW. Symptomatic intracranial atherosclerosis: outcome of patients who fail antithrombotic therapy [comment]. Neurology 2000;55: 490–7.

3. Wityk RJ, Lehman D, Klag M, et al. Race and sex differences in the distribution of cerebral atherosclerosis. Stroke 1996;27:1974–80.

4. Feldmann E, Daneault N, Kwan E, et al. Chinese-white differences in the distribution of occlusive cerebrovascular disease. Neurology 1990;40:1541–5.

5. Yadav JS, Abou-Chebl A. Intracranial angioplasty and stenting. J Interv Cardiol 2009;22:9–15.

6. Chimowitz MI, Lynn MJ, Howlett-Smith H, et al. Comparison of warfarin and aspirin for symptomatic intracranial arterial stenosis. N Engl J Med 2005;352:1305–16.

7. Failure of extracranial-intracranial arterial bypass to reduce the risk of ischemic stroke. Results of an international randomized trial. The EC/IC bypass study group. N Engl J Med 1985;313:1191–200.

8. Kasner SE, Chimowitz MI, Lynn MJ, et al. Predictors of ischemic stroke in the territory of a symptomatic intracranial arterial stenosis. Circulation 2006;113:555–63.

9. Abou-Chebl A, Steinmetz H. Critique of "Stenting versus aggressive medical therapy for intracranial arterial stenosis" by Chimowitz et al in the new England journal of medicine. Stroke 2012;43:616–20.

10. Chimowitz MI, Lynn MJ, Derdeyn CP, et al. Stenting versus aggressive medical therapy for intracranial arterial stenosis. N Engl J Med 2011;365: 993–1003.

11. Gupta R, Schumacher HC, Mangla S, et al. Urgent endovascular revascularization for symptomatic intracranial atherosclerotic stenosis. Neurology 2003;61:1729–35.

12. Connors JJ III, Wojak JC. Percutaneous transluminal angioplasty for intracranial atherosclerotic lesions: evolution of technique and short-term results. J Neurosurg 1999;91:415–23.

13. Liebeskind DS, Cotsonis GA, Saver JL, et al. Collaterals dramatically alter stroke risk in intracranial atherosclerosis. Ann Neurol 2011;69:963–74.

14. Mori T, Fukuoka M, Kazita K, et al. Follow-up study after intracranial percutaneous transluminal cerebral balloon angioplasty. AJNR Am J Neuroradiol 1998;19:1525–33.

15. Jiang WJ, Cheng-Ching E, Abou-Chebl A, et al. Multi-center analysis of stenting in symptomatic intracranial atherosclerosis. Neurosurgery 2012; 70:25–30.

16. Foley DP, Serruys PW. Provisional stenting–stent-like balloon angioplasty: evidence to define the continuing role of balloon angioplasty for percutaneous coronary revascularization. Semin Interv Cardiol 1996;1:269–73.

17. Knight CJ, Curzen NP, Groves PH, et al. Stent implantation reduces restenosis in patients with suboptimal results following coronary angioplasty. Eur Heart J 1999;20:1783–90.

18. Abou-Chebl A, Krieger DW, Bajzer CT, et al. Intracranial angioplasty and stenting in the awake patient. J Neuroimaging 2006;16:216–23.

19. Jiang WJ, Yu W, Du B, et al. Wingspan experience at beijing tiantan hospital: new insights into the mechanisms of procedural complication from viewing intraoperative transient ischemic attacks during awake stenting for vertebrobasilar stenosis. J Neurointerv Surg 2010;2:99–103.

20. Mazighi M, Yadav JS, Abou-Chebl A. Durability of endovascular therapy for symptomatic intracranial atherosclerosis. Stroke 2008;39:1766–9.

21. Lee TH, Choi CH, Park KP, et al. Techniques for intracranial stent navigation in patients with tortuous vessels. AJNR Am J Neuroradiol 2005;26:1375–80.

22. SSYLVIA Study Investigators. Stenting of Symptomatic Atherosclerotic Lesions in the Vertebral or Intracranial Arteries (SSYLVIA): study results. Stroke 2004;35:1388–92.

23. Bose A, Hartmann M, Henkes H, et al. A novel, self-expanding, nitinol stent in medically refractory intracranial atherosclerotic stenoses: the wingspan study. Stroke 2007;38:1531–7.

24. Diener HC, Bogousslavsky J, Brass LM, et al. Aspirin and clopidogrel compared with clopidogrel alone after recent ischaemic stroke or transient ischaemic attack in high-risk patients (match): randomised, double-blind, placebo-controlled trial. Lancet 2004;364:331–7.

25. Bhatt DL, Flather MD, Hacke W, et al. Patients with prior myocardial infarction, stroke, or symptomatic peripheral arterial disease in the charisma trial. J Am Coll Cardiol 2007;49:1982–8.

26. Rasmussen PA, Perl J, Barr JD, et al. Stent-assisted angioplasty of intracranial vertebrobasilar atherosclerosis: an initial experience. J Neurosurg 2000; 92:771–8.

27. Alazzaz A, Thornton J, Aletich VA, et al. Intracranial percutaneous transluminal angioplasty for arteriosclerotic stenosis. Arch Neurol 2000;57:1625–30.

28. Abou-Chebl A, Bashir Q, Yadav JS. Drug-eluting stents for the treatment of intracranial atherosclerosis: initial experience and midterm angiographic follow-up. Stroke 2005;36:e165–8.

29. Weber W, Mayer TE, Henkes H, et al. Stent-angioplasty of intracranial vertebral and basilar artery stenoses in symptomatic patients. Eur J Radiol 2005;55:231–6.

30. Kim DJ, Lee BH, Kim DI, et al. Stent-assisted an-gioplasty of symptomatic intracranial vertebrobasi-lar artery stenosis: feasibility and follow-up results. AJNR Am J Neuroradiol 2005;26:1381–8.

31. Higashida RT, Meyers PM, Connors JJ III, et al. Intracranial angioplasty & stenting for cerebral atherosclerosis: a position statement of the amer-ican society of interventional and therapeutic neuroradiology, society of interventional radiology, and the american society of neuroradiology. AJNR Am J Neuroradiol 2005;26:2323–7.

32. Jiang WJ, Wang YJ, Du B, et al. Stenting of symp-tomatic m1 stenosis of middle cerebral artery: an initial experience of 40 patients. Stroke 2004;35:1375–80.

33. Abou-Chebl A, Krieger D, Bajzer C, et al. Intracra-nial angioplasty and stenting in the awake patient. J Neuroimaging 2006;16(3):216–23.

34. Lee JH, Kwon SU, Lee JH, et al. Percutaneous transluminal angioplasty for symptomatic middle cerebral artery stenosis: long-term follow-up. Cere-brovasc Dis 2003;15:90–7.

35. Marks MP, Wojak JC, Al Ali F, et al. Angioplasty for symptomatic intracranial stenosis: clinical outcome. Stroke 2006;37:1016–20.

36. Mori T, Kazita K, Chokyu K, et al. Short-term arterio-graphic and clinical outcome after cerebral angio-plasty and stenting for intracranial vertebrobasilar and carotid atherosclerotic occlusive disease. AJNR Am J Neuroradiol 2000;21:249–54.

37. Mori T, Mori K, Fukuoka M, et al. Percutaneous transluminal cerebral angioplasty: serial angio-graphic follow-up after successful dilatation. Neuroradiology 1997;39:111–6.

38. Lylyk P, Cohen JE, Ceratto R, et al. Angioplasty and stent placement in intracranial atherosclerotic ste-noses and dissections. AJNR Am J Neuroradiol 2002;23:430–6.

39. Gupta R, Al-Ali F, Thomas AJ, et al. Safety, feasi-bility, and short-term follow-up of drug-eluting stent placement in the intracranial and extracranial circu-lation. Stroke 2006;37:2562–6.

40. Fiorella D, Levy EI, Turk AS, et al. Us multicenter experience with the wingspan stent system for the treatment of intracranial atheromatous disease: periprocedural results. Stroke 2007;38:881–7.

41. Zaidat OO, Klucznik R, Alexander MJ, et al. The nih registry on use of the wingspan stent for symptom-atic 70-99% intracranial arterial stenosis. Neurology 2008;70:1518–24.

42. Levy EI, Turk AS, Albuquerque FC, et al. Wingspan in-stent restenosis and thrombosis: incidence, clin-ical presentation, and management. Neurosurgery 2007;61:644–50.

43. Abou-Chebl A. Intracranial stenting with wingspan: still awaiting a safe landing. Stroke 2011;42:1809–11.

44. Zaidat OO, Castonguay AC, Fitzsimmons BF, et al. Design of the Vitesse Intracranial Stent Study for Ischemic Therapy (VISSIT) Trial in symptomatic intracranial stenosis. J Stroke Cerebrovasc Dis 2012. [Epub ahead of print].

45. Reigel MM, Hollier LH, Sundt TM Jr, et al. Cerebral hyperperfusion syndrome: a cause of neurologic dysfunction after carotid endarterectomy. J Vasc Surg 1987;5:628–34.

46. Abou-Chebl A, Yadav JS, Reginelli JP, et al. Intra-cranial hemorrhage and hyperperfusion syndrome following carotid artery stenting: risk factors, pre-vention, and treatment. J Am Coll Cardiol 2004;43:1596–601.

47. Abou-Chebl A, Krieger D, Bajzer C, et al. Multi-modal therapy for the treatment of severe ischemic stroke combining gpiib/iiia antagonists and angio-plasty after failure of thrombolysis. Stroke 2003;34.

48. Fiorella D, Albuquerque FC, Han P, et al. Strategies for the management of intraprocedural thromboem-bolic complications with abciximab (reopro). Neuro-surgery 2004;54:1089–97 [discussion: 1097–98].

49. Smith WS, Sung G, Saver J, et al. Mechanical throm-bectomy for acute ischemic stroke: final results of the multi merci trial. Stroke 2008;39:1205–12.

50. Bose A, Henkes H, Alfke K, et al. The penumbra system: a mechanical device for the treatment of acute stroke due to thromboembolism. AJNR Am J Neuroradiol 2008;29:1409–13.

51. Saver JL, Jahan R, Levy EI, et al. Solitaire flow restoration device versus the merci retriever in pa-tients with acute ischaemic stroke (swift): a rando-mised, parallel-group, non-inferiority trial. Lancet 2012;380:1241–9.

52. Nogueira RG, Lutsep HL, Gupta R, et al. Trevo versus merci retrievers for thrombectomy revascu-larisation of large vessel occlusions in acute is-chaemic stroke (trevo 2): a randomised trial. Lancet 2012;380:1231–40.

53. Ahn JY, Chung YS, Lee BH, et al. Endovascular rescue from arterial rupture and thrombosis during middle cerebral artery stenting. Neuroradiology 2003;45:570–3.

54. Khatri R, Ansar M, Sultan F, et al. Requirements for emergent neurosurgical procedures among pa-tients undergoing neuroendovascular procedures in contemporary practice. AJNR Am J Neuroradiol 2012;33:465–8.

55. Meyers PM, Higashida RT, Phatouros CC, et al. Ce-rebral hyperperfusion syndrome after percuta-neous transluminal stenting of the craniocervical arteries. Neurosurgery 2000;47:335–43.

56. Abou-Chebl A, Reginelli J, Bajzer CT, et al. Inten-sive treatment of hypertension decreases the risk of hyperperfusion and intracerebral hemorrhage following carotid artery stenting. Catheter Cardio-vasc Interv 2007;69:690–6.

Current Reperfusion Strategies for Acute Stroke

Panagiotis Papanagiotou, MD[a],*,
Wolfgang Reith, MD, PhD[b], Andreas Kastrup, MD[c],
Christian Roth, MD[a]

KEYWORDS

- Thrombectomy • Brainstem • Reperfusion • Stent

KEY POINTS

- In anterior circulation strokes the impact of successful thrombectomy is greater in the first 3 to 4.5 hours after stroke than in late recanalization after 5 to 8 hours. In posterior circulation and brainstem strokes caused by vertebral or basilar artery (BA) occlusion, recanalization of occluded vessels has a therapeutic window up to 24 h after symptom onset.
- Multimodal computed tomography (CT) includes unenhanced CT, CT angiography (CTA), and CT perfusion. Noncontrast CT can identify intracranial (IC) hemorrhage and detect early signs of acute ischemic stroke. CTA can identify the occlusion site, detect arterial dissection, and grade collateral blood flow, whereas CT perfusion can differentiate between *tissue at risk* and irreversibly damaged brain tissue.
- CT perfusion helps distinction of the infarct core from the penumbra. In the penumbra, autoregulation is preserved, mean transit time (MTT) is prolonged, but cerebral blood volume (CBV) is preserved because of vasodilatation and collateral recruitment as part of the autoregulation process. In the infarct core, autoregulation is lost, MTT is prolonged, and CBV is down.
- In the authors' experience, the most effective reperfusion strategy today is the stent-retriever-based thrombectomy, in cases of large thrombus load, in combination with plain aspiration through a large distal access catheter (DAC). In special groups of patients with extracranial carotid occlusion, arterial dissection, and IC stenosis acute stenting is necessary.
- Complications that can occur during or after the procedure include distal embolization to the same or other vessel territories, dissection of the arteries, and subarachnoid or intracerebral hemorrhage.

 Videos of direct clinical examination of a patient with left side hemiplegia due to an MCA occlusion, examples of "hard" thrombi, brachial artery access, recanalization of MCA occlusion with stent-retriever, and treatment of acute atherosclerotic extracranial ICA occlusion accompany this article at http://www.interventional.theclinics.com/

INTRODUCTION

Stroke is the most common cause of permanent disability, the second most common cause of dementia, and the third most common cause of death in the Western world.[1] The World Health Organization estimates that 5.7 million people die from stroke each year. Each year, ≈795,000 people experience a new or recurrent stroke (ischemic or hemorrhagic) in the United States and 1 million people in the European Union. Those who survive

[a] Clinic for Diagnostic and Interventional Neuroradiology, Klinikum Bremen-Mitte/Bremen-Ost, St. Jürgen Str. 1, Bremen 28211, Germany; [b] Clinic for Diagnostic and Interventional Neuroradiology, Saarland University Hospital, Kirrbergerstr, Homburg 66421, Germany; [c] Clinic for Neurology, Klinikum Bremen-Mitte/Bremen-Ost, St. Jürgen Str. 1, Bremen 28211, Germany
* Corresponding author.
E-mail address: papanagiotou@me.com

Intervent Cardiol Clin 3 (2014) 145–167
http://dx.doi.org/10.1016/j.iccl.2013.09.008

interventional.theclinics.com

are often burdened with exorbitant rehabilitation costs, lost wages and productivity, limitations in their daily social activity, and significant residual disability.[2] Given that the aging population of the world is increasing, the statistics of stroke incidence and prevalence will also climb proportionately.

Timely treatment and intervention can minimize long-term disability by salvaging the at-risk penumbra and, consequently, reducing the associated morbidity and mortality. The only known drug therapy for acute ischemic stroke is thrombolysis with recombinant tissue plasminogen activator (t-PA), which has been proved in many clinical trials to be effective in improving clinical outcome and reducing subsequent disability.[3] The only improvement in this therapy has been the extension of the 3-h time frame to 4.5 hours in which it can be safely administered.[4] The number needed to treat, even with the extended window of 3 to 4.5 hours, is still 14.

A key advantage of intravenous (IV) t-PA is that it can be started rapidly after clinical assessment and CT of the brain without the use of contrast material. However, fewer than 15% to 40% of patients with acute stroke arrive at the hospital early enough to receive thrombolytic treatment, and only 2% to 5% of patients actually receive it.[5] Limitations of IV t-PA include dependence on available serum plasminogen, the resistance of a large thrombus to fibrinolysis, and the risks of systemic and cerebral hemorrhage.[6,7]

About 20% of strokes are due to large-artery occlusions causing severe strokes. IC arterial occlusion is independently associated with poor functional outcomes and high mortality rates. The treatment of these patients still remains a challenge because IV thrombolysis often reaches its limit of effectiveness. IV thrombolysis on its own leads to a good clinical outcome (modified Rankin Scale [mRS] ≤2) in only 15% to 25% of these cases compared with 40% good clinical outcome in minor strokes.[8,9] For this reason, patients with IC occlusion are considered to be candidates for additional or primary intra-arterial (IA) therapies.[10]

IA treatments for ischemic stroke that are approved by guidelines include IA fibrinolysis until 6 h after onset and mechanical thrombectomy until 8 h after onset.[11]

INDICATIONS AND PATIENT SELECTION

Important features of the patient's clinical presentation that influence endovascular treatment decisions include clinical status, time of presentation, and imaging characteristics.

Clinical Status

The National Institutes of Health Stroke Scale (NIHSS), a quantitative measure of the severity of the stroke, should be used for assessment during the initial examination in all patients with stroke, but especially in patients being considered for IV t-PA.[11] Strokes that are graded 0 to 3 on the scale are considered minor; 4 to 7, mild; 8 to 15, moderate; and greater than 15, severe. Patients with scores greater than 20 are less likely to benefit from any reperfusion treatment.[1,12] Patients with scores between 8 and 20 are more likely to benefit from reperfusion, making them better candidates for treatment.[2,13] Patients with minor to mild symptoms (NIHSS score <8) and an existing IC large-vessel occlusion can also be treated by mechanical thrombectomy; in these patients, the decision to perform additional IA therapy is based on the operators experience and the estimated risk of the procedure.

Time of Presentation

IV t-PA and IA reperfusion therapies have both been shown to improve patient outcome. However, the time window for treatment of both approaches is limited. IV thrombolysis can be given up to 4.5 hours after stoke onset; additional or primary IA therapies can be used up to 8 hours after stroke onset. However, outcome depends on the length of time between onset of symptoms and revascularization.[3,14,15] Analysis of pooled data from six large randomized t-PA trials showed greater neurologic improvement at 90 days with earlier t-PA treatment.[4,16] The therapeutic benefit of t-PA is greatest when given early after ischemic stroke onset and declines over 3 to 4.5 hours.[4,5]

In anterior circulation strokes, the impact of successful thrombectomy is greater in the first 3 to 4.5 hours after stroke, compared to late recanalization after 5 to 8 hours.[6,7,17] Posterior circulation and brainstem strokes caused by vertebral or BA occlusion may be less susceptible to the hemorrhagic complications of reperfusion therapy. Safe recanalization of occluded posterior circulation vessels has been reported up to 24 h after brainstem infarction.[8,9,18]

Imaging of Acute Stroke

Imaging in patients with acute stroke should be targeted toward assessment of the brain parenchyma, pipes, perfusion, and penumbra, as described by Rowley[10,19] and summarized in **Table 1**. This approach enables the detection of IC hemorrhage, differentiation of infarcted tissue from salvageable tissue, identification of arterial occlusion, selection

Table 1
Goals of acute stroke imaging

Parenchyma	Assess early signs of acute stroke, rule out hemorrhage
Pipes	Assess extracranial circulation and intracranial circulation for evidence of intravascular thrombus
Perfusion	Assess CBV, CBF, and MTT
Penumbra	Assess tissue at risk of dying if ischemia continues without recanalization of intravascular thrombus

Abbreviation: CBF, cerebral blood flow.

of the appropriate therapy, and prediction of the clinical outcome. A comprehensive evaluation may be performed with multimodal CT or multimodal magnetic resonance imaging (MRI) techniques.

The major advantages of CT compared to MRI are that CT is widely available and that a stroke imaging protocol that consists of unenhanced CT, CTA, and CT perfusion imaging can be executed in 5 minutes for the comprehensive evaluation of the extracranial and IC circulation, the amount of infarcted brain tissue, and the penumbra.

CT

With its widespread availability, short scan time, non-invasiveness, and safety, CT has been the traditional first-line imaging modality for the evaluation of acute ischemic stroke.

Multimodal CT includes unenhanced CT, CTA, and CT perfusion. Noncontrast CT can identify IC hemorrhage and detect early signs of acute ischemic stroke. CTA can identify the occlusion site, detect arterial dissection, and grade collateral blood flow, whereas CT perfusion can differentiate between tissue at risk (the so-called penumbra) and irreversibly damaged brain tissue.[11,20,21] Multimodal CT offers rapid data acquisition and can be performed with modern CT equipment.

Noncontrast CT In the acute ischemic stroke setting, noncontrast CT is typically used to rule out IC hemorrhage (a contraindication to thrombolysis), or other stroke mimics (eg, tumor, infection, etc) that preclude the use of thrombolytic therapy, and to detect early CT signs such as insular ribbon sign, obscuration of the lentiform nucleus, or hyperdense artery sign (**Fig. 1**A, B).[11,22,23] Although these early ischemic changes can be helpful in stroke detection, they are subtle and difficult to detect. Moreover, noncontrast CT cannot reliably

differentiate between irreversibly damaged brain tissue and penumbra. In contrast to these early ischemic changes, hypodensity is highly specific for irreversible tissue damage, and its extent is predictive of the risk of hemorrhagic transformation (see **Fig. 1**C).[24,25] Nevertheless, it is critical to determine the tissue at risk before irreversible tissue damage occurs and frank hypodensity appears, as this is essential to prevent hemorrhagic transformation. In the European Cooperative Acute Stroke Study trials (ECASS I and II), involvement of more than one-third of the middle cerebral artery (MCA) territory on noncontrast CT was utilized as the criterion for patient exclusion for reperfusion therapy because of the potential increased risk for hemorrhagic transformation.[26]

CTA CTA is widely available, with fast, thin-section, volumetric spiral CT images acquired during the injection of a time-optimized bolus of contrast material for vessel opacification. The entire region from the aortic arch up to the circle of Willis can be covered in a single data acquisition. CTA allows a detailed evaluation of the IC and extracranial vasculature.[27,28] Its utility in acute stroke lies in its ability to detect large-vessel occlusion within IC vessels and to evaluate the carotid and vertebral arteries in the neck (**Fig. 2**).

CTA can also depict the leptomeningeal collaterals and can identify large-vessel occlusions with *good* and *poor* collaterals (**Figs. 3** and **4**). Collateral circulation likely improves neurologic outcome by limiting the extent of brain infarction. Therefore, a favorable pattern of leptomeningeal collaterals as visualized on CTA correlates with improved functional outcomes in patients with acute ischemic stroke.[29] Although clinical data are missing, it can be hypothesized that patients with good collaterals can profit from an IA reperfusion therapy, even in an extended time window. On the contrary, patients with poor collaterals are unlikely to profit from a reperfusion therapy, even if the treatment is performed in a good time window (**Table 2**).

CT perfusion CT perfusion involves dynamic acquisition of sequential CT slices on a cine mode during rapid IV administration of nonionic iodinated contrast material. CT perfusion allows rapid, noninvasive, and quantitative evaluation of cerebral perfusion. CT perfusion imaging can be used to measure the following perfusion parameters: CBV (ie, the volume of blood per unit of brain tissue, normal range, 4–5 mL/100 g); cerebral blood flow (CBF) (ie, the volume of blood flow per unit of brain tissue per minute, normal range in gray matter, 50–60 mL/100 g/min); MTT, defined

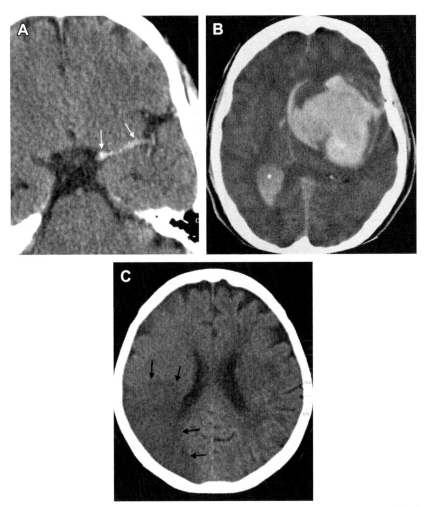

Fig. 1. Hyperdense artery sign (*white arrows*) (*A*). CT with intracerebral hemorrhage (*B*). CT with subacute infarction (hypodensity, *black arrows*) (*C*).

as the time difference between the arterial inflow and venous outflow; and time to peak enhancement, which represents the time from the beginning of contrast material injection to the maximum concentration of contrast material within a region of interest.[30,31]

MTT maps are more sensitive, whereas CBF and CBV maps are more specific for distinguishing

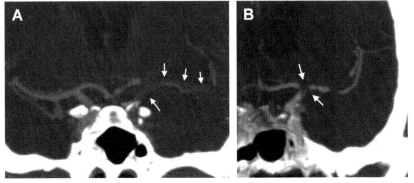

Fig. 2. CTA depicts occlusion of left terminal internal carotid artery (ICA) and MCA (*white arrows*) (*A*). CTA shows a short thrombus in the bifurcation of ICA (*white arrows*) (*B*).

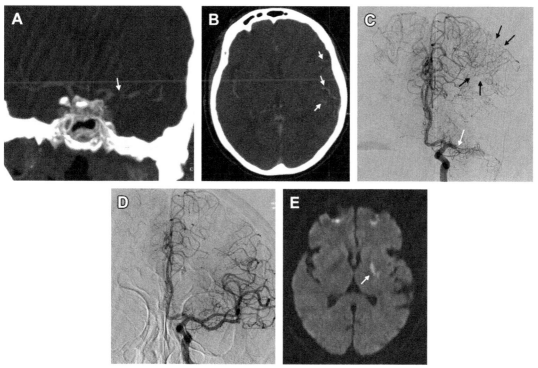

Fig. 3. MCA occlusion (*white arrow* in *A*, *C*) with good leptomeningeal collateral status on CTA and angiography (*white arrows* in *B*, *black arrows* in *C*). After successful thrombectomy (*D*), only a small infarction is seen in MRI (*white arrow* in *E*).

ischemia from infarction.[32] CT perfusion distinction of the infarct core from the penumbra is based on the concept of cerebral vascular autoregulation. In the penumbra, autoregulation is preserved, MTT is prolonged, but CBV is preserved because of vasodilatation and collateral recruitment as part of the autoregulation process. In the infarct core, autoregulation is lost, MTT is prolonged, and CBV is decreased.[33] Thus, using appropriate MTT and CBV thresholds, infarct core and penumbra can be distinguished on CT perfusion maps (**Fig. 5**).[34] Direct assessment of an individual patient's ischemic penumbra ("penumbra is brain") may allow for more personalized, appropriate selection of candidates for intervention than generalized time criteria ("time is brain"), because individuals may have different timelines for evolution of penumbra into infarct.

MRI

A thorough evaluation of acute stroke can be performed by using a combination of conventional MRI, magnetic resonance (MR) angiography, and diffusion- and perfusion-weighted MRI techniques.

Conventional MR sequences can rule out hemorrhage. Acute infarcts may be seen early on conventional MR images, whereas diffusion-weighted

MR imaging is more sensitive for detection of hyperacute ischemia. Like CTA, MR angiography is useful for detecting intravascular occlusion due to a thrombus and for evaluating the carotid bifurcation in patients with acute stroke. MR angiography is commonly used to evaluate the IC and extracranial circulation. A mismatch between findings on diffusion and perfusion MR images may be used to predict the presence of a penumbra.[31]

Relevant Anatomy

The normal anatomy of the aortic arch and cervical arteries that supply the brain is subject to considerable variation. Three aortic arch morphologies are distinguished based on the relationship of the brachiocephalic (innominate) arterial trunk to the aortic arch (**Fig. 6**A, B). Type I aortic arch is characterized by the origin of all 3 major vessels in the horizontal plane defined by the outer curvature of the arch. In Type II, the brachiocephalic artery originates between the horizontal planes of the outer and inner curvatures of the arch. In Type III, it originates below the horizontal plane of the inner curvature of the arch. In addition to aortic arch anatomy, the configuration of the great vessels varies.

The distal common carotid artery typically bifurcates into the internal and external carotid arteries

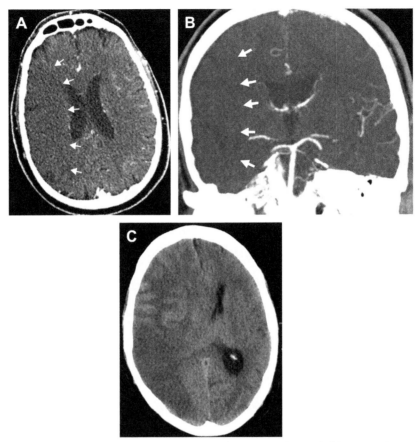

Fig. 4. CTA shows *poor collaterals* in the right hemisphere after MCA occlusion (*white arrows* in A, B), resulting in large infarction even after recanalization of the occluded vessel (*C*).

at the level of the thyroid cartilage, but anomalous bifurcations may occur up to 5 cm higher or lower (see **Fig. 6**C). The carotid bulb, a dilated portion at the origin of the internal carotid artery (ICA), usually extends superiorly for a distance of approximately 2 cm, where the diameter of the ICA becomes more uniform. The length and tortuosity of the ICA are additional sources of variation, with undulation, coiling, or kinking in up to 35% of cases, most extensively in elderly patients.

The IC portion of each carotid artery begins at the base of the skull, traverses the petrous bone, and enters the subarachnoid space near the level of the ophthalmic artery (see **Fig. 6**D). There, the artery turns posteriorly and superiorly, giving rise to the posterior communicating artery, which connects through the circle of Willis with the posterior cerebral artery that arises from the vertebrobasilar circulation. The ICA then bifurcates into the anterior cerebral and middle cerebral arteries. The anterior cerebral arteries connect with the circle of Willis through the anterior communicating artery. The configuration of the circle of Willis is also highly variable, with a complete circle in fewer than 50% of individuals (see **Fig. 6**E, F).

PREPROCEDURE PLANNING

Despite the fact that the efficacy of IV thrombolysis decreases over time, less than one-third of the patients meet the goal of a *door-to-needle time* of 60 min or less because of in-hospital delays.[35]

Table 2
Predictors for clinical outcome in patients who received thrombectomy

Predictors for Favorable Clinical Outcome	Predictors for Unfavorable Clinical Outcome
Young age	Old age
NIHSS <20	NIHSS >20
Symptoms onset <4.5 h	Symptoms onset >6 h
Good leptomeningeal collaterals	Poor leptomeningeal collaterals
Penumbra on CT perfusion	CT perfusion without tissue at risk

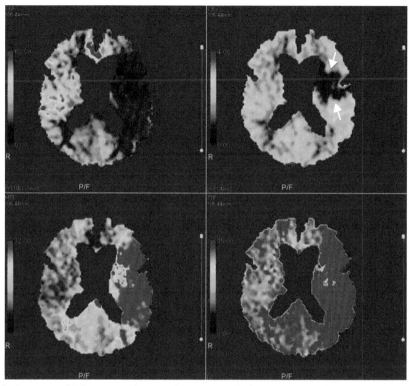

Fig. 5. CT perfusion map of left MCA occlusion. The area in which CBV is less (*white arrows*) corresponds to the infarct core. There is a penumbra because there is a large area of the MCA territory in which MTT is prolonged and CBV is preserved. R, right; P/F, posterior.

Improvements in prehospital and in-hospital stroke management can translate into increased eligibility for thrombolysis and more prompt treatment.[36] Therefore, in every stroke center, optimized stroke management must be established to reduce the *door-to-therapy* time. The offering of a 24 × 7 × 365, on-demand, stroke service, including reperfusion therapies, is also required.[13]

Optimized Systems-Based Stroke Management

Emergency services are instructed to bring patients with a suspected stroke directly to the stroke treatment room in the authors' facility, which is located next to the CT scanner. After neurologic examination, the native CT scan is acquired. To reduce the time-to-treatment decision in patients with stroke, point-of-care laboratory analysis is performed. This analysis has been shown to significantly reduce the time-to-treatment decision compared with a setup in which the laboratory workup is performed by a centralized laboratory.[37] If an intracranial hemorrhage (ICH) can be ruled out, CTA and CT perfusion are performed. Within the 4.5-h time window, patients are treated with IV thrombolysis directly within the CT scanner after

exclusion of clinical and neuroradiological contraindications. If an occlusion of a large IC vessel is found, the decision to perform additional or primary endovascular therapy is based on the clinical condition of the patient, the time window (up to 6 hours after stroke onset), as well as imaging criteria of CTA and CT perfusion (presence of leptomeningeal collaterals and ischemic penumbra). If the decision of endovascular therapy is made, the patient is transferred immediately to the angiography suite, which is located on the same floor.

At this point, the decision regarding treatment under sedation or intubation and ventilation is made, depending on the patient's clinical condition. The authors perform about 80% of the procedures under conscious sedation. One advantage of this approach, when compared with general anesthesia, is the ability to start the procedure immediately. Another major advantage is to control the clinical status of the patient during the procedure and to evaluate the success of treatment (Video 1). A disadvantage of sedation is the patient's movements, which require experienced operators for a safe and successful procedure.

With this optimized stroke protocol, the authors defined in a prospective study (ReFlow Study) the door-to-device (D2D) time (time from arrival at the

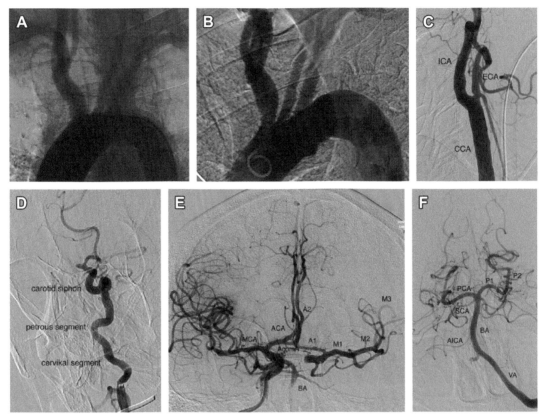

Fig. 6. Aortic arch Type I (*A*) and Type III (*B*). Anatomy of extracranial and intracranial arteries (*C–F*). A1 and A2, segments of the ACA; ACA, anterior cerebral artery; AcomA, anterior communicated artery; AICA, anterior inferior cerebellar artery; BA, basilar artery; CCA, common carotid artery; ECA, external carotid artery; ICA, internal carotid artery; M1, M2, and M3, segments of the MCA; MCA, middle cerebral artery; P1 and P2, segments of the PCA; PCA, posterior cerebral artery; SCA, superior cerebellar artery; VA, vertebral artery.

hospital until the thrombectomy device is placed in the target lesion). D2D time of less than 100 min resulted in a favorable outcome in 66% of patients, compared with a favorable result in 44% of patients with a D2D time of more than 100 min.[38] Just as reduced door-to-balloon time influences the outcome of patients with ST-segment elevation myocardial infarction, the D2D time likely also plays an important role in the outcome of these patients with acute stroke. Physicians, hospitals, and health care systems should work to reduce the D2D time, as has been done for *door-to-balloon* time in ST-segment elevation myocardial infarction.[39]

DESCRIPTION OF THE PROCEDURE
Evolution from IA Thrombolysis to Flow Restoration Devices (Stent Retriever)

Early recanalization and restoration of flow is the goal in treatment of patients with acute ischemic stroke due to a large-vessel occlusion. A meta-analysis of 52 studies on IV thrombolysis outcome in 2066 patients showed that the chance of an independent life after stroke increases by 4.4 times for patients with successful recanalization compared to patients without recanalization; the mortality rate decreases 4-fold.[14] That said, recanalization rates achieved with IV t-PA for large-vessel arterial occlusion are low, ranging from 4% to 32% depending on the vessel (4% for ICA occlusions and 32% for MCA occlusions).[8,9] Most failures of IV thrombolysis are because of presence of hard or white thrombus (Video 2) or the large volume of clot (**Fig. 7**).

Naturally, these patients are considered to be candidates for additional or primary IA therapies to increase the recanalization rates. IA treatments include IA thrombolysis and mechanical thrombectomy. IA thrombolysis has been used for nearly 3 decades. In the past decade, mechanical recanalization devices have been developed to achieve better results than IA thrombolysis, and they represent the only treatment option for patients with contraindications to thrombolytics. The Merci (Concentric Medical, Mountain View, USA) device

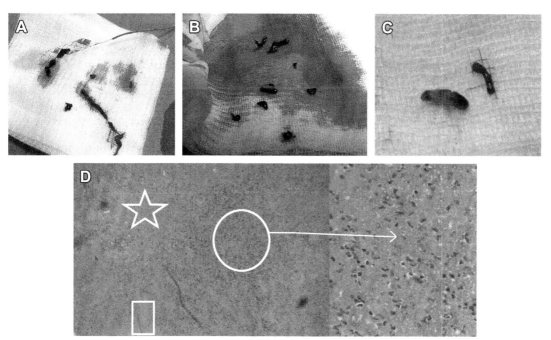

Fig. 7. Large amount of thrombi retrieved with stent retriever (*A, B*). Fibrin-rich, hard thrombus (*C*). Histology of the thrombus shows the fibrin components (*star*), erythrocytes (*circle*), and leucocytes (*rectangle*) (*D*) (hematoxylin-eosin, original magnification ×300).

and the Penumbra aspiration system were the first devices for which large clinical experiences have been reported.[40,41] However, the breakthrough in interventional treatment of acute stroke was achieved by the use of a new technique—the combination of flow restoration and mechanical thrombectomy showed very promising clinical results. For this technique, self-expandable, stent-like thrombectomy devices are used (stent retriever).[42,43] The stent retriever devices enable higher success rate and reduced time to recanalization and are associated with low complication rates.[44]

In the authors' experience, the most effective reperfusion strategy today is stent-retriever-based thrombectomy, in combination with simple aspiration through a large distal access catheter. In special groups of patients with extracranial carotid occlusion, arterial dissection, and IC stenosis, permanent stenting is necessary. These reperfusion techniques are described in detail below.

IA Thrombolysis

For IA thrombolysis the thrombolytic agent is applied with a microcatheter directly into the occluding thrombus. Prourokinase and t-PA are used as thrombolytic agents. Although IA fibrinolysis has been used for nearly 3 decades and has shown apparent benefit in case series, Prolyse in Acute Cerebral Thromboembolism II trial

(PROACT II)[12] is the only randomized trial to date documenting the safety and efficacy of IA fibrinolysis in acute ischemic stroke. In this study, 12,323 patients with stroke were evaluated to identify 180 eligible patients with proximal MCA occlusions (1.4% of screened patients). The patients were randomized to a treatment regime with IA prourokinase in combination with IV heparin versus IV heparin alone. PROACT II achieved recanalization in 66% and good neurologic outcomes in 40% and remains the benchmark by which newer endovascular methods are judged. However, in this study, standard medical therapy was not IV thrombolysis, which has since then become the standard therapy in acute ischemic stroke. Disadvantages of IA thrombolysis are the low recanalization rates and the long and complex interventions. Moreover, it cannot be applied in patients with contraindications.

Merci Device/Penumbra System

Mechanical thrombectomy techniques are widely used in case of failed recanalization after IV thrombolysis or in patients with contraindications to thrombolytic therapy. In the past decade, a variety of devices have been developed. The Merci device and the Penumbra aspiration system were the first devices for which large clinical experiences have been reported. However, the outcomes remain relatively poor. The MERCI trial improved flow to Thrombolysis in Myocardial Infarction (TIMI) grade 2 or 3 in only 69% of the cases.[45] Use of the Penumbra system, an aspiration device, showed high target vessel recanalization rates (80%). However, associated favorable functional outcome (mRS≤2 at 90 days) was low (29%), even in patients with successful recanalization.[46] Importantly, successful recanalization was typically defined as a TIMI flow grade of 2 (partial) or 3 (complete) within the target vessel on angiography after the procedure; flow into the distal vascular territory was not assessed. The more detailed rating scale *thrombolysis in cerebral infarction* (TICI) emphasizes flow in the periphery of the target vessel. One may assume that the recanalization rates of the MERCI and Penumbra trials would have been much lower if rated with the TICI scale (**Table 3**). Disadvantages to these devices are that clots may adhere to the intima and become refractory to mechanical disruption or retrieval. Another major disadvantage is the high rate of IC bleeding, which resulted in high mortality in these studies. Symptomatic IC hemorrhage was reported in 10% of patients with the MERCI retriever and in 11% with the Penumbra system. Mortality rates in the MERCI and Penumbra trials ranged from 32.5% to 44%.[41]

Flow Restoration Devices/Stent Retriever Technique

To achieve better angiographical and clinical results self-expanding stents were used. The application of self-expanding stents in acute stroke seems to have several advantages compared with other interventional techniques. First, stenting has a high reported rate of successful recanalization.[47,48] Second, whereas other techniques often take hours to achieve recanalization, permanent implantation of a self-expanding stent seems to produce immediate flow restoration. Recent studies have reported positive outcomes with self-expanding stents in patients with acute IC occlusions. The first prospective trial of stent-assisted recanalization in acute ischemic stroke demonstrated a 100% recanalization rate in 20 patients. Beyond the high recanalization rates, the safety profile was reasonable.[49]

However, there are important disadvantages in the use of stenting to treat acute stroke. The clot is only pressed to the vessel wall and not removed from the vessel, so there are concerns about early rethrombosis. Furthermore, the placement of an IC stent may induce late in-stent stenosis. Finally, implantation of a permanent IC self-expanding stent requires aggressive antiplatelet therapy after placement.

Table 3	
TICI score overview	
Grade 0	*No perfusion.* No antegrade flow beyond the point of occlusion.
Grade 1	*Penetration with minimal perfusion.* The contrast material passes beyond the area of obstruction but fails to opacify the entire cerebral bed distal to the obstruction for the duration of the angiographic run.
Grade 2	*Partial perfusion.* The contrast material passes beyond the obstruction and opacifies the arterial bed distal to the obstruction. However, the rate of entry of contrast into the vessel distal to the obstruction and/or its rate of clearance from the distal bed are perceptibly slower than its entry into and/or clearance from comparable areas not perfused by the previously occluded vessel, eg, the opposite cerebral artery or the arterial bed proximal to the obstruction.
Grade 2a	Only partial filling (two-thirds) of the entire vascular territory is visualized.
Grade 2b	Complete filling of all the expected vascular territory is visualized, but the filling is slower than normal.
Grade 3	*Complete perfusion.* Antegrade flow into the bed distal to the obstruction occurs as promptly as into the obstruction and clearance of contrast material from the involved bed is as rapid as from an uninvolved other bed of the same vessel or the opposite cerebral artery.

Stent retrievers are self-expandable stentlike devices that are fully recoverable. Therefore, these devices combine the advantages of prompt flow restoration and mechanical thrombectomy. Because the stent can be removed, there are no concerns about early rethrombosis and late in-stent stenosis and there is no need for aggressive antiplatelet therapy.[42]

The first dedicated combined flow restoration and thrombectomy device for acute stroke treatment was the Solitaire FR (Covidien, Mansfield, MA, USA). The device is basically the Solitaire

AB Neurovascular Remodeling Device, originally developed for stent-assisted treatment of wide-necked IC aneurysms. The first clinical results that were published in 2010 were promising. In a retrospective study with 22 patients, the authors demonstrated that deployment and withdrawal of the unfolded Solitaire stent seems to be a safe and technically feasible method to achieve high recanalization rates. A recanalization rate of TICI 2a/b or 3 flow was achieved in 20 of 22 patients (90.9%). About 50% of patients had a good clinical outcome with an mRS score of 2 or less after 30 and 90 days. The mortality rate was 18.1%.[44] The results of the prospective ReFlow Study showed high rate of favorable clinical outcome at 3 months (60%), a low rate of symptomatic hemorrhage (2.5%), and low mortality (12.5%).[38] The low mortality reflects the low incidence of symptomatic ICH and demonstrates the safety of flow restoration devices compared with the Merci device and the Penumbra system.[38]

Since 2010, much clinical experience has been reported and numerous variants of this device type are currently developed (Trevo, Concentric Medical Inc, Mountain View, CA, USA; ReVive, Micrus Endovascular LLC, San Jose, CA, USA; Aperio, Acandis GmBH & Co. KG, Pforzheim Germany; pRESET, Phenox GmBH, Bochum, Germany; Catch plus, Balt Extrusion, Montmorency, France; and Solitaire FR, Covidien, Mansfield, MA, USA) (**Fig. 8**).

Two randomized trials comparing flow restoration devices (Solitaire and Trevo) with the Merci retriever showed better clinical and recanalization results with the use of stent retrievers.[50,51] The improved clinical outcome with flow restoration devices is due to rapid and effective clot removal and the possibility of temporarily restoring flow to the periphery between retrieval attempts, a feature that is impossible with the devices used in the MERCI, Multi-MERCI, and Penumbra trials.

As a result of these recent clinical experiences, stent retrievers have all but replaced IA thrombolysis and Merci retriever as the treatment of choice for direct recanalization.

Stent Retriever Recanalization Technique: Step by Step

Vascular access
The common femoral artery is the typical vascular access site, with placement of a 6F sheath. The brachial artery can also be used in cases in which the puncture of the femoral arteries is not possible because of peripheral atherosclerotic disease (Video 3) or tortuous anatomy. In some cases with tortuous vessel anatomy it can be difficult or even not possible to reach the IC vasculature. Pre-procedural CTA provides the necessary information and can predict the accessibility of the IC vasculature.

Catheter and sheaths
To perform an IC thrombectomy, it is necessary to place of a long (90–100 cm) 6F sheath or an 8F guide catheter into the ICA or vertebral artery (VA). The authors prefer to use a long sheath; to place the tip of the sheath into the target vessel a 125-cm-long catheter is required. Two catheters that can be used are the linear multipurpose catheter and the SIM2 catheter for types II and III aortic arch configurations (**Fig. 9**). Primary use of the SIM2 catheter is preferred because it allows

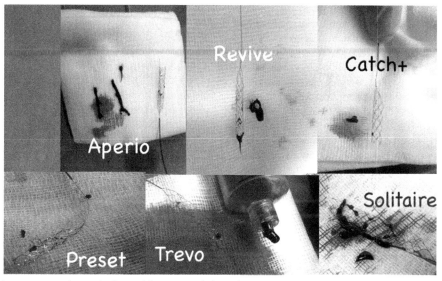

Fig. 8. Various stent retriever devices with extracted thrombi.

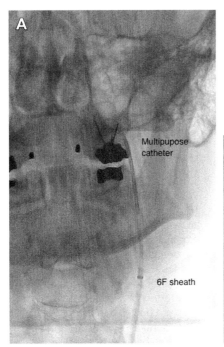
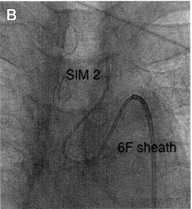

Fig. 9. Multipurpose catheter (*A*) and SIM2 catheter (*B*).

access to the target vessel in most cases. For placement of the sheath into the ICA or VA, the telescope technique is used with a coaxial system of a 0.035″ guide wire (eg, a Terumo Radifocus Guide wire, Terumo Medical Corporation, Somerset, NJ, USA), the 125-cm-long catheter, and the 6F sheath (see Video 3).

DAC and balloon guide catheter
DAC can be used to achieve a more distal access to the occlusion site. The size of the catheter can be 5F or 6F with an inner lumen of up to 0.72″, allowing retrieval of the recanalization device with sufficient aspiration. The DAC usually is advanced over a standard 0.035″ guide wire or coaxially with the microcatheter into the petrous segment, in some cases as far as the carotid siphon or M1, or V4 segment of the BA (see Video 3). DACs provide stable access and reduce friction, which is especially important with tortuous anatomy. A disadvantage of DAC's is the smaller lumen compared long sheath, which can result to thrombus disruption and distal embolization during the retrieval maneuver. The authors recommend that DACs are not necessary in cases in which the sheath can be placed up to the distal cervical segment of the ICA or the V3 segment of the VA (**Fig. 10**A). However, they are often necessary in cases with elongated ICA as well as in cases with failed recanalization due to a hard thrombus or due to massive thrombus load, where they serve as an aspiration catheter (see **Fig. 10**B, C, Video 3).

The use of balloon guide catheters is also controversial. Balloon guide catheters can be used instead of the long sheath and placed into the ICA or VA. The goal is to achieve flow arrest during the retrieval maneuver, which should prevent embolization of any lost clot in other vessels (see **Fig. 10**D).[52] However, the disadvantage of the balloon guide catheter is that distal access into the ICA or VA is often not possible and contrast visualization during the procedure is more limited.

Microwires, microcatheters, and retriever devices
For IC navigation, typically a 0.014″ microwire is used; based on the size of the thrombectomy device, a microcatheter between 0.018″ and 0.027″ is used. The size of the stent retriever devices range from 3 × 15 mm up to 6 × 30 mm. The size of the used retriever device is based on the size of the occluded artery. Typically, a 4- to 4.5-mm device is used for the MCA or BA and a 6-mm device is used for occlusions in the terminal ICA (tICA). However, 6-mm devices are also used for the MCA and BA if the smaller devices fail to recanalize the vessel (**Box 1**).

IC Recanalization Procedure

After the placement of the long, 6F sheath or the distal catheter either in the VA or in the ICA the occlusion of the target vessel is verified angiographically. The target vessel is navigated with

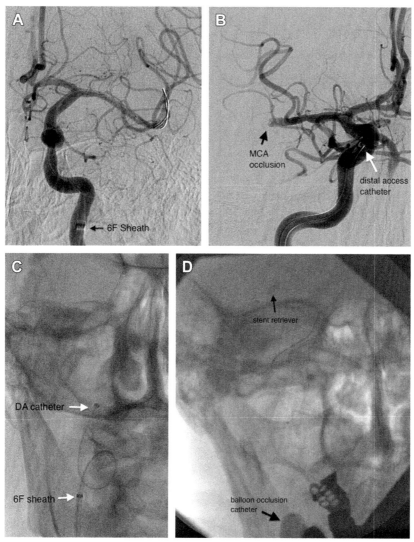

Fig. 10. Placement of 6F sheath into the distal cervical segment of the ICA (*A*); in this case a distal access (DA) catheter is not necessary. Placement of DA catheter into the carotid siphon (*B*). The 360° loop of the ICA; in this case, a DA catheter is necessary to perform the thrombectomy (*C*). Use of balloon occlusion catheter in an MCA occlusion (*D*).

a 0.014″ microguidewire and a microcatheter. The thrombus is passed with the microwire, and the microcatheter is placed distal to the thrombus. Because the anatomy distal to the occlusion is not known, there is a potential danger of vessel injury with the relatively stiff tip of the microguide-wire. The authors recommend shaping the tip of the microguidewire with a J-form or hockey stick configuration so that it can form a loop that allows atraumatic passage of the occlusion site (**Fig. 11**). The other benefit of this technique is that because of the relatively large diameter of the loop the wire is likely to advance into the largest vessel of the MCA bifurcation or basilar tip, usually following the way of the thrombus. The retriever device is

then advanced through the microcatheter; the microcatheter is pulled back until the self-expandable stentlike device completely unfolds. The device is placed with the proximal third within the thrombus. A control angiogram is performed after successful unfolding of the stent device to evaluate reestablishment of flow. After a short period, the device is pulled back in its unfolded state under continuous aspiration with a 50-mL syringe together with the microcatheter into the guiding sheath. After removal of the device and microcatheter, another 20 to 50 mL is aspirated from the guiding sheath to prevent reembolization of the potentially lost clot. If the subsequent con-trol angiogram shows a TICI score less than 2,

---

Box 1
Basic materials for intracranial thrombectomy

A 90- to 100-cm-long sheath or 8F guiding catheter

A 125-cm-long multipurpose or SIM2 5F catheter

A 0.035″ guide wire

Distal access catheter (optional)

Balloon occlusion catheter (optional)

A 0.014″ microwire

Microcatheter between 0.018″ and 0.027″

Stent retriever device between 3 × 15 mm to 6 × 30 mm

5F reperfusion aspiration catheter (optional)

---

the procedure is repeated until a TICI score of 2b or 3 is reached (**Figs. 12–14**; see Videos 4 and 5).

Technique of the Aspiration Procedure: Step by Step

Aspiration indications

Despite the impressive results of the stent retriever devices (up to 95% recanalization), there are some vessel occlusions and thrombi that are resistant to this technique even after repeated recanalization attempts. These vessel occlusions include cases of tICA occlusions and distal BA occlusions. Moreover hard thrombi in other locations, such as the MCA, can also be resistant to the stent retriever technique. For these cases, direct aspiration of the thrombus can be used as primary or second-line technique.

Aspiration systems

The most common aspiration catheters that are used for these purposes are 5F system, for example, the Penumbra 5Max Aspiration Catheter (Penumbra Inc, Alameda, CA, USA), which has a 0.54″ inner lumen; alternatively, 6F systems, with better aspiration capacity (0.70″–0.72″ inner lumen), can be used if they can be navigated through the carotid siphon.

Technique

After the placement of the long, 6F sheath, the target vessel is navigated with a 0.014″ microwire, a microcatheter, and the aspiration catheter. The thrombus is passed with the microwire and microcatheter, and the aspiration catheter is placed directly into the thrombus. The microwire and the microcatheter are removed. Entrapment of the thrombus is indicated by the absence of backflow. The catheter is then retrieved with constant negative pressure to avoid loss of thrombus. After each retrieval of clot fragments, the procedure is repeated (**Figs. 15 and 16**).[53] If the aspiration catheter cannot be navigated through the carotid siphon using the technique described above, it is possible to place a stent retriever in the M1 or P1 segment. By then pulling the device slowly backward without using too much force so that it will actually be retrieved the vessels are straightened a little bit; this makes it in most of the cases easier to bring up the 5F or 6F aspiration catheter into the M1 or basilar tip.

Extracranial ICA Occlusion

The treatment of extracranial ICA occlusions is a challenge because treatment with standard IV thrombolysis alone leads to a good clinical outcome in only 17% of the cases; death rate is as high as

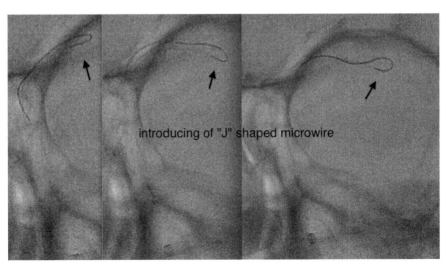

introducing of "J" shaped microwire

Fig. 11. J-shaped microwire technique.

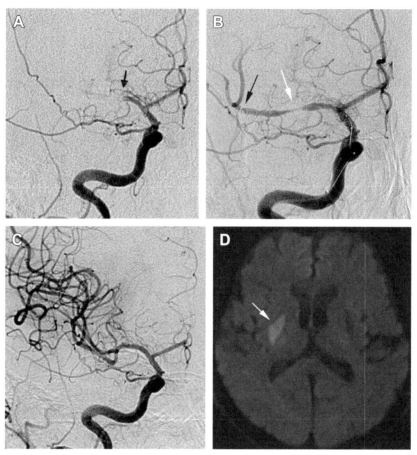

Fig. 12. Acute MCA occlusion (*black arrow* in *A*), and placement of the stent retriever with immediate flow restoration distal end of the device (*black arrow*); the thrombus is pressed to the vessel wall (*white arrow* in *B*). Successful recanalization of the artery (*C*); only a small infarction is seen in MRI (*white arrow* in *D*).

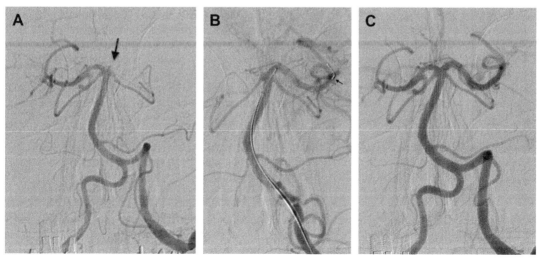

Fig. 13. Acute BA/ posterior cerebral artery occlusion (*black arrow* in *A*); placement of the stent retriever with immediate flow restoration distal marker of the device (*black arrow* in *B*). Successful recanalization of the artery (*C*).

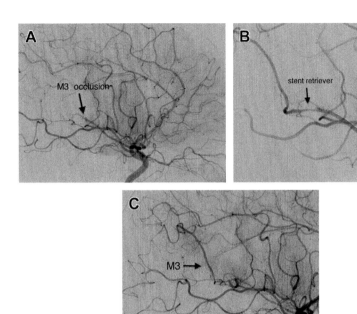

Fig. 14. Occlusion of M3 segment of the MCA in a patient with high-grade hemiparesis (*A*). Because of the severe symptoms, the decision of thrombectomy was made. After placement of a stent retriever, immediate flow restoration was achieved (*B*). Successful recanalization of the M3 segment (*C*).

55%. Acute extracranial ICA occlusion resulting in ischemic stroke is different from other forms of acute occlusions of the cerebral vessels. The pathophysiologic process involved in acute occlusion of the extracranial ICA, similar to that observed in acute occlusion of the coronary arteries, is predominantly ruptured atherosclerotic plaque and superimposed thrombus. Therefore, large contributions of atherosclerotic plaque and platelet activation do not provide an ideal substrate for thrombolytics.[54] In these patients, acute stenting of the extracranial ICA is performed to recanalize the vessel.[55]

Interventional treatment consists of 2 steps. The first step is extracranial revascularization of the ICA with stent implantation, as in the treatment of atherosclerotic stenosis. The second step is IC mechanical recanalization of the occluded vessel, if necessary.

Extracranial revascularization

Once an acute occlusion of the ICA is identified, a long 6F guide sheath is placed in the distal common carotid artery. A long 0.014″ or 0.018″ microwire is used to pass the occlusion. If this is unsuccessful, a 0.035″ guidewire is used together with a 4F multipurpose catheter. Once the wire has successfully passed the occlusion, the catheter is advanced into the occluded vessel segment and contrast medium is injected to verify the intraluminal position of the catheter and rule out the

possibility of having caused a dissection by the manipulation. To remove the 4F catheter, a long 0.014″ wire is introduced if necessary. A self-expanding carotid stent is then placed in the area of the occlusion to appose the stent to the vessel wall, and to eliminate a residual stenosis, balloon angioplasty is performed. Typically, a Wallstent (Boston Scientific Corporation, Natick, MA, USA) is used because the closed-cell design of the stent makes it easier to place a catheter in the distal ICA for IC recanalization if necessary. After emergency stent implantation, antiplatelet medication is necessary to prevent acute stent thrombosis. In the acute-phase, administration of IV aspirin, if available, or IV glycoprotein IIb/IIIa receptor antagonist, such as abciximab, would be possible.[56] However, the ideal medical regimen in carotid artery stenting (CAS) for acute stroke is not known, and it must be borne in mind that aggressive anticoagulation, especially in combination with thrombolytics, may increase the risk of ICH. To minimize this risk, thrombolysis may be ceased in this special group of patients.[55]

After successful CAS of an ICA occlusion, further recanalization measures may be taken if there remains an additional occlusion in the terminal segment of the ICA or the MCA. A mechanical approach with the use of stent retriever should be the first option to treat these lesions (**Fig. 17**, see Video 6).

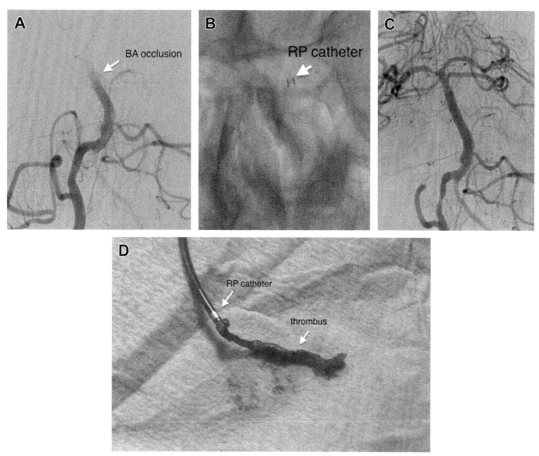

Fig. 15. Occlusion of the distal segment of the BA (*A*). A penumbra reperfusion (RP) aspiration catheter 054 was placed into the thrombus (*B*). The catheter was then retrieved with constant negative pressure and removed the thrombus (*C, D*).

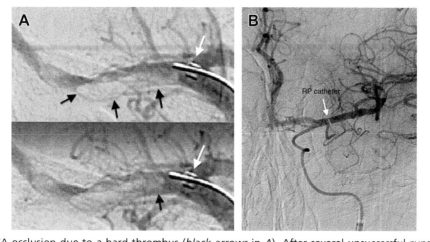

Fig. 16. MCA occlusion due to a hard thrombus (*black arrows* in *A*). After several unsuccessful runs with stent retriever devices, an aspiration catheter was placed into the M1 segment (*white arrow* in *A*); the catheter was then retrieved with constant negative pressure and removed the thrombus. Placement of a Penumbra RP 054 catheter in the MCA in another patient (*B*).

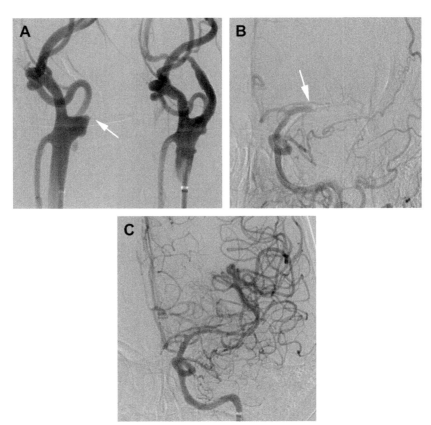

Fig. 17. Acute atherosclerotic occlusion shortly beyond the origin of the ICA (*white arrow* in *A*). Following stent placement, normal ICA outflow is visible (*A*). Additional intracranial MCA occlusion (*white arrow* in *B*). After stent retriever withdrawal, the vessel is fully recanalized (*C*).

IC Occlusion due to ICA Dissection

Acute dissection of the ICA can result in occlusion of the vessel with severe stroke symptoms, with or without additional IC occlusion. Similar to the atherosclerotic ICA occlusion, acute stenting of the dissection and, mechanical recanalization of IC occluded vessel(s), if necessary, is performed (**Fig. 18**). Care must be taken to ensure that wires and catheters are within the distal true lumen and not advanced into subintimal dissection planes.

POTENTIAL COMPLICATIONS/MANAGEMENT

Complications that can occur during or after the procedure include distal embolization to the same or other vessel territories, dissection of the arteries, and subarachnoid or intracerebral hemorrhage.

In case of distal embolization, the management depends on the relevance of the occluded branch. If the patient is not intubated, clinical examination can show the importance of the branch occlusion. If deemed appropriate to recanalize, a stent retriever can be used even in the M3 branches of

the MCA or in the A2 segment of the ACA (see **Figs. 14** and **18**B–D).

Dissections mostly occur in the ICA or VA and are associated with use of DACs. Dissections without significant stenosis do not require any therapy. For those with flow-limiting stenosis, stenting can be performed.

Small subarachnoid hemorrhages are often seen on the control CT and do not require any therapeutic measures. Intracerebral hemorrhage can occur during the procedure or within 48 hours after the procedure as a result of reperfusion injury. Blood pressure control is a critical element of post-procedure management. Any worsening of neurologic status should be considered a possible sign of ICH, warranting immediate clinical evaluation and emergency CT scan of the brain. Should ICH be found, reversal of all antithrombotic agents should be carried out.

CLINICAL RESULTS IN THE LITERATURE

The most important studies on mechanical IA therapies are summarized in **Table 4**.

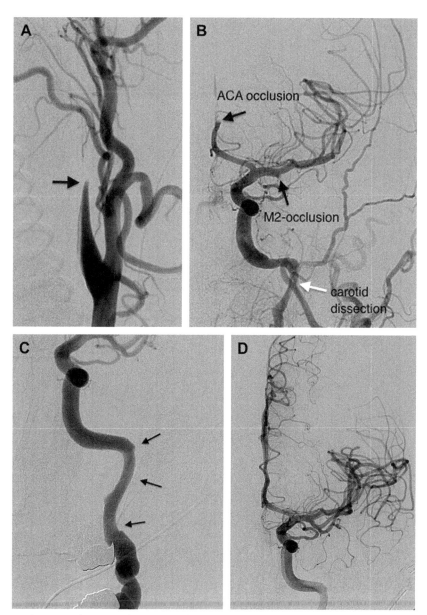

Fig. 18. Acute occlusion in the cervical segment of the ICA (*black arrow* in *A*). The occlusion passed with a wire and a microcatheter and was advanced into petrous segment, and contrast medium was injected to verify the intraluminal position of the catheter. Angiography showed a dissection of the ICA in the distal cervical segment (*white arrow* in *B*). A self-expanding stent is placed in the area of the dissection (*black arrows* in *C*). Additional intracranial occlusion of the ACA and M2 segment of the MCA were also present (*black arrows* in *B*). After placement and stent retriever withdrawal, the vessels were fully recanalized (*D*).

A large number of prospective registers on mechanical thrombectomy have been published. Until recently, there were no randomized trials comparing recanalization devices with standard therapy. Recently, the results of the Interventional Management of Stroke III (IMS III) trial show no benefit of endovascular therapy after the use of IV thrombolysis over IV thrombolysis alone in the treatment of moderate to severe acute ischemic stroke.[57] However, there were major weaknesses in this study. First was the issue of patient selection: CTA was not required, which led to inclusion patients who had no proven IC large-vessel occlusion. Second, the current iteration of reperfusion devices (stent retrievers), which have demonstrated much greater success, were used only in 5 patients. Finally, unlike with IV thrombolysis, there was no time limit for the beginning of the

Table 4
Major clinical studies for IA therapies of acute ischemic stroke

	Method/Device	Patients (N)	Age (y)	NIHSS	Recanalization (%)	90-d mRS≤2	90-d Mortality (%)	Symptomatic ICH (%)
PROACT II IA t-PA[12]	IA t-PA	121	64	17	66	40	25	10.9
PROACT II control[12]		59	64	17	18	25	27	2
MELT IA t-PA[58]	IA t-PA	57	67	14	73	49.1	5.3	9
MELT control[58]		57	67	14		38.6	3.5	2
MERCI 2[45]	Merci device	141	67	20	48	27.7	43.5	7.8
Multi-MERCI[41]	Merci device	164	68	19	68	36	34	9.8
Penumbra Pivotal[46]	Penumbra system	125	64	18	82	25	32.8	11.2
IMS III endovascular[57]	IA t-PA; Merci device; Penumbra system; Solitaire retriever	434	69	17	74	40.8	19.1	6.2
IMS III IV t-PA[57]	IV t-PA	222	68	16		38.7	21.6	5.9
ReFlow[38]	Solitaire retriever	40	70	16	95	60	12.5	2.5
STAR[59]	Solitaire retriever	202	72	17	79	57.9	6.9	1.5
SWIFT Solitaite device[50]	Solitaire retriever	58	67	17	61	58	18	2
SWIFT Merci device[50]	Merci device	55	67	17	24	33	44	11
TREVO 2 Trevo device[51]	Trevo retriever	88	67	18	85	40	34.1	7
TREVO 2 Merci device[51]	Merci device	90	67	18	66	21.8	24.1	9

Abbreviations: IMS, Interventional Management of Stroke; MELT, the middle cerebral artery embolism local fibrinolytic intervention trial; Star, Solitaire FR Thrombectomy for Acute Revascularisation; SWIFT, SOLITAIRE FR With the Intention For Thrombectomy; TREVO, Thrombectomy REvascularization of Large Vessel Occlusions in Acute Ischemic Stroke.

mechanical thrombectomy; thus, in 40% of patients, endovascular therapy was delayed and was not initiated until more than 90 minutes after receiving IV thrombolysis. It is possible that if these fundamental flaws were corrected, endovascular therapy for appropriately selected patients would be superior.

SUMMARY

Large-artery occlusions cause severe strokes. The treatment of affected patients is a challenge because IV thrombolysis is often ineffective. IV thrombolysis on its own leads to a favorable clinical outcome in only 15% to 25% in patients with large-artery occlusion. Current IA reperfusion therapies enable high recanalization rates, high rate of favorable clinical outcome, and low complication rates. However, to achieve good clinical results, appropriate patient selection and the use of an optimized stroke management system are obligate.

Additional randomized trials are needed to establish the role of mechanical thrombectomy in stroke treatment. In such trials, flow restoration devices should be used for mechanical thrombectomy and in-hospital stroke management should be used in which a limit of D2D time should be defined.[38]

VIDEOS

Videos related to this article can be found online at http://dx.doi.org/10.1016/j.iccl.2013.09.008.

REFERENCES

1. Rothwell PM, Coull AJ, Silver LE, et al. Population-based study of event-rate, incidence, case fatality, and mortality for all acute vascular events in all arterial territories (Oxford Vascular Study). Lancet 2005;366:1773–83.
2. Go AS, Mozaffarian D, Roger VL, et al. Executive summary: heart disease and stroke statistics–2013 update: a report from the American Heart Association. Circulation 2013;127:143–52.
3. Tissue plasminogen activator for acute ischemic stroke. The National Institute of Neurological Disorders and Stroke rt-PA Stroke Study Group. N Engl J Med 1995;333:1581–7.
4. Hacke W, Kaste M, Bluhmki E, et al. Thrombolysis with alteplase 3 to 4.5 hours after acute ischemic stroke. N Engl J Med 2008;359:1317–29.
5. Lichtman JH, Watanabe E, Allen NB, et al. Hospital arrival time and intravenous t-PA use in US Academic Medical Centers, 2001-2004. Stroke 2009; 40:3845–50.
6. Albers GW, Olivot JM. Intravenous alteplase for ischaemic stroke. Lancet 2007;369:249–50.
7. Lees KR, Bluhmki E, von Kummer R, et al. Time to treatment with intravenous alteplase and outcome in stroke: an updated pooled analysis of ECASS, ATLANTIS, NINDS, and EPITHET trials. Lancet 2010;375:1695–703.
8. Bhatia R, Hill MD, Shobha N, et al. Low rates of acute recanalization with intravenous recombinant tissue plasminogen activator in ischemic stroke: real-world experience and a call for action. Stroke 2010;41:2254–8.
9. Tomsick T, Broderick J, Carrozella J, et al. Revascularization results in the interventional management of stroke II trial. AJNR Am J Neuroradiol 2008;29:582–7.
10. Rubiera M, Ribo M, Pagola J, et al. Bridging intravenous-intra-arterial rescue strategy increases recanalization and the likelihood of a good outcome in nonresponder intravenous tissue plasminogen activator-treated patients: a case-control study. Stroke 2011;42:993–7.
11. Adams HP, del Zoppo G, Alberts MJ, et al. Guidelines for the early management of adults with ischemic stroke: a guideline from the American Heart Association/American Stroke Association Stroke Council, Clinical Cardiology Council, Cardiovascular Radiology and Intervention Council, and the Atherosclerotic Peripheral Vascular Disease and Quality of Care Outcomes in Research Interdisciplinary Working Groups: the American Academy of Neurology affirms the value of this guideline as an educational tool for neurologists. Circulation 2007;115:e478–534.
12. Furlan A, Higashida R, Wechsler L, et al. Intra-arterial prourokinase for acute ischemic stroke. The PROACT II study: a randomized controlled trial. Prolyse in Acute Cerebral Thromboembolism. JAMA 1999;282:2003–11.
13. White CJ. Acute stroke treatment: carotid "stenters" to the rescue. J Am Coll Cardiol 2011;58:2370–1.
14. Rha JH, Saver JL. The impact of recanalization on ischemic stroke outcome: a meta-analysis. Stroke 2007;38:967–73.
15. Saver JL. Time is brain–quantified. Stroke 2005;37: 263–6.
16. Hacke W, Donnan G, Fieschi C, et al. Association of outcome with early stroke treatment: pooled analysis of ATLANTIS, ECASS, and NINDS rt-PA stroke trials. Lancet 2004;363:768–74.
17. Nogueira RG, Liebeskind DS, Sung G, et al, MERCI. Predictors of good clinical outcomes, mortality, and successful revascularization in patients with acute ischemic stroke undergoing thrombectomy: pooled analysis of the Mechanical Embolus Removal in Cerebral Ischemia (MERCI) and Multi MERCI Trials. Stroke 2009;40:3777–83.

18. Hacke W, Zeumer H, Ferbert A, et al. Intra-arterial thrombolytic therapy improves outcome in patients with acute vertebrobasilar occlusive disease. Stroke 1988;19:1216–22.

19. Rowley HA. The four Ps of acute stroke imaging: parenchyma, pipes, perfusion, and penumbra. AJNR Am J Neuroradiol 2001;22:599–601.

20. Wintermark M, Maeder P, Thiran JP, et al. Quantitative assessment of regional cerebral blood flows by perfusion CT studies at low injection rates: a critical review of the underlying theoretical models. Eur Radiol 2001;11:1220–30.

21. Heiss WD, Sobesky J, Hesselmann V. Identifying thresholds for penumbra and irreversible tissue damage. Stroke 2004;35:2671–4.

22. Truwit CL, Barkovich AJ, Gean-Marton A, et al. Loss of the insular ribbon: another early CT sign of acute middle cerebral artery infarction. Radiology 1990;176:801–6.

23. Tomsick TA, Brott TG, Chambers AA, et al. Hyperdense middle cerebral artery sign on CT: efficacy in detecting middle cerebral artery thrombosis. AJNR Am J Neuroradiol 1990;11:473–7.

24. von Kummer R, Bourquain H, Bastianello S, et al. Early prediction of irreversible brain damage after ischemic stroke at CT. Radiology 2001;219: 95–100.

25. Larrue V, von Kummer R, Müller A, et al. Risk factors for severe hemorrhagic transformation in ischemic stroke patients treated with recombinant tissue plasminogen activator: a secondary analysis of the European-Australasian Acute Stroke Study (ECASS II). Stroke 2001;32:438–41.

26. Hacke W, Kaste M, Fieschi C, et al. Intravenous thrombolysis with recombinant tissue plasminogen activator for acute hemispheric stroke. The European Cooperative Acute Stroke Study (ECASS). JAMA 1995;274:1017–25.

27. Lev MH, Farkas J, Rodriguez VR, et al. CT angiography in the rapid triage of patients with hyperacute stroke to intraarterial thrombolysis: accuracy in the detection of large vessel thrombus. J Comput Assist Tomogr 2001;25:520–8.

28. Lell MM, Anders K, Uder M, et al. New techniques in CT angiography. Radiographics 2006;26(Suppl 1): S45–62.

29. Lima FO, Furie KL, Silva GS, et al. The pattern of leptomeningeal collaterals on CT angiography is a strong predictor of long-term functional outcome in stroke patients with large vessel intracranial occlusion. Stroke 2010;41:2316–22.

30. Tomandl BF, Klotz E, Handschu R, et al. Comprehensive imaging of ischemic stroke with multisection CT. Radiographics 2003;23:565–92.

31. Srinivasan A, Goyal M, Al Azri F, et al. State-of-the-art imaging of acute stroke. Radiographics 2006; 26(Suppl 1):S75–95.

32. Schaefer PW, Grant PE, Gonzalez RG. Diffusion-weighted MR imaging of the brain. Radiology 2000;217:331–45.

33. Provenzale JM, Jahan R, Naidich TP, et al. Assessment of the patient with hyperacute stroke: imaging and therapy. Radiology 2003;229:347–59.

34. Liu G, van Gelderen P, Duyn J, et al. Single-shot diffusion MRI of human brain on a conventional clinical instrument. Magn Reson Med 1996;35: 671–7.

35. Fonarow GC, Smith EE, Saver JL, et al. Timeliness of tissue-type plasminogen activator therapy in acute ischemic stroke: patient characteristics, hospital factors, and outcomes associated with door-to-needle times within 60 minutes. Circulation 2011;123:750–8.

36. Fonarow GC, Smith EE, Saver JL, et al. Improving door-to-needle times in acute ischemic stroke: the design and rationale for the American Heart Association/American Stroke Association's target: stroke initiative. Stroke 2011;42:2983–9.

37. Walter S, Kostopoulos P, Haass A, et al. Point-of-care laboratory halves door-to-therapy-decision time in acute stroke. Ann Neurol 2011;69:581–6.

38. Roth C, Reith W, Walter S, et al. Mechanical recanalization with flow restoration in acute ischemic stroke: the ReFlow (mechanical recanalization with flow restoration in acute ischemic stroke) study. JACC Cardiovasc Interv 2013;6: 386–91.

39. Blankenship JC, Scott TD, Skelding KA, et al. Door-to-balloon times under 90 min can be routinely achieved for patients transferred for ST-segment elevation myocardial infarction percutaneous coronary intervention in a rural setting. J Am Coll Cardiol 2011;57:272–9.

40. Grunwald IQ, Walter S, Papanagiotou P, et al. Revascularization in acute ischaemic stroke using the penumbra system: the first single center experience. Eur J Neurol 2009;16:1210–6.

41. Smith WS, Sung G, Saver J, et al. Mechanical thrombectomy for acute ischemic stroke: final results of the Multi MERCI trial. Stroke 2008;39: 1205–12.

42. Papanagiotou P, Roth C, Walter S, et al. Treatment of acute cerebral artery occlusion with a fully recoverable intracranial stent: a new technique. Circulation 2010;121:2605–6.

43. Pérez MA, Miloslavski E, Fischer S, et al. Intracranial thrombectomy using the Solitaire stent: a historical vignette. J Neurointerv Surg 2012;4:e32.

44. Roth C, Papanagiotou P, Behnke S, et al. Stent-assisted mechanical recanalization for treatment of acute intracerebral artery occlusions. Stroke 2010;41:2559–67.

45. Smith WS, Sung G, Starkman S, et al. Safety and efficacy of mechanical embolectomy in acute

ischemic stroke: results of the MERCI trial. Stroke 2005;36:1432–8.

46. Penumbra Pivotal Stroke Trial Investigators. The penumbra pivotal stroke trial: safety and effectiveness of a new generation of mechanical devices for clot removal in intracranial large vessel occlusive disease. Stroke 2009;40:2761–8.

47. Brekenfeld C, Schroth G, Mattle HP, et al. Stent placement in acute cerebral artery occlusion: use of a self-expandable intracranial stent for acute stroke treatment. Stroke 2009;40:847–52.

48. Samaniego EA, Dabus G, Linfante I. Stenting in the treatment of acute ischemic stroke: literature review. Front Neurol 2011;2:76.

49. Levy EI, Siddiqui AH, Crumlish A, et al. First food and drug administration-approved prospective trial of primary intracranial stenting for acute stroke: SARIS (stent-assisted recanalization in acute ischemic stroke). Stroke 2009;40:3552–6.

50. Saver JL, Jahan R, Levy EI, et al. Solitaire flow restoration device versus the Merci Retriever in patients with acute ischaemic stroke (SWIFT): a randomised, parallel-group, non-inferiority trial. Lancet 2012;380(9849):1241–9.

51. Nogueira RG, Lutsep HL, Gupta R, et al. Trevo versus Merci retrievers for thrombectomy revascularisation of large vessel occlusions in acute ischaemic stroke (TREVO 2): a randomised trial. Lancet 2012;380:1231–40.

52. Dávalos A, Pereira VM, Chapot R, et al. Retrospective multicenter study of Solitaire FR for revascularization in the treatment of acute ischemic stroke. Stroke 2012;43:2699–705.

53. Gralla J, Brekenfeld C, Mordasini P, et al. Mechanical thrombolysis and stenting in acute ischemic stroke. Stroke 2012;43:280–5.

54. Qureshi AI. Endovascular revascularization of symptomatic acute extracranial internal carotid artery occlusion. Stroke 2005;36:2335–6.

55. Papanagiotou P, Roth C, Walter S, et al. Carotid artery stenting in acute stroke. J Am Coll Cardiol 2011;58:2363–9.

56. Kapadia SR, Bajzer CT, Ziada KM, et al. Initial experience of platelet glycoprotein IIb/IIIa inhibition with abciximab during carotid stenting: a safe and effective adjunctive therapy. Stroke 2001;32:2328–32.

57. Broderick JP, Palesch YY, Demchuk AM, et al. Endovascular therapy after intravenous t-PA versus t-PA alone for stroke. N Engl J Med 2013;368:893–903.

58. Ogawa A, Mori E, Minematsu K, et al. Randomized trial of intraarterial infusion of urokinase within 6 hours of middle cerebral artery stroke: the middle cerebral artery embolism local fibrinolytic intervention trial (MELT) Japan. Stroke 2007;38:2633–9.

59. Pereira VM, Gralla J, Dávalos A, et al. Prospective, multicenter, single-arm study of mechanical thrombectomy using solitaire flow restoration in acute ischemic stroke. Stroke 2013;380(9849):1241–9.

Index

Note: Page numbers of article titles are in **boldface** type.

Intervent Cardiol Clin 3 (2014) 169–173
http://dx.doi.org/10.1016/S2211-7458(13)00100-4
2211-7458/14/$ – see front matter © 2014 Elsevier Inc. All rights reserved.

Moving?

Make sure your subscription moves with you!

To notify us of your new address, find your **Clinics Account Number** (located on your mailing label above your name), and contact customer service at:

Email: journalscustomerservice-usa@elsevier.com

800-654-2452 (subscribers in the U.S. & Canada)
314-447-8871 (subscribers outside of the U.S. & Canada)

Fax number: 314-447-8029

Elsevier Health Sciences Division
Subscription Customer Service
3251 Riverport Lane
Maryland Heights, MO 63043

*To ensure uninterrupted delivery of your subscription, please notify us at least 4 weeks in advance of move.

Printed and bound by CPI Group (UK) Ltd, Croydon, CR0 4YY

03/10/2024

01040367-0019